Hughes' Outline of
Modern Psychiatry

Fifth Edition

Hughes' Outline of Modern Psychiatry

Fifth Edition

David Gill
Consultant Psychiatrist
Lister Hospital
Stevenage: Hertfordshire Partnership NHS Trust

John Wiley & Sons, Ltd

Other Wiley Editorial Offices

John Wiley & Sons Inc., 111 River Street, Hoboken, NJ 07030, USA

Jossey-Bass, 989 Market Street, San Francisco, CA 94103-1741, USA

Wiley-VCH Verlag GmbH, Boschstr. 12, D-69469 Weinheim, Germany

John Wiley & Sons Australia Ltd, 33 Park Road, Milton, Queensland 4064, Australia

John Wiley & Sons (Asia) Pte Ltd, 2 Clementi Loop #02-01, Jin Xing Distripark, Singapore 129809

John Wiley & Sons Canada Ltd, 6045 Freemont Blvd, Mississauga, Ontario, L5R 4J3

Wiley also publishes its books in a variety of electronic formats. Some content that appears in print
may not be available in electronic books.

Anniversary Logo Design: Richard J. Pacifico

Library of Congress Cataloging-in-Publication Data

Gill, D. (David), Dr.
    Hughes' outline of modern psychiatry / David Gill. – 5th ed.
        p. ; cm.
    Rev. ed. of: Hughes' outline of modern psychiatry / Jennifer Barraclough and David Gill. 4th ed. c1996.
    Includes bibliographical references and index.
    ISBN 978-0-470-03392-0 (pbk. : alk. paper)
    1. Psychiatry–Handbooks, manuals, etc.   I. Barraclough, Jennifer. Hughes' outline of modern
psychiatry.   II. Title.   III. Title: Outline of modern psychiatry.
    [DNLM: 1. Mental Disorders–Handbooks. WM 34 G475h 2007]
    RC456.H84 2007
    616.89 – dc22

                      2007010266

British Library Cataloguing in Publication Data

A catalogue record for this book is available from the British Library

ISBN 978-0-470-03392-0

Typeset in 10½ / 12½ pt Minion by SNP Best-set Typesetter Ltd., Hong Kong
Printed and bound in Great Britain by TJ International, Padstow, Cornwall
This book is printed on acid-free paper responsibly manufactured from sustainable forestry in which at
least two trees are planted for each one used for paper production.

Dedication

I am grateful to all my teachers, especially Roger Chitty, Neil Davies and Chris Bass, and to my colleagues and patients.

For Mandy and Bertie.

Contents

Preface

I am most grateful to Dr Jennifer Barraclough for inviting me to help with the previous edition of this book. Following her retirement from clinical psychiatry, I am grateful to her and to John Wiley for the opportunity to prepare a new edition. Any good qualities it may have are hers; its many faults are mine alone.

For reasons of confidentiality, the clinical examples are made up of composite case histories and do not refer to real individual patients.

Some of the references are to internet sites; these may be open to criticism as being potentially impermanent, but they have the merit of availability and they are free at point of access.

Part I The nature and assessment of psychiatric disorder

1 Classification

Psychiatry is the branch of medicine that deals with mental, emotional, and behavioural disorders. In psychiatry, as in other branches of medicine, classification of disease is useful for the following:

- *Informing clinical practice.* By placing a given patient's disorder into a recognized diagnostic category, the clinician is able to make an appropriate choice of treatment, and judge the probable future outcome. Using a classification system in this way does not, of course, remove the need to consider and respect those features that are unique to each individual case.

- *Communication between professionals.* A universally understood classification system permits efficient communication, whether in everyday clinical practice when colleagues are discussing a case, or in the national and international literature.

- *A basis for research.* Research workers require a classification system in order to investigate the causes, clinical features, natural history, and response to treatment of the various psychiatric disorders.

- *Service planning.* The type of treatment services required in a given area will depend on the frequency of different disorders within the local population.

Hughes' Outline of Modern Psychiatry, Fifth Edition. David Gill.
© 2007 John Wiley & Sons, Ltd   ISBN 9780470033920

However, we must not forget that the existing classifications, in our present, highly imperfect state of knowledge, may be little more than a convenient shorthand, rather than a statement of fundamental scientific truth.

For example, we may say that a patient has a diagnosis of 'F45.4 persistent somatoform pain disorder' under ICD-10 (see below). This may sound very scientific. However, fundamentally, all it means is that the patient has chronic pain, unexplained by physical pathology, with some indication of underlying psychosocial problems. Hence, use of this term should not lead us to delude ourselves that we have a clear understanding of the cause of the patient's problems, let alone a specific effective treatment deriving from it.

The basis of classification

The most rigorous type of classification is one based on cause, such as a single-gene defect (e.g. Huntington's chorea) or a chromosomal anomaly (e.g. Down's syndrome caused by trisomy 21). However, for most psychiatric disorders, this is not applicable, and so official psychiatric classification systems largely consist of descriptive accounts of clinical syndromes, each with its characteristic symptoms, signs, and natural history.

Reliability and validity

Reliability

A diagnosis may be said to be reliable if the same observer reaches the same diagnosis in a repeat of the same clinical situation (test–retest reliability), or if two observers reach the same diagnosis in the same clinical situation (interrater reliability). Studies in clinical practice have often shown low reliability for psychiatric diagnosis because psychiatrists differ in the way they interview patients and interpret the information elicited. Diagnostic practices also vary between different parts of the world. Reliability is better for individual symptoms and signs. Reliability can be improved by using standardized interviews and questionnaires (Chapter 3), and by using the diagnostic criteria laid down in ICD-10 and DSM-IV (see below). This is necessary for research purposes, but it is too time-consuming to be a usual part of daily clinical practice.

Validity

The validity of a diagnosis is more difficult to ascertain than its reliability. If a classification is to be valid ('based on truth or correct reasoning'), the categories it contains should describe disorders, which really are separate from one another. Various types of validity have been distinguished, such as *face validity*, which is to do with whether the diagnosis 'looks right', that is, whether it appears, on inspection, to deal with the matters it says it is going to deal with.

Ways of testing the validity of diagnostic groupings include the following:

• examining the consistency of symptom patterns. Statistical techniques such as 'cluster analysis' and 'discriminant function analysis' facilitate this process

• demonstration of consistent genetic and biological correlates

• demonstration of a consistent natural history and long-term outcome

• demonstration of a consistent treatment response.

Limitations and problems of classification

Although a great deal of work has been devoted to making the official inter-national classification systems both reliable and valid, it must be acknowledged that they are still imperfect. The descriptive categories are continually being revised; for example, 'panic disorder' and 'post-traumatic stress disorder' were only recently listed as diagnoses, although the clinical phenomena have been recognized for many years.

The boundaries between some of the clinical syndromes are not absolute, as illustrated by the need for terms such as 'schizo-affective disorder' to describe an illness with mixed features of two supposedly discrete categories, 'schizo-phrenia' and 'affective disorder'. Some patients' symptoms do not fit well with any recognized category, and there is a danger that these may be forced into a residual or 'dustbin' category such as 'depression, not otherwise specified'. In insurance-based health systems, this may make the difference between receiving care or not, as insurers may restrict cover to certain 'hard' diagnostic categories.

Insensitive use of classification can lead to 'labelling' of patients. Classification systems are best used in a flexible and critical way, and clinical effort is often better directed toward relieving the patient's symptoms than excessive debate about the niceties of diagnosis.

Some mental health professionals prefer 'problem-based' to 'disease-based' care. Nurses, in particular, and also other non-medical professions such as social workers, have a tradition of a 'problem-oriented' approach. For example, if a social worker is trying to help a mental health patient find supported accommodation, so that they can leave hospital, the details of diagnosis will be less of a priority, than the patient's coping skills, attitude to illness, lifestyle, and likely cooperation with mental health services. The same applies to cognitive behavioural psychotherapy, where the approach depends upon developing a shared understanding between patient and therapists of what the problems are and how they should be addressed; the details of the precise ICD or DSM diagnosis would be of secondary importance.

Common terms in psychiatric classification

Organic and functional

Psychiatric conditions are sometimes divided into *organic brain disorders* and *functional mental illnesses*.

Organic conditions are caused by identifiable physical pathology affecting the brain, directly or indirectly, and include, for example, *learning disabilities* (formerly known as mental handicap) and the *dementias*.

Functional conditions have usually been attributed to some kind of psychological stress, although in many cases it would be more honest to say that their cause is not known. As knowledge advances, some 'functional' conditions are likely to be reclassified as 'organic' (as currently may be happening for schizophrenia), and for this reason the term 'organic' is not used in DSM-IV.

Psychosis and neurosis

These terms have largely been removed from the international classifications but are still used in clinical practice.

Psychoses (for example, schizophrenia, bipolar affective disorder)

Psychoses are characterized by the following:

- severe illness

- symptoms outside normal experience, such as delusions and hallucinations

- loss of insight; subjective experience mistaken for external reality.

Neuroses (for example, anxiety disorders, most cases of depression)

In comparison with psychoses, neuroses may be characterized as follows:

- more common

- often less severe

- symptoms possibly understandable as an exaggeration of the normal response to stress.

Psychiatrists also deal with conditions involving abnormalities of psychological development or behaviour, such as *personality disorders, alcohol and drug misuse, sexual dysfunction*, and *eating disorders*.

The descriptive study of abnormalities of mental functions such as mood, perception, thought, volition, memory, or cognition is called *psychopathology*. Definitions of some of the terms commonly used in psychopathology are given in the Glossary at the end of this book.

Classification systems

Classification systems include *categorical, dimensional*, and *multiaxial* types. In the *categorical* type of classification, each case is allocated to one of several mutually exclusive groups. This simple method is the most suitable one for clinical settings. Categorical systems are usually used in a hierarchical way, so that each case receives only one main diagnosis. Organic psychoses take precedence over functional psychoses, and functional psychoses over neuroses. This can lead to oversimplification of complex cases, and does not take account of 'comorbidity', in which two psychiatric diagnoses (for example, anxiety state and alcohol misuse) or a physical and a psychiatric diagnosis (for example, diabetes and depression) coexist.

In the *dimensional* type of classification, cases are rated on a continuous scale, or several separate continuous scales, for the characteristic(s) under study, as in, for example, depressed mood.

In the *multiaxial* type of classification, each case is rated on several separate categorical systems, each measuring a different aspect (for example, psychiatric illness, personality, intelligence).

The two main classification systems in international use, ICD and DSM, will now be summarized. Both systems are due to be published in revised editions shortly.

ICD-10 (World Health Organization, 1992)

The tenth edition of the *International Classification of Disease* (ICD-10), prepared by the World Health Organization, covers the whole of medicine, and also includes a Classification of Mental and Behavioural Disorders. This is the official classification used in the UK. It is available free at http://www3.who.int/icd/currentversion/fr-icd.htm. It is a descriptive classification, with main headings as follows:

F00–F09   Organic, including symptomatic, mental disorders
F10–F19   Mental and behavioural disorders due to psychoactive substance use
F20–F29   Schizophrenia, schizotypal and delusional disorders
F30–F39   Mood (affective) disorders
F40–F48   Neurotic, stress-related, and somatoform disorders
F50–F59   Behavioural syndromes associated with physiological disturbances and physical factors
F60–F69   Disorders of adult personality and behaviour
F70–F79   Mental retardation
F80–F89   Disorders of psychological development
F90–F98   Behavioural and emotional disorders with onset usually in childhood or adolescence
F99   Unspecified mental disorder.

Each of the main categories listed above has a number of subdivisions. Diagnostic guidelines for each condition are given in the ICD.

Some conditions relevant to psychiatry, such as suicide and self-inflicted injury or poisoning, are classified in other sections of the ICD. For example, 'factors influencing health status and contact with health services', codes Z00–Z99, is a neglected section of the ICD. Codes such as 'Z60.4 Social exclusion and rejection: Exclusion and rejection on the basis of personal characteristics, such as unusual physical appearance, illness or behaviour' seem to have a common-sense basis, and offer an antidote to the potential medicalization of some life problems through over-diagnosis of mental disorder. The Z codes to some extent fill the gap in the ICD left by the absence of the axes of the DSM, which cover aspects other than the presence or absence of mental illness (see next section).

DSM-IV (American Psychiatric Association, 1994)

The *Diagnostic and Statistical Manual of Mental Disorders*, Fourth Edition (DSM-IV) comprises the official classification system of the American Psychiatric Association, and has been influential in the UK. DSM-IV is a multiaxial system with five axes:

Axis I: Clinical syndromes
Axis II: Developmental disorders and personality disorders
Axis III: Physical disorders and conditions
Axis IV: Severity of psychosocial stressors
Axis V: Global assessment of functioning.

The strength of this approach lies in its requiring any clinical syndrome to be considered against the background of the permanent features, such as personality characteristics and intellectual level, of the person concerned. Each syndrome is defined by a set of practical criteria.

Comparison of DSM and ICD

DSM	ICD
USA	WHO, including UK
Symptoms must be 'more than an under-standable reaction' for diagnosis	No such test explicit
Mental health only	All of medicine
Subscription only	Free online
Guides only – need expert interpretation	
Consensus statements of committees – not immutable truths	

The chapter headings in this book do not follow either ICD-10 or DSM-IV exactly, because the arrangement of topics has been designed to accord with UK clinical practice rather than official classification systems.

Further reading

American Psychiatric Association (1994). *Diagnostic and Statistical Manual of Mental Disorders* (4th edn) (DSM-IV). Washington, DC: American Psychiatric Association.

World Health Organization (1992). *The ICD-10 Classification of Mental and Behavioural Disorders*. Geneva: WHO. http://www3.who.int/icd/currentversion/fr-icd.htm.

2 Causes and prevention

Causation in clinical practice

It is usual in everyday psychiatry to have multiple causes acting together, involving the interplay of constitutional and environmental factors, to produce an episode of illness – so-called multifactorial causation. These factors include genetic predisposition, personality characteristics, physical disorders, social circumstances, and life experiences.

The accepted way of considering these subsidiary causes in psychiatry is in terms of various *predisposing, precipitating,* and *perpetuating* factors.

Case illustration

For example, a person with a depressive illness may have been predisposed to develop it through an anxious personality, the illness being precipitated by relationship breakdown and perpetuated though alcohol misuse and inactivity.

A few psychiatric conditions are known to result directly from specific organic pathology, such as Down's syndrome caused by trisomy 21. But, even here, the overall outcome in functional terms may be profoundly influenced by social and family factors.

Hughes' Outline of Modern Psychiatry, Fifth Edition. David Gill.
© 2007 John Wiley & Sons, Ltd   ISBN 9780470033920

Historical background

Psychiatry goes through phases in which one or other of these various physical, social, or psychological models is regarded as most influential in psychiatric causation generally. In the early and mid-twentieth century, the psychological theories stemming from psychoanalysis (Freud) were dominant, especially in the USA. Later, 'biological' psychiatry was dominant, following the discovery – all in the 1950s – of effective mood stabilizers, antidepressants, and antipsychotic drugs.

Social factors were to the fore in the 1960s and 1970s, at the time of de-institutionalization and the 'anti-psychiatry' movement. However, ideas that psychiatric disability was mainly caused by social factors such as prejudice and 'stigma' have not been borne out.

Recently, psychological factors have staged something of a comeback, with the emergence of cognitive behavioural therapy; however, biological psychiatry, now emphasizing such factors such as 'receptors' and molecular genetics, remains influential.

The *bio-psycho-social model*, as originally derived for chronic pain patients, probably provides the most realistic overall model of causation, as we know enough to be sure that none of the above approaches is ever going to be capable alone of providing complete explanations.

This chapter outlines some general principles and research techniques. More detail regarding causation of individual disorders will be given in later chapters.

Genetics

Most psychiatric disorders show a tendency to run in families. This observation could be explained by genetic factors (nature) and/or by the influence of family and environment (nurture). Two long-established clinical research techniques have been used to distinguish these:

- *Twin studies*
  - *Comparison of monozygotic with dizygotic twins.* Any difference in the rates of illness between the types of twin can be attributed to the differences in the degree of sharing of genetic material between them.
  - *Comparison of monozygotic twins brought up together with those brought up apart.* Here the only difference is in the environment, so any differences in rates of illness between the two groups can be ascribed to the environment.

- *Adoption studies.* These examine rates of psychiatric disorder in children whose biological parents were affected but who were brought up by healthy adoptive parents, or vice versa.

Twin and adoption studies, many of which have been carried out in Scandinavia where comprehensive national records of individuals and their health are maintained, confirm a genetic predisposition for the majority of psychiatric conditions. The effect is strongest for conditions such as autism and attention deficit hyperactivity disorder (ADHD), in which there is a roughly 50-fold increase in risk in relatives; in schizophrenia, the increase is 10-fold; and in anxiety and unipolar depression, it is up to fivefold (for review, see Tandon and McGuffin, 2002).

The 'new genetics'

There have been prodigious investments of money and effort in this area. Since the last edition of this book in 1996, the human genome project has come and gone with great fanfare. However, there has as yet been little benefit to psychiatric practice. For single-gene disorders, such as Huntington's disease, research at least has a clear starting point. There is now understanding of the genetic abnormality at the chemical level; efforts at 'gene therapy', however, have yet to bear fruit.

However, long before the advent of these new techniques, studies of inheritance patterns had made it clear that the hereditary component of the major psychiatric conditions is polygenic: that is, not due to one gene, but to small contributions from a number of genes. A recent review describes some of the various techniques being used to hunt this collection of needles in a haystack: 'coordinated pathway genotype analysis, genome-wide linkage scans . . . genome-wide association studies' (Aitchison et al., 2005).

Use is made of quantitative trait loci (QTLs), which are genetic markers associated with the characteristics in question. The task facing researchers is huge: 'Between 100 000 and 1 000 000 markers may be required for an exhaustive sweep of the genome for all QTLs contributing to a disorder' (Aitchison et al., 2005).

The localization of defective genes and identification of their DNA sequences and biochemical products may have various clinical applications, including the following:

• *Diagnosis of affected or at-risk individuals*, perhaps at a presymptomatic stage: that is, screening. There are obvious implications for ethics and insurance, however.

• *Treatment possibilities*, mainly theoretical at present as regards psychiatry, including:
  – development of specific drugs

– 'gene therapy', where genes are introduced through viruses into affected individuals, as already being trialled in malignancies and in immune deficiency states.

The new techniques may bring marked clinical benefit, but they also raise ethical problems. There is a danger of patients' hopes being falsely raised, particularly by media stories about 'discovery of the gene for . . .', and doctors are already seeing possible negative effects.

Case example

A man consulted his GP in distress, having just found out that his divorced wife had Huntington's disease. He knew this disease is inherited, and that a test had recently become available to diagnose it in the presymptomatic stage. What, if anything, should he tell their 23-year-old daughter who lived with him, and who knew nothing of her mother's illness? The GP referred the man to a genetic counsellor. After prolonged discussion, in which it was explained that a test was available but preventive or symptomatic treatment was not, he decided against telling his daughter. He felt that the possibility of her finding out, through testing, that she was to develop such a disease in later life might blight her young adulthood. However, he felt that he would wish to review this decision should she later consider starting a family. He was left with the strain of carrying a secret.

Neurochemistry

Disturbance of brain biochemistry, especially involving monoamine transmitters, appears to be present in most psychiatric disorders, although it cannot be assumed that a chemical abnormality is the cause of the disorder rather than its result. Direct studies on the brains of living patients are limited for both practical and ethical reasons. Indirect techniques of investigation include the following:

• *Post-mortem brain studies.* These require brains to be harvested and frozen within a few hours of death. Findings may be influenced by recent medication, and the condition that caused the death, as well as by the psychiatric disorder of interest.

- *Analysis of cerebrospinal fluid (CSF), blood, or urine* for precursors or metabolites of neurotransmitters. The findings are affected by many factors such as diet and exercise, and may not give an accurate reflection of concentrations in the brain itself.

- *Pharmacological studies.* Inferences about the biochemical defect present in a particular disorder may be made from studies, performed on patients or on animals, of the properties of drugs that are effective in treating that disorder.

Neuroradiology

Modern brain-imaging techniques (Chapter 3) show abnormalities of structure and function associated with major psychiatric illness, such as ventricular enlargement in chronic schizophrenia, and altered patterns of glucose uptake in the manic and depressed phases of bipolar affective disorder.

Epidemiology

Epidemiological studies investigate the frequency of psychiatric disorders, their relationship to social factors, and their natural history. They are carried out on whole populations rather than individual patients. Sources of information include the following:

- *population surveys,* in which every member of a defined population, or a random sample of it, is studied by interview or questionnaire

- *GP consultation* records

- *case registers,* which are kept in some health districts to provide information on all contacts with psychiatric services

- *hospital statistics.*

The frequency of a disorder may be expressed as *point prevalence* (the percentage of subjects with the disorder in question at one point in time) or *period prevalence* (the total percentage who receive the diagnosis during a defined period).

Incidence means the number of new cases within a defined population in a given period (rate). *Lifetime expectation* expresses the risk of an individual's developing the condition concerned sometime during their life.

The results of different surveys vary greatly. Community interview surveys find the highest rates, invariably detecting many psychiatric 'cases' that are not known to GPs, let alone to specialist services. GP and hospital statistics may be inaccurate because they reflect different definitions of a psychiatric 'case', or variations in local treatment policies. There remains a fundamental distinction between subjects who have presented themselves for medical attention, and therefore have identified themselves as patients, and those who have not so presented themselves.

Most community surveys report that 10–20 per cent of the population meet diagnostic criteria for psychiatric disorder at any one time, and that a person's lifetime risk of disorder may be as high as 50 per cent.

Several socio-demographic variables have an association with psychiatric morbidity, but the direction of cause and effect is not always clear-cut. For example, consider the following variables:

- *Sex.* Women have higher rates of most psychiatric disorders than men. This particularly applies to the common (non-psychotic) forms of anxiety and depression. Possible explanations include the following:
  - Women use health services of all kinds more frequently than men. They may be more willing to acknowledge emotional complaints and seek medical treatment, whereas men tend to express their distress through other means such as antisocial behaviour or alcohol misuse.
  - Doctors are more likely to diagnose women's symptoms as psychiatric.
  - Women suffer more psychosocial stress than men because of their role in society.
  - Biological differences, such as genetic constitution and sex hormone profile, play a role.

For other mental disorders, including schizophrenia, the sex ratio is equal.

- *Marital status.* For men, rates of psychiatric disorder are lower among the married than the single, divorced, or widowed. Possible explanations include the following:
  - Married life is beneficial for men's mental health.
  - Men with psychiatric disorder tend to remain single.
  - Psychiatric disorder results in marital breakdown.

- Widowhood and divorce are stressful life events that may lead to psychiatric disorder.

For women, the pattern is different than for men. Young working-class house-wives with several small children have high rates of depression and neurosis, whereas single women in paid employment have lower rates.

- *Residential area.* Urban areas, especially poor inner-city districts, have higher rates of psychiatric morbidity than rural areas. Possible explanations include the following:
  - The lack of stable social networks in inner-city areas contributes to psychiatric disorder.
  - The stresses of city life, such as overcrowding, high crime rates, and noise, contribute to psychiatric disorder.
  - Psychiatric disorder causes people to lose their jobs and social supports, and forces them to move to poorer areas.

- *Unemployment* is associated with psychiatric disorder. Possible explanations include the following:
  - The socio-economic adversity and loss of self-esteem of the unemployed contributes to psychiatric disorder.
  - Workers with psychiatric disorder are liable to lose their jobs.

- *Social class.* Manual workers show higher psychiatric morbidity than the pro-fessional/managerial classes. Possible causes include the following:
  - genetic factors
  - a stressful and unhealthy environment
  - 'drift down the social scale' caused by mental illness.

- *Nationality, and issues of 'transcultural' psychiatry.* Diagnostic statistics vary around the world. Organic brain syndromes and somatic presentations of 'functional' conditions are more common in developing societies. Suicide rates vary greatly between countries. Some of these observed differences are genuine. Others are artefactual, depending on what kinds of behaviour are considered abnormal in the culture concerned, and disappear when uniform diagnostic criteria are applied. For example, until the 1970s, the diagnosis of schizo-phrenia was made much more frequently in the USA than the UK. Yet, since introduction of more rigorous diagnostic criteria, it appears that schizophrenia and other major psychotic disorders occur about equally frequently in both countries, and also in most other parts of the world. *Migrants* show high psychiatric morbidity, being especially prone to develop a range of conditions including psychotic disorders and post-traumatic stress disorder (PTSD); refugees, who have been forced to migrate rather than doing so by choice, are most at risk. Possible explanations include the following:

- Pre-existing psychiatric disorder causes people to emigrate.
- Stressful circumstances in the country of origin precipitate both emigration and psychiatric illness.
- 'Culture shock' in the new country, including a strange language and customs, and discrimination against immigrants.
- Over-diagnosis occurs as a result of mental health professionals' unfamiliarity with the culture of immigrant groups and language difficulties.

Individual life experience

Adverse experiences in childhood, such as losing one's mother or father, or being sexually abused, would be expected to increase the risk of psychiatric disorder in adult life, and most research studies tend to confirm this long-term association. There is also evidence for a short-term effect whereby psychosocial stress in adult life can precipitate psychiatric illness in predisposed people. This effect applies both for individual *life events* of a common kind, such as family bereavement or divorce, and for extraordinary disasters (see Chapter 6 on PTSD). Chronic *social stresses*, such as marital difficulties or bad housing, can also contribute. In contrast, supportive *social networks*, and close confiding relationships with others, provide some protection against psychiatric disorder following adverse life events.

Life event experience may be measured by the following:

- *official records* in the case of certain major events like widowhood or divorce

- *questionnaires*, which are relatively easy to score but involve oversimplification

- *standardized interviews*, such as the Life Events and Difficulties Schedule (LEDS) developed by Brown and Harris.

The effects of life experiences can be satisfactorily investigated only by prospective follow-up of people subjected to adversity, but such studies take many years to complete and are expensive. Many published studies have therefore used retrospective methods, and their interpretation is subject to error for the following reasons:

- *Mistaking the direction of causality.* An event apparently precipitating an illness (such as losing a job) may really be the result of changes in the patient's behaviour during the prodromal phase of that illness.

- *Effort after meaning.* Some patients unwittingly exaggerate their experience of life event stress in order to explain the illness. For example, a woman who has given birth to a baby with a congenital abnormality will be more likely than a control to report adverse events during pregnancy.

- *Inaccurate recollection of timing of life events in relation to illness onset.*

- *Recall bias.* For example, depressed persons naturally tend to recall negative memories in preference to positive ones; this means they are intrinsically more likely to recall adverse life events than control subjects.

Kindling refers to a presumed process whereby repeated applications of a stimulus produce an escalating response. This theory has been used to try to understand the course, for example, of recurrent unipolar depression, in which the time between episodes tends to decrease, and the role of life events in provoking an episode becomes less prominent (see Chapter 5).

Prevention of psychiatric disorder

A cynic might say that a work called *Prevention of Psychiatric Disorder* would be in danger of winning a prize for the world's shortest book. But this would be too negative a view. In fact, most mental health professionals spend most of their time on prevention in the sense of *secondary* prevention.

Secondary prevention is reduction of severity of existing disease and prevention of relapse by means of early detection and treatment. Prevention of relapse may be achieved by drug therapy, psychotherapy, and/or social support for patients who have recovered from an episode of mental illness. This most important work is done by trying to optimize the care of existing psychiatric patients.

Tertiary prevention, so called, means reduction of the handicaps that may result from established disease, as in rehabilitation programmes to prevent patients from becoming needlessly disabled for employment and community services to reduce the burden on families. It really merges with secondary prevention in the community mental health team environment; for example, if the patient's family are involved in the care of the patient, they will be entitled to a 'carer's assessment' under the terms of the Care Programme Approach. And links can be forged with local schemes for returning people to work, such as Employment Direct, Job Centre Plus, etc.

The value of early detection of relapse in existing patients is not in dispute. Education of patients and carers is vital. When education extends to organized campaigns directed at other health professionals and the general public, however (as in the Royal College of Psychiatrists' recent 'Defeat Depression' campaign), it becomes more controversial. It is clearly in the interests of the drug companies who tend to pay for such campaigns that diagnosis of depression should be increased. Increased prescription of antidepressant medication will then follow. However, there is a danger of medicalizing normal states of distress.

Use of screening questionnaires (Chapter 3) in medical settings, has been advocated. However, screening has not so far, at least in the case of depression, met standard UK criteria for introduction on a routine basis (Gilbody *et al.*, 2006).

Primary prevention is prevention of disease from developing in the first place. The following list of measures might be important for psychiatry, although hard evidence of effectiveness is not available for all of them:

- *medical and public health measures* to avert damage to the brain:
  - genetic counselling and prenatal diagnosis (Chapter 19)
  - improved care during pregnancy and childbirth
  - improved infant welfare services including immunization
  - control of infections, such as meningitis and HIV disease
  - avoidance of nutritional deficiencies
  - reduction of alcohol and drug misuse
  - reduction of pollution such as atmospheric lead
  - prevention of accidents, and hence of head injury, as, for example by using seat belts and crash helmets
  - provision of adequate housing.

- *psychological approaches*:
  - counselling for the bereaved, divorced, and other groups known to have a high risk of illness
  - crisis intervention for victims of major trauma has been advocated in the form of debriefing; however, contrary to expectations, this has been found to be harmful in some cases. It appears that most people cope better from

their own resources; perhaps being forced to talk about the experience again serves to retraumatize (Rose *et al.*, 2002).
- social work with disturbed families with particular emphasis on counterbalancing adverse effects on children.

Many of the measures noted above under primary prevention are outside the sphere of influence of psychiatrists. Concentrating on secondary and tertiary prevention is more practical and has the additional benefit of focusing services on those most in need.

References

Aitchison, K., Gonzalez, F. J., Quattrochi, L. C. *et al.* (2005) Psychiatry and the 'new genetics': hunting for genes for behaviour and drug response. *Br J Psychiatry* **186**, 91–92.

Gilbody, S., Sheldon, T. and Wessely, S. (2006). Should we screen for depression? *BMJ* **332**, 1027–1030.

Rose, S., Bisson, J and Churchill, R. *et al.* (2002). Psychological debriefing for preventing post traumatic stress disorder (PTSD). *Cochrane Database Syst Rev* **2**, 10.1002/14651858. CD000560.

Tandon, K. and McGuffin, P. (2002). The genetic basis for psychiatric illness in man. *Eur J Neurosci* **16**, 403–407.

3 Assessment

Reaching a diagnosis in a psychiatric patient relies on an accurate case history, often including information from relatives or other sources, and the mental state examination. Laboratory investigations are helpful in a minority of cases only. Previous psychiatric notes should be obtained. This can be easier if the notes are in electronic form. The GP records, which build up a sequential medical history because of universal NHS registration, are vital in medico-legal cases.

Circumstances of referral

If the referral is from a GP, it can be very helpful to speak to the GP by telephone before the interview; similarly, in an emergency situation, much useful information can be obtained from police officers, ambulance personnel, and other informants.

It is also useful to ask oneself not only why the patient has been referred, but *why now?* For example, a patient may be seen with a long-standing condition, and there may appear to have been little change from an objectively medical point of view. Non-medical factors such as disruption of networks of informal care, accommodation problems, financial crisis, or arrest, are commonly the precipitating factors for referral.

Hughes' Outline of Modern Psychiatry, Fifth Edition. David Gill.
© 2007 John Wiley & Sons, Ltd   ISBN 9780470033920

The psychiatric interview

The psychiatric interview is designed to obtain detailed information about past life, physical health, personality, relationships, and social circumstances, as well as past and present psychiatric symptoms. Such background information can help in making the diagnosis, choosing appropriate treatment, deciding whether the case should be managed on an inpatient or outpatient basis, and setting realistic goals.

In addition, experience of psychiatry affords a good opportunity to improve the practitioner's own interviewing and communication skills; training in consultation and interview skills may include the use of video recordings.

The first interview plays an important part in establishing the relationship between patient and psychiatrist, and therefore has a therapeutic function as well as an information-gathering one. The interviewer must reach the best compromise between listening to the patient's own concerns, and asking the requisite factual questions. Some patients, such as those who are very anxious, need some time to talk freely before they can cooperate with more structured enquiry. Open-ended questions ('How have you been sleeping lately?') are preferable to leading ones ('Have you been waking up early?').

The interview should start with the presenting complaint, though the order of the other components may vary. It is important to include all the sections, but a common-sense approach is called for; there is little use exploring the fine details of symptomatology but failing to find out that the patient has just been evicted from his accommodation or is about to appear in court. It is usual to take notes during the interview since there is too much material to recall accurately afterward.

Assessment may take place in an outpatient clinic, a general practice, the patient's home, a general hospital, or another site such as a police station. Occasionally, one may be asked to interview a patient across a video link; for example, the criminal justice system has a well-developed system allowing an inmate at a prison to be seen by a doctor, lawyer, or other party who attends by arrangement at a local police station. However, this is not fully satisfactory, as it is not a completely professional setting; it would be important, if it were used, that it be backed up by a face-to-face interview as soon as possible.

Privacy is important, and most psychiatrists prefer to see the patient alone, although occasional exceptions are necessary, for example, if the patient is potentially violent or likely to make allegations against the practitioner. Examination candidates are traditionally allowed 1 hour to assess a new case. Complex cases ideally need longer than this, whereas emergencies may have to be assessed more quickly.

If the patient is too ill or uncooperative to give a history, one should concentrate on the mental state examination. It is necessary to use the limited time available wisely; if it is a case of delirium caused by, say, acute infection, the interview will mainly consist of the mental state examination and physical examination. The history will be incoherent, and the priority is finding and diagnosing the underlying acute physical problem. By contrast, in a patient with neurosis, there may be little abnormality on the mental state examination, and physical examination will probably not be done. Therefore, the assessment will concentrate mainly on the history. A patient with psychosis will come somewhere in the middle; the history will be important to have, but more time will be spent on the mental state examination, and neurological or other physical examination may also be needed.

The assessment is often regarded as incomplete until another informant, usually a relative or friend, has been interviewed; this is especially true for cases of psychotic illness or organic brain disease. The patient's prior consent is required except in special circumstances. Where language barriers exist, the help of an interpreter may be required.

A letter summarizing the assessment interview is normally sent to the patient's GP, copies being filed in the case notes and sometimes sent to other professional agencies. Issues of confidentiality may cause problems, so it is important to ensure that the patient knows about the letter, who will receive a copy, and whether any sensitive personal material is to be included.

The status of medical notes has changed. For example, patients now have the right to read their medical notes. There never has been a place for pejorative or personal remarks about patients in the medical notes; this practice is now completely unsustainable.

Many mental health organizations now have computerized notes; there is a plan to have a national NHS information technology (IT) network, containing all patients' notes (although what the plan is intended to achieve, apart from enriching IT companies, is at present unclear). Many psychiatrists have reservations about these developments, but they are happening anyway. Inevitably, this means that there may be a trend toward highly sensitive information not being recorded in medical notes, as these are seen as less confidential than previously.

History

Begin by explaining who you are, and outlining the purpose, format, and length of interview. For example, shake hands, invite the patient to sit down, and say, 'My name is Paula Johnson. I am a psychiatrist working with your consultant,

Dr Jones. We have about an hour to get an idea of your problems and what help we could offer.' The material may then be presented as follows:

- *introduction*: name, age, marital status, occupation, where seen, and how referred; for inpatients, legal status: whether informal or on a 'section' of the Mental Health Act 1983 (if so, which one)

- *complaints*: in patient's own words

- *history of present illness*:
  – symptoms, including changes in sleep, appetite, mood, energy, and concentration
  – duration
  – possible precipitating factors
  – effect of illness on lifestyle, relationships, and working ability
  – treatment so far.

(*Note*: if the disorder is a recurrent one, concentrate on the latest episode here, leaving the rest for 'past psychiatric history'.)

- *past psychiatric history*: previous episodes of illness with dates, precipitating factors, symptoms, diagnosis, and treatment, plus previous 'sections' under the Mental Health Act, hospital admissions, and episodes of deliberate self-harm

- *substance use*: alcohol, illegal drugs; any psychological or physical dependency on substances or binge use. Tobacco and caffeine may be enquired into; their use tends to be higher in psychiatric patients, but they are seldom directly relevant to diagnosis or treatment of mental disorder.

- *medical history*: past illnesses, present physical symptoms, and medication

- *forensic history*: previous offending behaviour, with any cautions or convictions; attitude to this and presence or absence of remorse; previous sentences if applicable; and any currently outstanding matters, including whether the patient is on probation, parole, or bail, and whether he is subject to an injunction or arrest warrant.

- *family history*:
  – parents' and siblings' ages, occupation, health, and relationship with patient. If dead, cause of death, age at death, and patient's age at the time.
  – family history of psychiatric illness (the term 'nervous breakdown' may be useful), suicide, or alcoholism.

(*Note*: this section is concerned with family of origin. Spouse and children come later.)

- *childhood*:
  - complications during pregnancy or birth, serious illness in infancy, or delays in development
  - home environment: place of birth, subsequent changes of residence, emotional atmosphere and practical circumstances at home, and outstanding events
  - school: academic achievements, ability to mix with other children, attitude to teachers.

- *work*: training and qualifications, jobs held, reasons for change, extent of satisfaction with work and ability to cope, relations with workmates and employers.

- *sex and marriage*:
  - sexual practice: hetero- and homosexual experience, extent of satisfaction, sexual difficulties, and past history of sexual abuse
  - marital: duration of marriage/cohabitation; partner's age, occupation, health, and relationship with patient. For any previous marriages or long-term relationships, record duration and reasons for ending
  - children: names, ages, health, and relationships with patient
  - for women: live births, stillbirths, miscarriages, abortions, contraceptive practice, and menstrual pattern.

(*Note*: use judgement about the extent of questioning on sexual topics. For some patients, detailed questioning is not relevant and may cause offence.)

- *premorbid personality*:
  - social relations: ability to make friends and relate to those in authority
  - mood: cheerful or despondent, anxious or placid, tendency to mood swings, way of expressing anger, and response to stress
  - character: confident or diffident, independent or reliant on others, conscientious or casual, and impulsive or cautious
  - level of energy and activity
  - ways of coping with stress
  - attitude to religion, politics, membership of societies, and hobbies.

In some patients, the presenting disturbance is an exaggeration of long-standing personality problems. In others, recent alteration of mood and behaviour suggest psychiatric illness.

(*Note*: many patients cannot describe their previous personality accurately and an account from another informant is often useful.)

- *present circumstances*: type of accommodation, people in household, and financial or practical problems.

(*Note*: parts of the history not concerned with the present illness are called the 'personal history'.)

Mental state examination

As an objective assessment of the patient's present condition, made by a trained observer, this is especially important if there is any doubt as to the completeness or reliability of the history.

- *Introduction.* Mention quality of rapport and interview; for example, 'This was a difficult interview because the patient was unforthcoming, and we did not establish a warm rapport.'

- *Appearance and general behaviour.* Use factual descriptions rather than judgemental comments:
  - whether cooperative
  - striking physical features (such as extremes of height or weight, or deformities)
  - type of dress
  - standard of self-care
  - degree of activity
  - abnormalities of movement or gait: this would include, for example, the bizarre posturing of patients with catatonia, the jerking and writhing of tardive dyskinesia, or the stiffness and shakiness in Parkinsonism or due to antipsychotic drugs. Repetitive touching or checking movements may indicate compulsive rituals of obsessive-compulsive disorder (OCD), although these may not be apparent at interview.

- *Mood.* Include both patient's own description and interviewer's observations.
  - mood states of depression, euphoria, anxiety, perplexity, fear, or suspicion

- lability of mood: mood fluctuating during interview
- mood incongruence: inappropriate to circumstances or thought content
- somatic symptoms such as those affecting appetite and energy level
- suicidal ideation/plans.

- *Speech.* Obviously, it is from people's speech that we gain information about their thoughts. By convention, however, the section of the mental state covering speech is confined to the loudness of speech, and to the presence or absence of any difficulty with the production of speech, such as dysarthria or stammering.

- *Thought.* Again, by convention, we refer to four aspects of thought:
  - *Speed.* This refers to the speeded-up thoughts of a patient with, for example, mania (pressure of thought), or the slowed-up thoughts of a patient with, for example, retarded depression.
  - *Possession.* This refers to certain experiences in schizophrenia. For example, patients may relate that their thoughts are not their own: 'someone else's thoughts are in my mind'; this is so-called *thought insertion.* Related experiences of *thought withdrawal* and *thought broadcasting* are also seen (see Chapter 4 on schizophrenia).
  - *Form.* This refers to disruption in the proper connection between thoughts. For example, in mania, pressure of speech may proceed to the point that the patient is jumping from topic to topic, irrationally; this is the so-called flight of ideas. In psychosis, there may be bizarre connections between thoughts, the so-called knight's move thinking. In extreme cases, speech may become a jumble of words or even syllables, the so-called word salad.
  - *Content.* In schizophrenia or retarded depression, there may be little or no spontaneous speech, and this may be termed 'poverty of thought'. Abnormal beliefs may also occur, either 'overvalued ideas', where the patient can still be reasoned with, or frank delusions, where the patient holds to the idea in spite of all evidence and reasoned argument.

A delusion can be defined as a belief, usually but not always false, that is inappropriate, bearing in mind, the person's educational and cultural background, and that is not amenable to reasoned argument. Bizarre delusions – for example, that Martians are interfering with TV transmission – are suggestive of psychosis, particularly schizophrenia; persecutory delusions – for example, that there is a conspiracy to poison the patient's water supply – are seen in paranoid states including paranoid schizophrenia; grandiose delusions – for example, that the patient has special powers – are seen in mania; nihilistic delusions – for example, that the patient's bowels have turned to stone – are seen in psychotic depression.

Occasionally, a patient may become deluded about something that is real – for example, he may believe he is being persecuted by visits from the Gas Board. But the Gas Board may in reality be trying to get in, in order to cut off his gas if he has not paid the bill; it is the quality of the reasoning, or lack of it, behind the belief of persecution that decides whether or not the belief is a delusion or not.

Under content of thought must also be noted any subjects which preoccupy the patient, such as the negative thoughts of a patient with depression, or obsessional ruminations in OCD.

- *Perception.* This involves perceptual disorders, including hallucinations (false perceptions) and illusions (false interpretations of real perceptions). (*Note*: these terms are defined in the Glossary.) Auditory hallucinations, which are common in psychiatric inpatients, can be approached by direct enquiry about whether the patient has ever heard anyone speaking when there was no one around, or some such question. Sometimes, problems arise with such an approach when patients are repeatedly interviewed and may eventually get so fed up over being asked the question that they say yes, even though they are not experiencing auditory hallucinations. If hallucinations were truly present, they would usually be apparent to the observer without direct enquiry; for example, the patient mutters under his breath, apparently conversing with unseen voices.

- *Cognitive function.*
  - *Conscious level.* This is not recorded in most cases as it is obviously normal, but if there is a possibility of organic (physical) factors affecting the mental state, it must be recorded whether the patient is clearly conscious, is slightly drowsy, or is lapsing into unconsciousness. Intoxication by alcohol or other substances would be the commonest cause of this, although acute confusional states and neurological conditions including head injury must also be considered.
  - *Orientation.* Is the patient oriented in time (day, date, and time of day), place, and person (identifying the interviewer or ward staff)? Problems in this basic information indicate that the patient may have either learning disability or an organic mental state such as delirium or dementia.
  - *Attention and concentration.* There are various tests of this, including digit span (normally at least seven forward and five backward). Subtracting 'serial sevens' from 100 (93, 86, 79, 72, etc.) is often advocated, but this is a quite

difficult test – less than 50 per cent of normal subjects score perfectly, two or even three errors being not necessarily abnormal. If the patient scores poorly on digit span, it might be more realistic to proceed straight to an easy test such as 'name the months of the year backward, starting with October'.

- *Memory*. Even patients with early dementia can often give a good history of their early life; this is sometimes referred to as *biographical memory*. This is not what *long-term memory* means for present purposes, however. Long-term memory means things that have happened recently, such as political or sporting events that most people would remember. It can be assessed by asking about recent news events, soccer, etc., and the name of the monarch or prime minister. Tests of *short-term memory* include the name-and-address test: the patient is asked to repeat a name and address that the examiner writes down (to avoid trusting his own fallible memory), together with the time of starting. The patient's inability to repeat it after the examiner indicates a deficit of registration (psychologists may refer to this as 'immediate recall'). Then the patient is asked to remember it, and the interview continues, preferably on neutral subjects so that the patient does not become upset and hence forget. After 5 minutes (use an alarm, such as that on a mobile phone, so as not to forget to retest!), a patient with normal memory should remember it with only trivial errors. The three-object recall test is an easier one, more appropriate for cases of possible dementia; this can be made easier by using objects physically in front of the patient (e.g. pen, desk, phone).

(*Note*: do not neglect cognitive testing, which may reveal unsuspected defects pointing to organic cerebral dysfunction. Cognitive testing should always be done in examinations. It is a very valuable skill in patients with a neurological aspect, such as dementia or head injury, and in medico-legal work. Sometimes, important discrepancies can be found and documented, such as the ability to give a minutely detailed history, but very poor scores on name and address testing.)

- *Insight*. The final category of the mental state examination, denoted 'insight', sounds somewhat unimportant, but, in fact, it is crucial, as it is shorthand for all of the following:
  - the patient's understanding of the illness
  - its cause
  - its effect upon his life

– his attitude to treatment
– the outcome he expects.

Patients who feel they are going to get better and take ownership of the process of treatment and rehabilitation tend to do better than pessimistic patients who rely entirely on the outside world to effect a cure. Insight is therefore closely linked to prognosis. Avoid meaningless statements such as 'partial insight present', but consider practical questions such as, does the patient believe an illness is present, or does he attribute all the symptoms to an external cause (such as poisoning by rays)? Will he accept treatment?

(*Note*: not all patients referred to psychiatrists are mentally ill! Apparent paranoid delusions, for example, may reflect real persecution. And not everyone involved in an accident receives an injury.)

Physical examination

All inpatients should have a physical examination, including a thorough neurological one. For outpatients, the responsibility for physical examination is generally accepted as remaining with the referrer; however, it is good practice to check for physical signs relevant to the case; for example, to look for signs of thyrotoxicosis in a patient with symptoms of anxiety, for injection marks in a patient with suspected intravenous drug use, or for extrapyramidal signs in a patient on antipsychotic drugs. Examination candidates should always check for selected physical signs such as these.

Summary (formulation)

The summary of a new case includes the following:

- the *positive features* of history and examination

- any *relevant negative features*, such as absence of a family history

- *differential diagnoses*, starting with the most likely possibility, and giving evidence for and against each one. A definite diagnosis cannot always be made from the first interview, so listing two or three possibilities is quite acceptable.

- *aetiology*, considering predisposing, precipitating, and perpetuating factors, and the question of why the disorder has developed at this stage in the patient's life

- plan of *investigation*; for example, interview with informant, selected laboratory tests

- plan of *management*

- comments on *prognosis*.

Case example 1

A single man aged 26, who has been unemployed since he dropped out of art college 5 years ago, and who lives with his mother, was admitted to the psychiatric hospital under Section 2 of the Mental Health Act 1983, after trying to jump from an Underground platform but being pulled back by another passenger. He did this because he kept hearing two voices talking to each other, saying 'foul things' about him. He says his problems began 6 months ago when he saw the girl he wanted to marry (though he had never spoken to her) going into a pub with another man. Since then, he has felt low in mood, lost interest in everything, stayed in his room most of the day, had both early and late insomnia, and not wanted to eat because the food tasted different. He admits to smoking cannabis several times a week for several years.

On examination, he was a thin man, casually dressed. He seemed suspicious, and several times he suddenly stopped talking in midsentence and looked round as if he had heard something behind him. He described depressive symptoms and third-person auditory hallucinations as above.

The differential diagnosis includes schizophrenia; depressive illness; and drug-induced psychosis.

Predisposing factors include genetic loading for psychiatric disorder, because the patient's father has had several admissions to a mental hospital and now has injections from a community nurse.

Further investigations should include a physical examination, urine screen for drugs, an interview with the patient's mother, and perusal of his father's notes. Initial management will include close observation in the ward setting, bearing in mind a possible continuing suicide risk.

Case example 2

A 37-year-old married man was referred to psychiatric outpatients from the gastroenterology clinic where he has been attending for 2 years with a diagnosis of irritable bowel syndrome. Recent physical investigations have not shown any new pathology. His symptoms of abdominal pain and diarrhoea have been worse over the past 6 months since he was made redundant from work. During this time, he has also developed low mood, poor appetite with weight loss, loss of libido, and insomnia with early waking. On mental state examination, he appeared anxious and depressed; borborygmi were audible during the interview, and the patient had to leave at one point to visit the lavatory.

The most likely diagnosis is depressive illness, with associated anxiety symptoms, and exacerbation of his functional bowel disorder. The diagnosis of anxiety disorder alone would not cover his 'biological' symptoms of depression. Another possibility is organic bowel disease, but this seems unlikely in view of his recent normal investigations. He appears predisposed to psychological disorder by an anxious personality, and this present episode appeared precipitated by his redundancy and perpetuated by his continuing unemployment.

An interview with his wife confirmed the likely diagnosis of depression, and suggested that the patient had been particularly affected by his loss of role as breadwinner for the family, because his wife had recently been promoted in her own work.

Further physical investigation seems unnecessary, and might even prove unhelpful by adding to the patient's worries about his physical health. Antidepressant medication would be the quickest way to help this man, and amitriptyline would be suitable with its additional sedative, anxiolytic, and hypnotic properties. He could also be offered training in psychological techniques of anxiety management.

Structured interviews and questionnaires

These instruments are used mainly in research work. Their purpose is collection of data in a reliable standard form, minimizing the bias, which can arise from variation in individual interview technique. They can be administered by trained personnel other than psychiatrists.

Well-known examples of structured interviews are the Present State Examination (PSE) and its later development, the Schedules for Clinical Assessment in Neuropsychiatry (SCAN), which is analysed by computer (CATEGO program) to produce a diagnosis; the Standardized Psychiatric Interview (SPI) or Clinical Interview Schedule (CIS), developed for use in general practice and concerned largely with neurotic symptoms; and the Structured Clinical Interview for DSM–IV (SCID).

A widely used questionnaire is the General Health Questionnaire (GHQ), a self-rating instrument used to detect probable cases of psychiatric disorder in general practice settings or community surveys. Many other questionnaires, both self-rating and observer rating, exist for specific parameters such as depression, anxiety, or cognitive impairment.

Computer programs for direct self-assessment of patients have been used in research projects and found to be valid, acceptable, and cost-effective for certain psychiatric conditions, but seem unlikely to replace clinical interviews in everyday practice.

Interview with informant

It is customary to use the word 'informant', although, of course, this does not imply that the communication with this person is secret. On the contrary, it would be unethical and antitherapeutic to speak with a third party without the patient's consent, unless it is an emergency. A separate interview with an informant, usually the nearest relative, is essential if the patient is too disturbed, confused, or uncooperative to give a full history. In other cases, it often adds useful information, too, especially on the premorbid personality and the extent to which the illness has disrupted the patient's life.

Further assessments

Most general psychiatry is now done as part of a Community Mental Health Team (CMHT). Mild cases may be seen by just the psychiatrist. More severe or complex cases, or where the nature of the problems is unclear, may also be seen by a CMHT member as well as the psychiatrist. Often, CMHT staff work 'generically', so that the patient may be seen by a community psychiatric nurse, a social worker, or a member of another discipline such as an occupational therapist. By talking to the patient, preferably at home, and interviewing (with the patient's agreement) relatives, friends, neighbours, or workmates, the professional can obtain additional information about the psychiatric history and any other relevant problems, such as those concerning marriage, family, work, and finance.

This is then fed back and discussed at a team meeting, and a plan of management is formulated.

Most CMHTs have a psychologist, or access to one, and the main way in which this resource is used is in various forms of treatment. This usually depends on the psychologists forming an independent assessment of their own, which is very useful as part of the overall formulation of the case, even if the patient is deemed unsuitable for psychotherapy.

Psychometric tests, measuring such parameters as intelligence, memory, perception, behaviour, and personality, may be useful aids to assessment in patients with organic brain damage, or in assessing child or learning-disability patients. However, they are not routinely used in general psychiatry, because the clinical psychologists who used routinely to administer them have now – probably rightly – become more concerned with therapy than with diagnostic assessment.

Psychological tests that quantify the type and severity of impairments, and identify those abilities that still remain intact, are helpful in planning rehabilitation programmes, and also provide a baseline for monitoring long-term progress.

In medico-legal cases, especially those involving head injury, scores on memory testing can be reduced, owing either to genuine reduction in intellectual capability or to poor effort in testing. *Effort testing* allows assessment of the effort the patient brings to cognitive testing, by examining the pattern of scores on tests of varying degrees of difficulty. Someone making a good effort scores well on tests that are in fact easy (even though they may look hard), and scores lower on more difficult tests (http://www.wordmemorytest.com). Effort testing is important in medico-legal and disability assessments.

Physical investigations

The aim of physical investigation is to find a treatable lesion and/or make an aetiological diagnosis. 'Routine' laboratory tests seldom yield abnormal results in young adult psychiatric patients, unless there are physical symptoms or signs, or a history of alcohol misuse. Therefore, screening of younger patients who appear to be in good physical health is clearly not cost-effective, although many units do carry out blood tests on all new admissions, and these reveal occasional cases of unsuspected organic disease, most commonly thyroid dysfunction in women.

Elderly patients, and patients of any age with symptoms or signs suggesting physical illness, do need investigation. Basic tests include blood count and erythrocyte sedimentation rate (ESR); urea and electrolytes; thyroid and liver function; vitamin B_{12} and folate; urine testing for glucose, protein, cells, and bacteria; and chest radiography (but skull radiography very seldom yields useful information). Other tests such as the electroencephalogram (EEG), brain scan, analysis of blood or urine for drugs, syphilis serology, and HIV testing may be done if clinical indications exist. (Except in very special circumstances, HIV testing should not be carried out unless the patient gives informed consent, and receives both pre- and post test counselling.)

The EEG

The EEG records the pattern of electrical activity from various parts of the brain. The main types of activity are called alpha, beta, delta, and theta. Most, but not all, patients with organic brain disorders show abnormalities on EEG. The main practical use of the EEG is in the diagnosis of epilepsy; for detecting focal brain lesions, computerized tomography (CT) or magnetic resonance imaging (MRI) scans are more helpful. Patients with untreated 'functional' psychiatric illness usually have normal EEGs, but treatment with psychotropic drugs and electroconvulsive therapy (ECT) alters the pattern.

Brain scans

- CT or CAT (computerized axial tomography) involves scanning from different angles with an X-ray tube and detector system, and reconstruction of cross-sectional or coronal pictures to provide views of both the brain and the ventricular system.

- MRI or NMR (nuclear magnetic resonance) works by recording the response to radio waves applied to the body within a magnetic field. Clear pictures of both white and grey matter may be obtained from any desired angle. MRI is superior to CT for some purposes, but less widely available.

- PET (positron emission tomography) works by detecting local concentrations of radioisotopes, and provides information about function, such as glucose or oxygen consumption and the activity of various neurotransmitters.

- SPECT (single photon emission computerized tomography) utilizes nuclear radiotracers to localize different receptors.

PET and SPECT are available in only a few centres in the UK, and are likely to remain research tools for the foreseeable future.

Further reading

Sims, A. C. P. (2002). *Symptoms in the Mind: An Introduction to Descriptive Psychopathology* (3rd edn). London: Baillière Tindall.

Part II Clinical syndromes

4 Schizophrenia

Definition

Schizophrenia is a psychotic illness that, in its active phase, includes delusions, hallucinations, and disruption of thinking, feeling, and many other mental functions. Many cases run a chronic course, leaving residual psychiatric symptoms and impaired social functioning, in respect of relationships, study, and work. On the positive side, however, the illness appears to be getting less frequent and milder, with severe 'classic' features of the disease such as catatonia (see below) now rare in the UK.

A patient with an acute episode is the general public's idea of a 'mad' person, and probably as a consequence, schizophrenia is often considered the most serious of all psychiatric conditions. It has gained more public prominence in recent years, since patients who would once have spent their lives in the old 'asylum' mental hospitals now live in the community. 'Care in the community' has generally been a success, but a few problem cases (for example, the tragic death of Jonathan Zito: www.zitotrust.co.uk) have tended to make the public think the opposite.

Frequency

As indicated, schizophrenia seems to have become less common and also less severe in recent years, at any rate in developed countries. The lifetime risk of

Hughes' Outline of Modern Psychiatry, Fifth Edition. David Gill.
© 2007 John Wiley & Sons, Ltd   ISBN 9780470033920

getting the condition is approximately 1 per cent. There are about 15 new cases per 100 000 population per annum.

Epidemiology

- *Age*: the condition usually begins in late adolescence or early adult life, although it can be before puberty in rare cases, and occasionally in later life.

- *Sex*: schizophrenia is equally common in men and women, but tends to start at a younger age in males.

- *Marital status*: patients are more likely to be single than the average members of the population, due both to problems in forming relationships and to increased relationship breakdown.

- *Fertility* is reduced, although it remains unclear whether there are additional biological factors responsible, or whether it is due to the aforementioned relationship difficulties.

- *Social class*: schizophrenia is commoner in lower socio-economic groups. This is probably due to the patient's drifting down the social scale, before the onset of the illness. The original social class of new patients with schizophrenia, as defined by father's occupation, is distributed according to the distribution of social class in the population.

- *Country*: the frequency of schizophrenia is roughly the same in most countries; in the countries where there is a different figure, this has generally been found to be due to different criteria for the diagnosis of the condition. In the 1970s, an international survey found that psychiatrists in the UK and a number of other countries diagnosed schizophrenia much less frequently than their counterparts in the USA, and also in Russia, where the communist regime misused psychiatry to confine dissidents.

Causation

Causation of the condition as a whole, and causation of an individual episode of it in a particular patient, will be described separately.

Causation of an acute episode

This is usually a readily understandable matter in clinical practice. The usual model of multifactorial causation applies, with predisposing, precipitating, and perpetuating factors. Important examples are as follows:

- poor compliance with medication; e.g. because of side-effects

- dropout from follow-up; e.g. after moving house

- substance misuse; e.g. alcohol or illegal drugs

- accommodation problems

- relationship problems

- contact with criminal justice system.

In most cases, the precipitating cause will be obvious; attention to the symptoms will be important, but the immediate problem causing the worsening of symptoms needs also to be addressed.

Causation of schizophrenia as a condition

As with the causation of an individual episode, many different factors contribute: genetic, environmental, psychological, and social. This may be disappointing to some, considering the huge amount of research that has gone into the question. However, a simple 'magic bullet' theory is never going to be sufficient to account for the complexity of the condition and its causation.

However, mental disorders are not different from physical disorders in being somewhat 'messy' as regards causation. Consider, for example, tuberculosis; we know that the tubercle bacillus is required to produce the clinical condition of tuberculosis. But we also know that other factors, such as heredity and socio-economic status, influence whether the bacilli go on to cause clinical tuberculosis.

Causation of schizophrenia: overall model

Although there is no agreement about the details, there is a general view that the condition reflects a combination of some or all of the following factors:

- There is genetic predisposition.

- There is subtle damage to the brain, perhaps through viral infection before birth.

- The condition 'lies dormant' in childhood (although prodromal signs such as clumsiness, developmental delay, and behavioural or emotional difficulties may later be recognizable, albeit retrospectively).

• The condition 'comes out' after puberty, in the context of the 'rewiring' or remodelling of the brain that is known to go on at adolescence.

• The condition 'comes out' especially if the person is subject to other pathogenic factors such as cannabis use.

'Is schizophrenia the price that *Homo sapiens* pays for language?' Such fascinating speculations (Crow, 2002) link the causation of schizophrenia with the evolutionary development of language, and the origins of cerebral dominance (left- or right-handedness). *Gender* differences are also important, males tending to develop the condition earlier, and to have a worse outlook than females.

Genetics

There is no doubt that the condition has a genetic aspect. *Twin studies* provide some of the strongest evidence, especially those comparing identical twins, who have entirely the same genes, with non-identical twins, who share only 50 per cent of their genetic material, and are no more alike genetically than two siblings from different pregnancies. If one twin has schizophrenia, about 50 per cent of the co-twins also have schizophrenia if they are identical, but only about 10 per cent if they are non-identical. Three points follow:

• There must be a genetic component of the causation of schizophrenia; otherwise, there is no way of explaining the differences in the 'concordance rates' between identical and non-identical twins.

• However, the condition is not completely genetic; otherwise, there would be 100 per cent concordance between identical twins for the condition.

• Therefore, environmental factors must also be important.

Hunting the gene for schizophrenia

The human genome project was trumpeted by its projectors as the fundamental answer to medical mysteries such as the causation of disease. Unravelling the DNA would thus lead to the discovery of the underlying biochemical abnormalities that, they presumed, were responsible for otherwise mysterious conditions such as schizophrenia. A new discipline of 'psychopharmacogenetics' (Tsapakis *et al.*, 2004) was even suggested, whereby genes would in some way guide drug treatment.

Unfortunately, like other reductionist movements in medicine, the so-called human genome project, even after the expenditure of enormous sums of money, has not led to major advances in understanding in medicine in general, let alone to practical advances for psychiatric patients. It has recently been decided that the answer in respect of schizophrenia, at least, is to sequence the entire human genome again, but this time in patients with the condition (http://www.schizophrenia.com/sznews/archives/003235.html); one hopes this will not be throwing good money after bad.

The overall pattern for the condition is that a first-degree relative of a patient with schizophrenia has an approximately 10 per cent chance of having the disease himself, as compared with approximately 1 per cent in the general population. Second-degree relatives have about a 3 per cent risk. If both the parents have schizophrenia, the risk in the children is about 50 per cent. Even if children with a genetic risk of schizophrenia are reared away from their biological families, as through adoption, there is not much reduction in their risk of getting the condition, confirming a genetic component in its aetiology.

Inheritance patterns

Here again, the picture is complex and confusing. Established techniques of genetic mapping have demonstrated that the patterns of inheritance differ between families. In some family trees, it looks as though a single gene might be responsible, although it is not expressed to full effect in every individual carrying it (so-called incomplete penetrance). In other pedigrees, however, the pattern is better fitted by smaller contributions from a number of different genes.

So far, therefore, it has not been possible to pinpoint one particular gene on one particular chromosome as the genetic key to the condition, either with traditional genetic mapping techniques or with more recent genome sequencing.

Brain biochemistry

Disturbance of the 'chemical balance' in the brain is frequently suggested as part of the background to mental illness. In the case of schizophrenia, the introduction of effective antipsychotic drugs in the 1960s, starting with chlorpromazine, gave rise to neurochemical theories of causation. When the drugs were introduced, they were dramatically effective, and allowed many long-term hospital inpatients to be discharged. They were known to be effective antihistamine drugs, but the previous generation of antihistamines did not have their powerful antipsychotic properties.

Studies were therefore done to see how these new drugs worked. It was found that they were probably working by action on the substance dopamine, which is a naturally occurring neurotransmitter in the brain. (A neurotransmitter is a chemical messenger that is released in small packets at the surface of one nerve cell – the synapse – allowing it to communicate with its neighbouring nerve cells by interaction with receptors on it.) For example, the potency of a drug per milligram, in blocking dopamine, was directly in proportion to its potency as an antipsychotic in clinical practice.

In line with this theory of how they work was the observed side-effect of antipsychotic drugs to produce stiffness and shakiness of the muscles, as in Parkinson's disease, which is itself known to be caused by a lack of dopamine in certain parts of the brain (the substantia nigra of the basal ganglia).

Other evidence supporting a role for dopamine includes the fact that drugs, such as amphetamines, which stimulate dopamine, can precipitate a schizophrenia-like condition (amphetamine psychosis). This point is somewhat vitiated, however, by the fact that such conditions can also be produced by other illicit drugs, including cannabis and LSD, which affect different neurotransmitter systems.

Some studies have shown changes in the number of dopamine receptors in the brains of patients with schizophrenia after death, but these are difficult to interpret because most of the patients will have received antipsychotic drugs, and it is not possible to be absolutely sure that the changes in dopamine receptors are not due to the effects of the drugs.

The subtype of D2 dopamine receptors has been particularly closely studied. Unfortunately, as with genetics, the continuation of research has caused simplistic theories of 'excessive D2 function = schizophrenia' to have to be abandoned. For example, clozapine is an extremely potent antipsychotic drug, but it has only weak D2 effects; this agent is powerful at 5HT2a receptors.

Other neurotransmitters, such as GABA, ACh, serotonin, and glutamate, have also been implicated. It seems clear that dopamine is concerned in the process, but also that this is not the whole story.

Brain structure

Abnormalities are apparent, both on naked eye (macroscopic) and microscopic examination, and on special investigation with brain scans (CT, MRI, and others). The brains of patients with schizophrenia tend to be smaller and lighter, and the normal fluid-filled spaces inside the brain (the ventricles) are larger. In particular, the temporal lobes of the brain (which are near the temple, and are to do with hearing) are smaller in schizophrenia; this establishes links with the possible source of auditory hallucinations, and ties in with the schizophrenia-like picture sometimes presented by patients who have temporal lobe epilepsy.

These structural changes are thought to reflect abnormal brain development in early life, but degeneration at a later date might also contribute. In support of the importance of brain damage are clinical observations that schizophrenia is associated with the following features:

• minor neurological signs (so-called soft signs)

• abnormalities on brain scan

• reduced intellectual function, including lower IQ and poor performance on tests of memory, concentration, and attention

• temporal lobe epilepsy of the dominant hemisphere

• birth complications, possibly involving mild brain damage due to lack of oxygen

• winter birth – possibly in association with the next feature

• maternal viral infection in pregnancy (although evidence for this is conflicting).

On *microscopic* examination, the neurons in this condition tend to be smaller and less richly connected to their neighbours; this would tie in with theories about 'neurodevelopment' as part of the pathological process.

Psychological aspects

Many psychological theories have been put forward over the years, particularly driving from psychoanalysis; however, concepts such as the 'schizophrenogenic mother' are no longer regarded as helpful.

In recent years, psychologists have used cognitive-behavioural models to try to understand and explain the psychotic phenomena seen in schizophrenia, suggesting, for example, that delusions may have their origin in a person's inbuilt tendency to jump to conclusions about things and to ignore conflicting evidence (this has led to the trial of cognitive-behavioural therapy in psychosis, although there is no clear evidence at present that it is effective, and it has yet to establish a place in routine clinical practice).

Personality

In about 50 per cent of patients, premorbid personality has 'schizoid' features such as social isolation and eccentricity, although this may represent a prodrome of the illness itself. Prospective cohort studies have shown that children who show such features have an increased risk of schizophrenia in later life.

Family and social factors

The work of R. D. Laing (*The Divided Self*) and many others, as in Bateson's 'double bind', has focused attention on family dynamics and on the attitude of society as primary causes of schizophrenia. In retrospect, the work of Laing and others seems to be more cultural than scientific, coinciding as it did with the 'anti-psychiatry' movement and wider criticism of the Western nuclear family.

The main survivor from these ideas has been the concept of 'expressed emotion' (EE), whereby patients with schizophrenia who come from families who react strongly to their behaviours are known to be at increased risk of relapse. Family therapy (Pilling *et al.*, 2002) can reduce the risk of relapse, but this result may not necessarily support the concept of EE, as the therapy could be operating in other ways.

Life events

As previously indicated, the occurrence of 'life events' frequently triggers an acute episode. This fact, although prosaic, is nevertheless important in the management of patients with this condition.

Clinical features

Clinically, schizophrenia is a highly heterogeneous condition.

Onset

Onset may be gradual and insidious, without obvious precipitating factors; however, it may be acute and seemingly associated with life events. Symptoms may include abnormalities of perception, such as hallucinations, abnormal beliefs, and delusions. There may be disruption of thought processes, so-called thought disorder, as well as behavioural and motor symptoms.

I will now discuss in detail the symptoms and signs of the condition, according to the standard headings of the mental state examination.

Appearance and behaviour

The patient may have a first presentation after contact with the criminal justice system or after failure to cope in a first job or at university, or may withdraw into their house or room. Deliberate self-harm and contact with drug and alcohol agencies are frequent.

Often the standard of self-care, as reflected in the appearance, may be reduced. In severe cases, where patients lose the ability to care for themselves, there may be self-neglect. More frequently, the patient's appearance will just be somewhat unusual. By saying this, of course, I do not mean that there is anything intrinsically unhealthy about the adoption of particular styles of appearance; it is just that clinical experience indicates that fairly outlandish styles of dress may be seen in newly presenting patients with schizophrenia. A misguided sense of 'political correctness' should not be permitted to lead one to ignore such matters. Tactful enquiry may therefore be necessary to find out the meaning to the patient, if, for example, they wear clothes of only one colour.

Presentations with abnormal movements and fixed posturing (*catatonia*) are classical, although now rare in developed countries. Catatonic features include mannerisms, stereotypies, imitation of the speech and behaviour of others (echolalia and echopraxia), negativism, mutism, stupor, hyperactivity, and prolonged maintenance of strange postures (waxy flexibility).

Speech

There is usually no abnormality in the production of speech itself.

Mood

Abnormalities of mood of some description are common. This is most often a flat or empty affect, especially in patients with an insidious onset and pronounced lack of will. There is not usually a pronounced and pervasive depression or elation of mood (if so, consideration of a primary mood disorder would be appropriate as an alternative diagnosis). Irritability and fear may also be present, as in response to delusions or hallucinations. The mood may be *incongruous*, for example, inexplicably cheerful, sometimes seeming to vary according to the content of auditory hallucinations.

Extreme mood changes of elation, depression, or rage may occur. Sustained depressive symptoms are found in at least 50 per cent of patients on follow-up, and are probably part of the schizophrenic process, although they may also represent side-effects of antipsychotic drug treatment, or a response to the realization of having such a serious disease.

Thought

Disorders of the possession of thought

These disorders include *thought insertion* (a sensation that some outside agency is putting thoughts into one's mind), *thought withdrawal* (the opposite experience), and *thought broadcasting* (the belief that one's thoughts are being communicated to other people). Strictly speaking, these could be considered to be delusions, although often the experience is described in such a matter-of-fact way by the patient that it seems to be a phenomenon that is real to them, and it is by custom classified separately. *Thought block* is the abrupt complete cessation of a train of thought.

Disorders of the stream of thought

· *Knight's move thinking* (asyndetic thinking, derailment of thought) is abrupt transition from one topic to another semi-related one.

· *Concrete thought* is inability to appreciate abstract concepts, although some patients show the opposite tendency and assume symbolic meanings that are not intended.

· *Poverty of thought* is one of the 'negative' symptoms characteristic of the chronic stages of the illness.

Of course, our only way of knowing about patients' thoughts is through their talk, which may be vague and difficult to follow. Sometimes, the patient will make sense in respect of individual sentences, but drift gradually off the point. They may seem to be articulate, and it may be some time before one appreciates that they are 'talking past the point' or are 'tangential' or 'over-inclusive'. There may be odd changes of topic, or the content may be incomprehensibly bizarre.

Some patients keep repeating the same words or phrases (verbigeration), use idiosyncratic words (neologisms), or, in very severe psychosis, speak in a jumble of words or even word fragments (word salad).

False beliefs (delusions)

The most common types of delusion in schizophrenia would probably be persecutory, but grandiose or nihilistic delusions are also common. At this point, it is worth noting that, strictly speaking, paranoid has a wider meaning than just persecutory: the derivation, I understand, is from Greek words meaning 'out of mind', and paranoid has been used to cover, for example, the grandiose or sexual content of delusions also.

As previously described, a delusion is a false belief that is unshakable by reasoned argument, and that is inappropriate, bearing in mind the patient's cultural and religious background. Delusions, are almost always false, although occasionally they may be true; perhaps, for example, the police may really be 'after' the person. It is the reasons for the belief that are irrational, and fundamentally define the belief as delusional – for example, that the patient knows the police are after him because they are wearing blue uniforms.

Onset of schizophrenia may be preceded by a *delusional mood* in which the patient feels perplexed because the environment seems subtly changed. This feeling may be suddenly followed by a *primary delusion* (*autochthonous delusion*), usually linked with an ordinary sense perception (*delusional perception*). For example, one patient saw a yellow car drive by and took this to mean that he was Christ reincarnated. Delusions are most often paranoid, but may be of any kind. A complex system of secondary delusions may be elaborated from the primary one.

Hallucinations

Hallucinations can affect any sensory modality, but most commonly hearing (auditory). Indeed, hallucinations affecting vision or smell would give rise to a suspicion that the patient might have an organic (physical) condition affecting the brain, and appropriate examinations and investigations (e.g. MRI of the brain) would then be considered. Nevertheless, visual hallucinations and tactile hallucinations are seen in patients with very extreme schizophrenic states.

Detailed enquiry into the possible hallucinatory experiences is vital at a first presentation. It is all too easy for phenomena to be labelled as 'auditory hallucinations' when, in fact, they do not satisfy criteria for this. The problem is that recording of auditory hallucinations in medical notes may immediately give rise to a diagnosis of psychosis/schizophrenia, so that the patient is placed on antipsychotic medication, and the symptoms and diagnosis repeated from year to year.

Patients with personality disorder may hear voices. 'They're inside me 'ead, Doc, they keep telling me to cut meself.' These are not true hallucinations, and they are sometimes referred to as 'pseudohallucinations'. In contrast, true auditory hallucinations in schizophrenia are experienced as coming from the outside world. They are real to the patient. It is a real voice to him, but there is no one there speaking.

It is necessary to find out the patient's explanation for this experience. Many patients, at least in the early stages, will find the hallucination completely terrifying. Other patients may regard it as 'part of the plan', as it will be part of a system of delusions. Still others will, as time goes by, get used to the idea that the voices are not real, even though they were undoubtedly psychotic phenomena in the early years, and remain so.

Voices discussing the patient in the third person are characteristic, but second-person voices which talk to the patient are common too.

Volition

Passivity feelings, in which emotions or actions are felt to be controlled by an outside agent, may be present. Bizarre urges out of keeping with the previous personality may occur. Some patients lack initiative and drive regarding the activities of daily life.

Cognition

One of the original (Kräpelinian) descriptions of the illness we now recognize as schizophrenia was 'dementia praecox'; in other words, presenile dementia. The patient would display a gradual onset of symptoms, characterized by loss of initiative, lack of interest in self-care, and general social withdrawal; delusions and hallucinations, although often present, were not the dominant part of the clinical picture. Stereotyped behaviour was common. These patients often ended up in long-stay care in institutions, and undoubtedly would show impairments on cognitive testing. However, such cases would be unusual in general psychiatric practice nowadays.

Regarding cognitive testing in patients with schizophrenia today, if they were in remission, it would be expected that 'bedside' tests of orientation, concentration, and memory would be roughly normal, although, if more subtle tests were done, it would be expected that they would underperform in comparison with control subjects.

As regards patients with current acute psychosis, obviously, it would not be expected that they would be unimpaired in such tests. The key point to remember, however, is that in most cases of schizophrenia, there is no substantial cognitive impairment, and there is no process of cognitive deterioration such as would be seen in presenile dementia due to cerebral pathology such as Alzheimer's disease.

Insight

Insight is the final heading in the mental state examinations as customarily set out. In schizophrenia, it is very important in management and is one of the main determinants of prognosis. It would be better if the term were replaced by some such phrase as 'patient's attitude to illness and treatment'. It is a complex matter, and questions such as 'does the patient believe he is ill?', and 'will the patient accept treatment?', are key; however, schizophrenic patients are often conflicted about these matters. For example, sometimes they will only come into hospital against their will on a section of the Mental Health Act; nevertheless, once in the hospital, they will seem to accept medication without dispute. Conversely, patients may say that they believe that they are ill, and that they will accept treatment when they leave the hospital; however, once out of the hospital, they refuse the treatment on the grounds that they do not believe that they are ill.

Accordingly, insight in schizophrenia is something of great practical importance. It can only really be assessed by trial and error, as it were, the proof of the pudding being in the eating.

Positive and negative symptoms

Symptoms of schizophrenia are sometimes divided into *positive*, such as delusions and hallucinations, and *negative*, such as poverty of thought and speech, lack of initiative, social withdrawal, slowness, unreliability, and poor self-care. Positive symptoms are prominent during acute episodes; negative symptoms are characteristic of the chronic stage.

A more recent subdivision of symptoms describes three groups: *reality distortion* (that is, delusions and hallucinations), *disorganization* (that is, disruption of the connection between thoughts, formal thought disorder), and *psychomotor poverty* (that is, negative symptoms).

Physical health

The physical health of patients with schizophrenia may be impaired by heavy smoking, substance misuse, unusual eating habits, excess fluid consumption leading to water intoxication, poor hygiene, lack of exercise, other forms of self-neglect, and the side-effects of antipsychotic drugs (see Chapter 23) on various body systems.

Metabolic problems

'Metabolic syndrome' is a combination of truncal obesity, abnormal blood lipids, disturbed insulin and glucose metabolism, and high blood pressure; it is associated with the development of diabetes mellitus and coronary heart disease. It is more frequent in patients with schizophrenia than in the general population. It may be particularly contributed to by antipsychotic medication, especially some of the newer 'atypical' agents such as olanzepine, which seems to have appetite-stimulating qualities.

Case example

A young man of 21 developed the belief that his computer games were communicating with him by messages through the screen that only he could see. Some of the messages were transmitted 'directly into my mind'.

He had been an above-average student in his early teens, but his performance had declined and he had left school at 18 without qualifications. He had then attended a local college sporadically, but had dropped out, and seemed to have been at home with his family.

Most of the time since then he seemed to have spent in his room, playing computer games for several hours per day; he also consumed a good deal of cannabis, and this seemed to be regarded as normal in his home.

Admission to hospital followed a disturbance at his home when he smashed up the television and his room.

On admission, he had delusions about being controlled by computer games; during admission, it became clear that he was subject to auditory hallucinations, but would never say anything about them.

He was tried on various medications, but was observed to deteriorate; he appeared to develop thought blocking such that it was impossible to have a conversation: he would volunteer no speech, and questions were answered, after a pause of a second or two, by an uncomprehending 'Eh?'

He showed no response to standard medications (haloperidol) or to 'atypical' medications (olanzepine); he was then tried on clozapine, which, in conjunction with a rehabilitation placement, resulted in partial symptomatic and functional improvement, so that he was able to be discharged eventually to supported – warden controlled – accommodation.

Clinical types

Much emphasis used to be placed on differentiating various subtypes of schizophrenia. It is important to be aware of the different terms. However, they are of limited practical usefulness. They do not seem to predict response to medication or overall prognosis.

Nor is it even clear that they are stable through time, so that, for example, a patient may display a picture of hebephrenic schizophrenia at one point but a picture of paranoid schizophrenia at another. Nevertheless, it is a matter of clinical experience that a patient does tend to have roughly similar patterns of symptoms and signs during each acute episode – the same behaviours, delusions, or hallucinations recur.

The following summary, based on the ICD–10 classification, depends on the description of clinical syndromes. These probably represent overlapping states, rather than distinct entities.

Paranoid schizophrenia

Paranoid schizophrenia has delusions, often accompanied by hallucinations, as a prominent symptom. Paranoid schizophrenia usually develops later in life than the other types, and schizophrenic illness starting after middle age nearly always takes this form. It is commoner in women, and in those with impaired hearing. Genetic factors may be less important than in other types of schizophrenia. Contrary to what the public sometimes seems to think, the term 'paranoid schizophrenia' does not necessarily mean the most serious or dangerous form of the illness.

Hebephrenic schizophrenia

Although the term 'hebephrenic schizophrenia' is seldom used in UK clinical practice, it may be applied to adolescents and young adults showing a clinical picture in which thought disorder and affective (mood) changes are prominent.

Catatonic schizophrenia

Catatonia was common in the 'classical' era of psychiatry, when such authors as Kräpelin and Bleuler were writing; it was frequently seen in the old mental hospitals, and remains common in developing countries. It is now rare in UK practice: I have not seen a full-blown case for several years. But it is important to be aware of, not least because it may pose diagnostic and management difficulty if staff have not encountered it before.

The patient's clinical picture is like no other; he may appear cut off from the external world, even though he has apparently an undiminished level of consciousness. This can progress to catatonic stupor. Patients may also have varying degrees of abnormal movement, especially the adoption of abnormal postures for prolonged periods of time; for example, keeping an arm outstretched for many hours in a way that would be impossible for most people. On examination, such a limb may exhibit the classical 'waxy flexibility'. This means an increase in muscle tone, which is continuous and progressive as the limb is passively moved. This is qualitatively different from the increased tone that is seen, for example, in upper motor neuron lesions such as stroke or Parkinsonism. The condition responds to medication and nursing care, but ECT may be necessary in emergencies.

Simple schizophrenia

'Simple schizophrenia' (another term now seldom used) is characterized by negative symptoms, with gradual deterioration of the personality, flattening of affect, withdrawal from reality, and loss of drive, resulting in a lifestyle of social isolation and self-neglect. Positive symptoms may be few; therefore, in some cases, it is debatable whether a diagnosis of schizophrenia is actually justified. However, such patients can be among the most disabled patients with schizophrenia, unable to function independently. Response to medication is often poor. They will clearly stand in need of mental health services such as supported accommodation. So the question of whether or not a particular diagnosis is appropriate may be somewhat academic.

Residual schizophrenia

'Residual schizophrenia' is again a term not frequently used in clinical practice. It refers to the 'defect state' when delusions and hallucinations have passed, but when the patient remains affected by negative symptoms such as lack of initiative, apathy, self-neglect, and emotional blunting. Reduction of medication and rehabilitation will be appropriate. Clozapine should be considered.

Related conditions

Schizotypal disorder

Schizotypal disorder is described in the ICD–10 as

> a disorder characterized by eccentric behaviour and anomalies of thinking and affect which resemble those seen in schizophrenia, though no definite and characteristic schizophrenic anomalies occur at any stage. The symptoms may include a cold or inappropriate affect; anhedonia; odd or eccentric behaviour; a tendency to social withdrawal; paranoid or bizarre ideas not amounting to true delusions; obsessive ruminations; thought disorder and perceptual disturbances; occasional transient quasi-psychotic episodes with intense illusions, auditory or other hallucinations, and delusion-like ideas, usually occurring without external provocation. There is no definite onset and evolution and course are usually those of a personality disorder.

Again, schizotypal disorder is not a diagnosis frequently used in UK clinical practice, in my experience. The ICD–10 avers that it excludes 'schizoid personality disorder', but does not give clear instructions as to how this disorder is to be differentiated. In practice, patients with the characteristics described would probably be regarded as having mild schizophrenia.

Delusional disorders

Delusional disorders are conditions where the patient just has delusions, with few other symptoms, and the personality is well preserved. These will be dealt with in a separate chapter.

Acute and transient psychotic disorders

Patients occasionally present having become acutely psychotic 'out of the blue', with no previous history. Delusions and hallucinations, with disturbed behaviour, may be prominent for a few days or so, and then completely resolve. Sometimes there are obvious precipitants, such as emotional distress, overwork, or physical illness. Some patients are never heard from again. Others go on to have further episodes. However, most UK psychiatrists would have reservations about accepting that stress, in the absence of predisposition, illicit drugs, or some other definite causative factor, can cause true psychosis.

Because of the difficulty in assessing and predicting further episodes, most psychiatrists would record a diagnosis of 'psychotic episode' after a first such psychotic episode, as the diagnosis of schizophrenia can be very upsetting for the patient, and can have worse consequences; for example, it may adversely affect insurance cover and work.

Schizo-affective psychosis

In schizo-affective psychosis, manic or depressive (affective) symptoms co-exist with schizophrenic ones, and the illness follows a course of relapses and remissions. The term often gives rise to confusion, however. Sometimes it refers to an episode in which the patient has a mixture of mood and psychotic symptoms; at other times, it denotes a patient who has an episode of mood symptoms and then an episode of psychotic symptoms, or vice versa. Both patterns occur.

Such patients would be assessed and treated according to the symptoms prominent at the time, but bearing in mind the overall temporal pattern of the disorder. If there were regular relapses with good recovery, it would resemble bipolar affective disorder; preventive treatment, for example, with a mood stabilizer, would be indicated even if the current symptoms were mainly psychotic.

Paraphrenia

If there are few other symptoms, and the general personality is well preserved, the condition may be called *paraphrenia* if it comes on in later life. This especially applies in older patients, often with social isolation (e.g. after being widowed) and deafness or other sensory impairments.

Diagnostic criteria

The current diagnostic criteria are purely clinical and not fully satisfactory. Controversies about the diagnosis of schizophrenia include the following:

- whether the term should be reserved for illnesses that result in permanent residual defects (*nuclear* or *process* schizophrenia) or may also be applied to acute episodes (*schizophreniform reactions*) that may resolve completely

- whether the different clinical types of 'schizophrenia' are variants of the same disease process or are separate conditions

- whether cases without positive symptoms should be included

- whether there is a valid distinction between schizophrenia and the affective psychoses.

When Kräpelin described the condition in 1896 under the term *dementia praecox*, he distinguished it from manic-depressive illness because of its worse prognosis. E. Bleuler, who coined the term 'schizophrenia' in 1911, considered that the essential features were loosening of associations in thought, flattening or incongruity of affect, ambivalence and autism (withdrawal from reality), and some permanent defect in personality.

As Bleuler's symptoms cannot be precisely defined, widely differing concepts of 'schizophrenia' developed in different centres; for example, schizophrenia was diagnosed more readily in the USA, which followed the looser Bleulerian approach, than in the UK, which adopted the tighter Kräpelinian view. The differences persisted until the later editions of the DSM, which came closer to the ICD view (see below).

In recent years, there have been attempts to standardize the definition. A popular criterion in Britain is that of *Schneider's first rank symptoms*. Schneider (1959) postulated the following set of symptoms, any one of which would be diagnostic of schizophrenia in a patient without organic brain disease:

- Two or more hallucinatory voices discuss the patient in the third person.

- Voices make a running commentary on his thoughts or actions.

- Voices repeat his thoughts aloud (*écho de la pensée*).

- There is thought insertion, or withdrawal.

- There is thought broadcasting.

- *Bodily (somatic) feelings of influence*: the patient has bodily symptoms which he feels are produced by some outside agency.

- *Passivity feelings*: the patient experiences his thoughts or actions as being controlled by some external agency.

- *Delusional perception*: a normal perception gives rise to a fully formed delusion; e.g. 'the red car has just gone past, so I am the Messiah.'

However, research has shown that Schneider's symptoms may occur in affective psychoses also; they do not necessarily predict long-term outcome. Nevertheless, they remain a useful diagnostic pointer.

The main systems in use today are the DSM–IV and the ICD–10. The current editions are now fairly similar (although widely different in the past). The main differences are in the *duration required* – in the ICD, 1 month; in the DSM, 6 months – and in *social or occupational dysfunction*, which is required in the DSM but not specified under ICD.

Differential diagnosis

- *Organic brain disease*, such as temporal lobe epilepsy, head injury, or any form of physical condition affecting the brain. HIV may produce similar pictures in developing countries.

- *Drug-induced psychosis*: relevant drugs include cannabis, LSD, amphetamines, cocaine, 'magic mushrooms', and MDMA ('Ecstasy'). This is a common diagnostic question – and management problem – in everyday clinical practice. The drugs involved vary from place to place and from time to time. In the UK, cannabis is the main culprit. Cannabis use is a frequent contributory cause of psychosis. Stimulants such as amphetamine and cocaine can produce major psychotic states, often with persecutory delusions and disturbed behaviour including aggression.

- *Affective psychosis*: in other words, schizophrenia needs to be distinguished from depressive psychosis, and from manic states in which there are delusions and hallucinations as part of the picture.

- *Obsessive-compulsive disorder*. In severe obsessional states, the behaviours and thoughts can almost take over the patient's life, and if they are of a bizarre nature may be difficult to distinguish from psychosis.

- *Personality disorder.*

- *Acute reactions to stress*, especially in adolescents.

- *Simulation* of mental illness: rare, but sometimes seen in forensic settings.

Some of these conditions may present as indistinguishable from schizophrenia, and the correct diagnosis can be made only after investigation of physical factors;

a period of observation, especially if the episode was triggered by drug misuse; and/or a trial of antipsychotic treatment.

Treatment

Medication

Antipsychotic drugs remain the mainstay of treatment. Medication is effective in controlling positive symptoms in about 90 per cent of acute cases. Oral administration is usually suitable, but severely disturbed patients may need intramuscular doses to start with. If there are worries that the patient may not be swallowing tablets, liquid preparations, or special tablets that dissolve quickly in the mouth, can be helpful, although such formulations are not available for all agents. Medication may need to be given for up to 4 weeks before improvement starts. If the patient requires sedation, the addition of a benzodiazepine such as lorazepam can be most helpful and will assist in avoiding excessive doses of an antipsychotic.

Choice of drug

There has been a great change in prescribing over recent years in the UK. Newer drugs, the so-called *atypicals*, have largely supplanted the original drugs such as chlorpromazine and haloperidol. There has been great enthusiasm for atypicals, which have been heavily promoted as having fewer side-effects, and therefore being more acceptable to patients and promoting better quality of life. They have undoubtedly been a success in commercial terms. However, as with any new drug, the adverse effects have taken a little time to come out, and we are now seeing the balance of risks and benefits of the new drugs, as against the older drugs, becoming clearer.

The National Institute for Health and Clinical Excellence (NICE) (5) recommends that in 'a person who has been newly diagnosed with schizophrenia, doctors should consider prescribing one of the following atypical (newer) oral antipsychotic drugs: amisulpride, olanzepine, quetiapine, risperidone or zotepine.' This has become accepted practice, and many patients do recover on such a regime. However, there is less agreement as to what should be done if the patient does not respond to, say, risperidone or olanzepine.

Experience indicates that the most severely psychotic patients often do not respond, or do not respond fully, to the newer drugs. It should be borne in mind that, in modern randomized, controlled trials of medication, the most severely affected patients are often excluded. This will be, for example, on the grounds that if a person is dangerously unwell, it would be wrong that they should be exposed to the risk of a placebo treatment.

The older drugs seem more powerful in such cases. Hence, if the patient is severely unwell, and has not responded to an atypical, one of the older drugs should be considered. The prescriber would then face a choice between either stopping the atypical, and starting one of the 'classic' medications, or adding the second drug and continuing with the atypical. In my practice, a typical example would be a patient who has been started on olanzepine, and has benefited from the sedative and hypnotic properties of that drug, but still has troublesome delusions and hallucinations. In such patients, I often see good results from adding a small dose of haloperidol, say, 1.5–5 mg daily.

In this connection, it should be remembered that medications such as halo-peridol gained their poor reputation for side-effects from having been used in excessively high doses over the years. Haloperidol 1.5 mg is a powerful antipsy-chotic regime in itself, and may be sufficient, for example, in elderly patients. If high doses of haloperidol are given, however, side-effects will increase, whereas antipsychotic effects may not.

Trials of atypical agents, compared with haloperidol or other older antipsy-chotics, have of course generally taken the opportunity to use large doses of the old drug, thereby helping to demonstrate greater acceptability to patients of the new agents.

Many patients do very well on small doses of haloperidol or trifluoperazine, and do not experience side-effects from them; NICE does not recommend changing patients who are well maintained on such regimes.

Side-effects of drugs

The older drugs cause extrapyramidal side-effects commonly, particularly increases in muscle tone (stiffness), and tremor; risperidone and the other atypi-cals can also cause these, though less frequently.

The main problem with the atypical medications has been weight gain, and olanzepine seems to be notable for this; it seems to have an appetite-stimulating effect, and cases of diabetes (Koro et al., 2002) have also been recorded. There is also a risk of stroke (Ballard et al., 2006) in elderly patients with Alzheimer's disease and behavioural problems, so that risperidone and olanzepine are now contraindicated in these patients. By extension, they would probably be best avoided in all elderly patients, and possibly also in all those with cerebral vascular risk factors of whatever age.

Maintenance treatment

Patients who have made a good recovery from a first episode of schizophrenia may be able to taper off their medication after a few months. Those who have persistent symptoms or frequent relapses will usually be advised to stay on long-term medication. However, long-term therapy carries a higher risk of side-effects, so it needs to be monitored carefully, and the dose kept at the minimum necessary for symptom control.

Patients who have done well on small doses of medication can be considered for a trial of seeing whether they can do without it completely. However, this will depend on what the patient wants; some patients who have been very unwell in the past, rightly fear the return of symptoms and prefer to carry on with long-term medication. If, however, they wish to see whether they can do without medication, they will require close monitoring during the trial period; it will be necessary to restart the medication straightaway if symptoms re-emerge.

In general, patients who have a clear history of schizophrenia, and who are doing well on a small dose of medication that is not causing side-effects, are probably best advised to stay on it indefinitely unless they have strong wishes to the contrary.

Depot medication

This refers to long-acting preparations of antipsychotic medication, so that a patient who, for whatever reason, does not take tablets regularly, can instead be offered an injection of antipsychotic medication every 2, 3, or even 4 weeks. The active drug is suspended in a tiny quantity of oil, from which it is gradually released into the bloodstream. This form of treatment serves to keep a large number of patients reasonably well.

Frequently, it is a somewhat paradoxical situation, with the patient not fully believing that they are unwell, and not being keen on taking tablets: nevertheless, they turn up for their injection every 2 weeks and stay reasonably well as a result. Since the medication has to be given by intramuscular depot injections, this also ensures that patients are seen regularly by a community nurse or GP.

Other drugs

Many patients with pronounced mood instability or depression – or more commonly flatness – of mood can be prescribed mood stabilizers or antidepressants. If the question arises, there is often a strong case for at least trying the effect of such medications; response is unpredictable. Sometimes there is an improvement. Even if there is no benefit, at least the practitioner will have tried, and will therefore have been seen to have listened to the patient, his family, and/or his care coordinator. This cannot but be helpful to the building up of a therapeutic relationship.

Clozapine   NICE is very positive about the use of this drug in treatment-resistant schizophrenia: 'In individuals with evidence of treatment-resistant schizophrenia (TRS), clozapine should be introduced at the earliest opportunity. TRS is suggested by a lack of satisfactory clinical improvement despite the sequential use of the recommended doses for 6 to 8 weeks of at least two antipsychotics, at least one of which should be an atypical' (http://www.nice.org.uk/page.aspx?o=TA043guidance). The disadvantages of clozapine include the fact that it can cause bone marrow suppression, and therefore frequent monitoring of blood tests is required; even with careful monitoring, occasional deaths occur. It can only be given by mouth, and often causes hypersalivation.

However, most practising clinicians would agree that these disadvantages are outweighed by the advantages, which are that it can produce improvements when other medications have failed to do so. It is very rewarding for all concerned when a patient who has been severely unwell in the hospital experiences symptomatic and functional improvement after clozapine treatment and can be discharged. The effect can take weeks or months to build up, and residual symptoms and impairments may continue to some extent. Nevertheless, this drug can offer dramatic improvements in symptoms and quality of life.

Psychiatric services and treatments

The key to the patient's remaining well is to have a good and continuing relationship with his psychiatrist, and his care coordinator, who will usually be either a community psychiatric nurse or a social worker.

There has recently been a good deal of development in services. *Assertive outreach teams* have been developed in community mental health services; these are concerned with patients who disengage with treatment, and they can be effective in reducing hospital admission and improving the lives of some of these severely affected ('revolving door') patients.

Crisis teams are designed to step in in emergencies and provide extra help; typically, this will be according to the results of a joint assessment with the community mental health team and other interested parties. They can be helpful in reducing hospital admissions; however, it is important that inpatient admission is not seen as a failure, let alone as a bad thing. On the contrary, hospital admission frequently achieves progress, even when the best efforts of community services have not.

The latest trend is for the introduction of *early intervention teams*; these are intended to identify and treat early or even prodromal cases. Their watchword is that, by reducing the duration of psychosis before treatment commences, prognosis can be improved (see Chapter 25 on services for more about organization of care).

The development of the foregoing teams, although largely driven from central government, is often in practice done 'within existing resources'. What this means in effect is that the new teams can take staff and resources from the existing community mental health teams, which can be depleted as a result. There may also be 'boundary problems', with patients having to be assessed repeatedly for the same fundamental problem, as they move from one team to another. Nevertheless, the prevailing direction of development of services at the moment is toward the setting up of specialized small teams. They can work well if adequately resourced, with a stable staff group.

ECT

ECT (see Chapter 24) is an effective treatment for acute psychotic states that have failed to respond to inpatient care and medication. It continues to be widely used in developing countries, and has been a first-line treatment in this setting. However, it is seldom used for schizophrenia now in the UK.

Psychological treatments (see Chapter 22)

There is evidence that 'psycho-educational' (Nadeem *et al.*, 2006) interventions, including individual and group sessions, are effective at reducing relapse.

- *Family therapy* of a structured kind, including elements of education of patient and relatives about the illness and the reduction of high 'expressed emotion' (EE), has been shown to improve outcome for patients who live in the family home. Support for relatives, provided by mental health care professionals and/or self-help organizations, is important.

- *Cognitive-behavioural therapy* has been the subject of a great deal of research. There are suggestions that it can improve some outcomes, such as insight, but the practical clinical significance of such changes remains unclear.

- Psychodynamic psychotherapy is not appropriate for schizophrenia.

Social aspects (see Chapter 25)

First episodes of schizophrenia have in the past routinely received inpatient treatment; however, some can be dealt with in the community if there are adequate community mental health services, supplemented perhaps by a crisis team. Emergency admission, sometimes under the Mental Health Act 1983, may be required for acutely disturbed patients.

After acute symptoms are under control, most patients will be able to be discharged home, and the aim should be to resume normal life including going back to work as soon as possible. Other patients with practical impairments in, for example, ability to look after themselves, may need a period of rehabilitation, including guidance in work, practical aspects of daily living, behavioural modification, and social skills.

In the past, many patients spent the rest of their lives in the chronic wards of large mental hospitals, but such institutions have now almost entirely closed down. Most patients are now managed by community mental health teams working in collaboration with primary care. Warden-controlled flats, hostels, or group homes provide a suitable environment for those who cannot live independently or with their families, and day centres or voluntary work offer rehabilitation activity.

Some patients, however, live rough, or in unsupervised lodgings, either because no suitable accommodation can be found for them, or because they reject offers of help. They are easily lost to follow-up especially in inner-city areas, and, in the absence of medical or social care, there is a serious risk of self-neglect, self-harm, and occasionally of violence to themselves or others.

Use of the *care programme approach* (see Chapter 25), in which high-priority cases are monitored through a register and each patient has a named key worker, should enable medical and social care to be coordinated and maintained.

Prognosis

About 25 per cent of patients make a good recovery from a first episode of schizophrenia. About 10 per cent require long-term care, as in supported accommodation or a long-stay ward. The rest, while able to live relatively independently, continue to suffer chronic symptoms and may experience intermittent acute relapses.

Poor prognostic factors include a premorbid personality of schizoid type, with poor social adjustment; onset of illness early in life; gradual onset of illness without precipitating life stress; predominance of negative symptoms such as affective flattening; and delay between onset of symptoms and starting drug therapy.

Suicide, often committed by a violent method and without warning, accounts for death in about 15 per cent of patients. There is an association between schizophrenia and violence to others, although homicide is fortunately rare. There is some evidence (Arango *et al.*, 2006) that adherence to medication is associated with a reduction of violence to others.

References

Arango, C., Bombín, I., González-Salvador, T. *et al.* (2006). Randomised clinical trial comparing oral versus depot formulations of zuclopenthixol in patients with schizophrenia and previous violence. *Eur Psychiatry* **21**, 34–40.

Ballard, C., Waite, J. and Birks, J. (2006). Atypical antipsychotics for aggression and psychosis in Alzheimer's disease. *Cochrane Database Syst Rev* Issue 1, Art. No. CD003476.

Crow, T. J. (2002). Handedness, language lateralisation and anatomical asymmetry: relevance of protocadherin XY to hominid speciation and the aetiology of psychosis. *Br J Psychiatry* **181**, 295–297.

Koro, C., Fedder, D. O., L'Italien, G. J. *et al.* (2002). Assessment of independent effect of olanzapine and risperidone on risk of diabetes among patients with schizophrenia: population based nested case-control study. *BMJ* **325**, 243–246.

Nadeem, Z. *et al.* (2006). Psychoeducational interventions. *Clinical Evidence* (15th edn), p. 1484. London: BMJ Books. http://www.clinicalevidence.com/ceweb/conditions/meh/1007/1007_132.jsp.

Pilling, S., Bebbington, P., Kuipers, E. *et al.* (2002). Psychological treatments in schizophrenia. I. Meta-analysis of family interventions and cognitive behaviour therapy. *Psychol Med* **32**, 763–782.

Tsapakis, E. M., Basu, A. and Aitchison, K. J. (2004). Clinical relevance of discoveries in psychopharmacogenetics. *Adv Psychiatr Treat* **10**, 455–465.

5 Mood disorders: depressive illness and mania

Mood disorders (affective disorders) include depressive illness and mania. These are episodic conditions, occurring only once or twice in a lifetime for some patients but recurring at frequent intervals for others, usually with good recovery between episodes.

- *Unipolar affective disorder*: single or recurrent depressive episode(s), without manic ones. This forms the vast majority of patients with affective disorders.

- *Bipolar affective disorder* (formerly called *manic depressive psychosis*): both depressive and manic episodes. This is much less common than unipolar depression, but is more serious in most cases.

Patients with manic episodes only are very rare. Mixed affective states can also occur, usually in the context of bipolar disorder.

The milder forms of depression are also considered in this chapter. In this book, anxiety disorders, although sometimes classed with mood disorders, will be considered with the neuroses (see Chapter 6).

Hughes' Outline of Modern Psychiatry, Fifth Edition. David Gill.
© 2007 John Wiley & Sons, Ltd   ISBN 9780470033920

Frequency

How common is depression? This obviously depends on how it is defined, immediately taking us into controversial areas. The standard answer to this question
starts with 'major depressive disorder', as defined in the DSM. Community
surveys have shown that extraordinarily high numbers of the general public
satisfy diagnostic criteria for 'major depression' at any one time; for example,
estimates of at least 10 per cent are often quoted, and it is held that 20 per cent
or more of the population will experience an episode of depression during their
lifetime.

Bipolar affective disorder is at least 10 times less frequent than depression.
This is not controversial.

However, regarding unipolar depression, only a few of this 10 per cent are
actually in receipt of a diagnosis of depression, let alone treatment for it.

This apparent paradox can be interpreted in various ways. Some would suggest
that these undiagnosed 'cases' represent a hidden burden of disease, which must
be identified and treated; it has even been suggested that, worldwide, depression
is the illness that 'causes the largest amount of non-fatal disability' (Üstün *et al.*,
2004).

This is clearly good news for the makers of antidepressant medications, who
have indeed prospered mightily since the definition of major depressive disorder
was promulgated from the 1980s onward.

Critics of this approach would point to the definition of major depression as
having been greatly widened; in other words, they say that the 'bar has been set
very low'. They would also suggest a fundamental difference between people
consulting a doctor for a health problem and people who may describe similar
experiences if they are approached and questioned by researchers, but who on
their own have not identified themselves as ill.

Controversy

Sceptics, such as Healy (http://www.healyprozac.com/), point out the close links
between the pharmaceutical industry and the psychiatric academic establishment, as seen, for example, in industry-sponsored 'public awareness' initiatives
such as the Defeat Depression campaign (http://www.rcpsych.ac.uk/campaigns/
defeat/index.htm).

This debate seems likely to run and run. Meanwhile, the NICE guidelines,
perhaps for present purposes, offer (http://www.nice.org.uk/page.aspx?o=236667)
a reasonable summary of figures on frequency of depression in the UK: 'The

estimated point prevalence for major depression among 16- to 65-year-olds in the UK is 21/1000 (males 17, females 25), but, if the less specific and broader category of "mixed depression & anxiety" (F41.2, ICD-10, WHO, 1992) was included, these figures rise dramatically to 98/1000 (males 71, females 124).'

Prevalence of depression: summary

In other words, major depression probably has a prevalence of about 2 per cent, but including milder patients with mixtures of anxiety and depression symptoms puts the total up to around 10 per cent of the population.

Epidemiology

- *Age*: affective episodes may occur at any age, including childhood, but tend to become more frequent in later life.

- *Sex*: depressive illness is diagnosed twice as often in women as in men, partly due to genuine excess, and partly due to women's more frequent GP consultation rates, which lead to higher detection. Mania has an equal sex incidence.

- *Marital status*: for men, rates of depressive illness are lower in the married than in the single, widowed, or divorced. For women, the protective effect of marriage is less marked. Young married women with children have high rates of depression; single women have low rates.

- *Social class and occupation*: community surveys find highest rates of depression among the lower socio-economic groups, but bipolar disorders referred to psychiatrists tend to come from the professional classes.

- *Residential area*: depression is more common in urban than rural districts.

Causes

As with most psychiatric disorders, a variety of factors contribute to the causation of depression and other mood disorders. This has well been expressed by NICE (http://www.nice.org.uk/page.aspx?o=236667):

> The enormous variation in the presentation, course and outcomes of depressive illnesses is reflected in the breadth of theoretical explanations for their aetiology,

including genetic, biochemical and endocrine, psychological and social processes and/or factors. . . . Most now believe that all these factors influence an individual's vulnerability to depression, although it is likely that for different people living in different circumstances, precisely how these factors interact and influence that vulnerability will vary between individuals.

Genetics

Genetic predisposition is proven, and exerts most influence for more severe mood disorders such as bipolar affective disorder.

If one identical twin has bipolar affective disorder, the co-twin will also develop it in about 60 per cent of cases. In non-identical co-twins, the risk is about 20 per cent. The only possible explanation for this difference in concordance rates is closer degree of genetic relation. Hence, this difference is proof of a genetic component in bipolar affective disorder. However, it will be noted that even in identical twins, the concordance rate is not 100 per cent, showing the importance of non-genetic, that is, environmental, factors.

There is also a higher risk of unipolar depression in the relatives of patients with bipolar affective disorder.

In general, it can be said that if an index patient has a mood disorder of any kind, their relatives are at higher risk than the general population of also having a mood disorder of any kind. The lifetime risk of illness in relatives of affected patients is about 10–20 per cent in first-degree relatives.

The more severe the disorder is in the index patient, the more likely that there will be relatives also affected.

The pattern of inheritance is polygenic. Much effort is going into the molecular genetic approach to this; however, clear conclusions as regards aetiology, let alone treatment, are still awaited.

Neurochemistry

Brain concentrations of monoamine neurotransmitters, and/or sensitivity of their receptor sites, appear to be altered in affective disorders. Noradrenaline (NA) and/or 5-hydroxytryptamine (5-HT, serotonin) are implicated in depressive illness; dopamine is implicated in mania. Evidence for neurotransmitter involvement includes the following points:

• Most drugs that are effective in treating depression increase the availability of NA and/or 5-HT in the brain.

- Antihypertensive drugs, such as reserpine, that deplete brain monoamine concentrations, can cause depression.

- Antipsychotic drugs, which block dopamine receptors, have a therapeutic effect in mania.

- Plasma concentration of tryptophan, a precursor of 5-HT, and the concentration of 5-HT in platelets are reduced in some depressed patients.

- Cerebrospinal fluid (CSF) concentrations of the amine metabolites 5-HIAA (5-hydroxyindole acetic acid), HVA (homovanillic acid), and MHGP (methoxy-hydroxy-phenylethylene glycol), as well as urine concentrations of MHGP, are reduced in some depressed patients.

- Post-mortems on depressed patients who died by suicide show low concentrations of 5-HT and 5-HIAA in the brain itself.

Such studies are difficult because delicate measurements are involved; concentrations of amine metabolites may reflect changes in the rest of the body rather than the brain itself; and findings may be affected by diet, exercise, and diurnal rhythms.

Drugs that affect other neurotransmitters such as NA are as effective as antidepressants as those that predominantly affect serotonin. Thus, simplistic theories of depression as a chemical imbalance ('your stores of serotonin are running out') are incompatible with the complexity of the various neurotransmitters and various receptors for them, as delineated by psychopharmacologists.

It seems likely that the neurochemical disturbance in depression is the route – or final common pathway – by which the depression is produced, rather than the ultimate origin of it.

Hormones

Deficiency of thyroid hormone or hormones from the adrenal gland is well recognized as a cause of depression. However, most patients with depression do not have conventional endocrine abnormalities. More subtle changes in hormones have nevertheless been proposed as the cause of depression, as in the response to stress of the adrenal gland. However, these have not so far led to major advances in treatment or understanding of the condition.

- Cortisol secretion in some patients with severe depression is increased up to twice normal values. Diurnal variation in cortisol levels is altered. The *dexamethasone suppression test* was proposed as an aid to the diagnosis of depression, but has seen found to be too non-specific to be clinically useful.

- Thyroid-stimulating hormone response to thyrotrophin-releasing hormone is changed in depression.

- In women, the occurrence of postpartum and premenstrual depression suggests that sex hormone balance can affect mood.

Socio-economic factors

In clinical practice, the predominant impression is of depression being linked to adverse life circumstances and to things that happen. The NICE guidelines go so far as to refer (http://www.nice.org.uk/page.aspx?o=236667) to the 'social origins of depression', and cite a study showing that up to 50 per cent of the difference between the rates of depression in neighbouring general practices could be explained by differing rates of unemployment, poverty, and related factors.

As well as long-term social difficulties, there is a well-established body of evidence indicating that patients with depression have experienced more adverse 'life events' than people without depression. These events, particularly so-called 'loss events', appear to be the precipitant of the majority of episodes of diagnosed depression. Such 'events, dear boy, events', seem to combine with the above-mentioned long-term difficulties, which include not only material poverty, but also absence of confiding relationships and family/social support, to produce the depressive episode.

Hence the medico-legal debate about the causation of an episode of depression following an accident, and the possible contribution of previously existing factors, such as social adversity, can be seen to have sound underpinnings in research on depression causation.

Psychological factors

Research has substantiated the clinical experience that patients with depression frequently have had adverse experiences in childhood, especially inadequate parenting or loss of a parent, especially the mother. This may lead to lack of confidence and low self-esteem as an adult, making the person more likely to have a depressive episode when they encounter, as we all inevitably do, adverse events.

The cognitive theory of depression was popularized by Beck. It proposes that depression of mood can be caused, or at least exacerbated, by a person's repeatedly and automatically thinking negative thoughts. For example, patients may 'run themselves down', or put everything that happens in the worst possible light. The corollary is that depression could be treated by training the patient to think positive thoughts, and there is indeed evidence that such training, in the form of cognitive therapy, can be effective.

Personality

It is probable that the effects of genetic loading, adversity in childhood, and psychological factors such as negative thinking come together in forming a particular type of personality that has a higher risk than the average of developing depressive illness. People with such a personality type include the anxious or dependent, those who have long term difficulties in coping with stress, and those with constitutional tendencies to gloom, sometimes referred to as dysthymia.

In younger people, mild depression tends to affect anxious or dependent personalities with poor tolerance of stress. Severe depressive illness in middle age tends to affect hard-working, conventional people with high standards and obsessional traits. Obsessional personalities can find it particularly difficult to adapt to stress or life changes, as in work or relationships, and this can 'come out' as depression.

There are frequent exceptions to these general impressions, and it is important to appreciate that patients in the throes of a depressive or manic episode may give distorted accounts of their previous personalities. Another postulated mechanism is that depression results from inability to express hostility and aggression, so that these emotions are directed inward to produce self-blame and guilt. The *learned helplessness* model postulates that depression results from repeated failure to overcome problems by personal effort. Bipolar disorder tends to develop in those of cyclothymic personality.

Social stress

Depressed patients report more 'life events', especially loss events, than general population controls during the few months before their illness onset. About 80 per cent of depressive episodes appear to be precipitated by life-event stress.

Chronic social difficulties, lack of confiding relationships, and absence of a supportive social network are important mediating factors.

The role of life events is strongest in respect of first episodes of depression. In subsequent episodes, the role of life events is less, and episodes of depressive illness can come on without life events (this is sometimes referred to as 'kindling'). In patients where there is a strong genetic component, the reduction in the importance of life events in triggering depressive episodes is seen early in the course of the illness ('pre-kindling'). In cases where there was a lesser genetic component, the reduction in the impact of life events occurred more gradually (Kendler *et al.*, 2001). In other words, patients can reach a state in which they are vulnerable to the occurrence of further episodes of depression in the absence of life events, either because of genetic vulnerability or because of the cumulative effects of previous depressive episodes.

There is also evidence that some social factors, such as the presence of a confiding relationship, can be protective.

Life events can also precipitate manic episodes.

Causation: summary

In conclusion, there is evidence that individuals may be *vulnerable* to the development of episodes of depression, and that this vulnerability can be made up of genetic, psychological, personality, and social factors (which probably overlap with each other in fundamental origin). The episode is *precipitated by life events* in most cases, but the role of life events may be less in cases which are recurrent and/or strongly familial.

Clinical features of depressive illness

The following description covers the key aspects of depressive illness in everyday psychiatric practice. These features can conveniently be thought of as either mental or physical.

Mental features of depression

The cardinal symptom of a depressive illness is of course a pervasive depression of mood. This must go beyond the everyday experience of, for example, 'I'm really depressed about the gas bill.' The mood must be low, flat, and empty, and not able to be cheered up by things that the patient formerly enjoyed.

There are those in psychiatry who feel that depression can be diagnosed without depression of mood being obvious to the patient or readily apparent to the psychiatrist. It is just conceivable that this may apply to prodromal or very mild cases of depression, or to patients with a mixture of anxiety and depression symptoms. However, generally speaking, it is necessary to do violence to the idea of clinical depression to consider that any significant case of depressive illness can exist without depression of mood.

Hence, if depression is diagnosed, there does need to be a proper description of the mood in the clinical notes. The essential feature is that there must be a pervasive depression of mood; that is, the mood must be low in respect of all aspects of the person's life, though not necessarily to the same extent throughout. There must also be loss of enjoyment of things the patient used to take pleasure in – the so called anhedonia.

If these features are not present, the proponent of a diagnosis of depression would be in a difficult position, although he might be able to establish the diagnosis, at least to the extent of a mild depressive condition, with the aid of associated symptoms.

In a true depressive illness, the patient has a negative view of himself, so that he feels guilty, and that he is a failure or a bad person. This will tend to be coupled with pessimism or hopelessness.

Accordingly, a diagnosis of depression cannot generally be based solely on anger, irritability, or hostility. Depression of mood, and negative view of self, should generally be present.

In any clinically significant depressive illness, the patient's intellectual function will seem to them to be affected. Perhaps because of lack of drive or preoccupation with negative ideas or both, the ability to concentrate will be reduced. This means that work becomes harder and takes longer; not infrequently, patients believe that they are losing their memory, whereas, in fact, they are not remembering things in the first place because they are not able to concentrate properly.

As with other mental disorders, the risk of suicide must be assessed. Patients often feel that 'it would be better if I was not around', or they think, 'I wish I was dead'. It is important to gauge whether the patient has gone beyond this, and has an active plan to kill himself. Thoughts of how they might do it are not uncommon as their subject of depressive rumination; patients can have prominent thoughts about methods of suicide, yet nevertheless give realistic, and apparently reliable assurances that they would not do this because of, for example, family responsibilities.

In severe depressive states, the patient may become psychotic. That is, he may develop delusions and hallucinations (psychotic symptoms). Typical depressive delusions include an unshakeable conviction that he is guilty of some dreadful crime, that his bowels have turned to stone, or some other hypochondriacal preoccupation. Typical hallucinations in psychotic depression include a voice addressing the patient (second person), saying, for example, 'You are a bad person, you deserve to die.'

What are sometimes referred to as 'biological' symptoms of depression are important because, in clinical practice in psychiatry, they are taken as one of the markers of a clinically significant depressive illness. Disturbance of sleep and appetite are the most frequent.

Sleep disturbances include difficulty in getting to sleep, so-called 'initial insomnia'; disturbed sleep with frequent wakening; and early-morning wakening. This last is a classic symptom of a depressive illness, and is often coupled with diurnal mood variation: that is, the patient wakes up early in the morning in a very depressed mood, which is then at its lowest point of the 24 hours. During the day, the mood gradually brightens as the patient gets going.

Traditional teaching has this pattern as indicative of an *endogenous* depressive illness, that is, one coming from within the patient, in contrast to an *exogenous* or *reactive* depression due to external causes, where the sleep disturbances were said to be more in the nature of initial insomnia. Perhaps unfortunately, research has not borne out these intuitively attractive patterns, and the endogenous/reactive classification of depressive illnesses is no longer regarded as useful for therapeutic or prognostic purposes, although, obviously, it remains an important aspect of assessment in respect of causation.

Classically, a depressive illness is accompanied by loss of appetite and loss of weight. Sometimes, however, especially in milder state of depression, there may just be a loss of interest in food with little change in weight; 'comfort eating' of junk and other food, with weight increase, is common also.

Physical (somatic, biological, vegetative) symptoms

Physical symptoms are just as common as psychological ones and often form the presenting complaint when depressed patients consult in general practice. Core symptoms of depression include pain and tiredness. These have been recognized since the early days of psychiatry. (Indeed, a more insightful way of looking at the problem would be to retreat from the somewhat arbitrary mind/body split in which, at any rate in Western societies, we view the experience of distress.)

Pain and fatigue and depressed mood can in fact be thought of as an army – or at any rate a platoon – that marches together; often, the depressed mood is the most prominent feature and the correct clinical diagnosis of a depressive illness is easily made.

Sometimes, however, if patients feel reticent about their emotional distress, the pain or the tiredness may be presented as the main problem. Depression of mood is the underlying problem in many patients given otherwise mystifying labels of 'chronic fatigue syndrome' or 'chronic pain syndrome'.

There may be effects on physical activity, with unwanted excessive movement – agitation (*agitated depression*) – or marked reduction of activity – the so-called retardation (*retarded depression*) – where the patient may take to bed or chair and become physically slow. This may progress to *depressive stupor*, although this is now very rare. Older patients may show marked intellectual impairment (*depressive pseudodementia*). Other physical symptoms include constipation or diarrhoea, disturbances of the menstrual cycle including cessation of the menstrual periods (amenorrhoea), loss of energy, and loss of interest in sex (loss of libido).

Types of depressive illness

The international classifications

The classification of depressive states is complex and controversial. The word 'depression' covers a wide range of conditions, from transient unhappiness to life-threatening psychiatric illness.

Various theories about types of depression, such as 'endogenous/ reactive' (see below), have had to be abandoned, as they have been found not to have predictive value in respect of treatment or prognosis. The current approach is atheoretical. ICD–10 (http://www3.who.int/icd/currentversion/fr-icd.htm?kf00.htm+) just lists the symptoms as follows:

> In typical mild, moderate, or severe depressive episodes, the patient suffers from lowering of mood, reduction of energy, and decrease in activity. Capacity for enjoyment, interest, and concentration is reduced, and marked tiredness after even minimum effort is common. Sleep is usually disturbed and appetite diminished. Self-esteem and self-confidence are almost always reduced and, even in the mild form, some ideas of guilt or worthlessness are often present. The lowered mood varies little from day to day, is unresponsive to circumstances and may be accompanied by 'somatic' symptoms, such as loss of interest and pleasurable feelings, waking in the morning several hours before

the usual time, depression worst in the morning, marked psychomotor retardation, agitation, loss of appetite, weight loss, and loss of libido.

Classification of depressive illness in the ICD

Depression in the ICD is just graded as mild, moderate, or severe, depending upon the number and severity of the symptoms.

F32.0 Mild depressive episode. Two or three of the above symptoms are usually present. The patient is usually distressed by these but will probably be able to continue with most activities.

F32.1 Moderate depressive episode. Four or more of the above symptoms are usually present and the patient is likely to have great difficulty in continuing with ordinary activities.

F32.2 Severe depressive episode without psychotic symptoms. An episode of depression in which several of the above symptoms are marked and distressing, typically loss of self-esteem and ideas of worthlessness or guilt. Suicidal thoughts and acts are common and a number of 'somatic' symptoms are usually present.

There are obvious problems with the practical use of ICD in daily clinical psychiatry, however. For example, there is no minimum time period. If one takes the description literally, a person who has a brief episode of, say, 'decrease in activity . . . and . . . marked tiredness after even minimum effort', and who is able to 'to continue with most activities' would nevertheless be diagnosable with a mild depressive episode.

The DSM–IV is slightly more rigorous, in that it does at least require, for a diagnosis of '*major depression*', all of the following:

- a 2-week minimum period
- five symptoms out of nine (see list below)
- at least one of the symptoms being either depressed mood or loss of interest or pleasure.

However, this continues to set the bar very low in order to contain a very wide potential diversity among different patients with the same diagnosis. DSM symptoms are as follows:

1. depressed mood, most of the day, nearly every day

2. diminished interest or pleasure in all or almost all activities most of the day, nearly every day

3. significant weight loss when not dieting, or weight gain

4. insomnia or hypersomnia nearly every day

5. agitation or retardation

6. fatigue or loss of energy

7. worthlessness or inappropriate guilt

8. reduced ability to think or concentrate

9. thoughts of death, or suicidal ideation or plan.

There is much more common ground between the subtype of major depression termed 'melancholia' in DSM–IV, and the 'severe depressive episode' of ICD–10. Patients with these diagnoses have a condition which has always been recognized by psychiatrists. It is the much larger numbers of milder cases where the potential for disagreement is greater.

Clinical classification of depression

The authors of the above classifications emphasize that they have to be interpreted by the experienced clinician. Their inherent problems in respect of depression have been alluded to briefly above. I therefore now proceed to give a clinical guide to depressive illness.

Severe depression is characterized by a pervasive depression of mood, which has a different quality from ordinary sadness, cannot be expressed by tears even if the patient wants to cry, and is unrelated to external circumstances. Somatic symptoms (early morning waking, diurnal variation of mood, anorexia, and weight loss) are often prominent, and psychotic features (delusions and/or hallucinations) may be present. Severe episodes usually respond best to physical methods of treatment (see below) rather than psychological therapies alone.

Case example

A 22-year-old man was brought to the GP by his girlfriend, who complained that over the previous few weeks he had become increasingly 'moody and withdrawn', and had been drinking too much. The GP, who had known him for years, was struck by his gaunt and miserable appearance, but was nevertheless surprised when, after his partner left the consulting room, the patient broke down in tears. There was a clear history of depressed mood, loss of interest in things which he usually found pleasurable, poor sleep with terminal insomnia, poor appetite with weight loss, and inability to concentrate, leading to problems at work.

The GP, noting a positive family history of bipolar affective disorder in the father, made a diagnosis of depressive illness. He prescribed lofepramine, and, with the patient's consent, involved the girlfriend in discussing the nature and prognosis of the illness.

After the consultation, the GP realized that he had not yet assessed suicidal risk, and decided to call on the patient on the way home.

Mild depression is more common, and the symptoms are more like an exaggeration of ordinary unhappiness. Somatic symptoms are not prominent, and delusions and hallucinations do not occur. There may be marked tearfulness, anxiety, irritability, and difficulty getting to sleep.

It is, however, probably an over-diagnosed condition these days, especially in general practice. This is not to criticize our colleagues in primary care. Patients have been encouraged to take their emotional difficulties to doctors; in previous eras, they might have been seen as tired and given a tonic, and in later times as anxious, and given benzodiazepines. Currently, the social and medical culture guides doctors and patients toward a diagnosis of depression and the prescription of an antidepressant.

Hence, it is a frequent experience for the psychiatrist to be referred patients who have been diagnosed and treated for depression, but who have truly never had the condition. Some are probably not best regarded as having had a mental illness at all; most of the rest have had adjustment reactions to changes in life circumstances.

The key point is the mood; the patient has to have a true depression of mood; that is, persistent low mood unrelieved by circumstances. If this is not present, depression is not present either. A natural reaction, an adjustment disorder, or dysthymia, is more likely.

Case example

A 22-year-old single mother was referred urgently to the community mental health team for treatment of what was described in the referral letter as 'severe refractory depression'. The patient was seen within a couple of days. It quickly emerged that the patient's 3-year-old daughter had had a convulsion, and had been admitted to hospital for investigation.

The patient had visited the GP to discuss this and had been tearful, upon which depression had been diagnosed and antidepressant medication prescribed. She was no better a month later and was referred by fax.

When the patient was seen, it emerged that she had been upset by her daughter's illness, but that she herself did not believe she was mentally ill. She did not have a truly depressed mood. She was under increasing stress because of accommodation problems, but had been improving.

She was reassured by the information that her feelings were an understandable reaction. When seen in follow-up 2 weeks later, she had been allocated a new flat, and had gone back to normal, and she was discharged.

Dysthymia is a chronic mild depression or unhappiness that may overlap with personality disorder. Recognizing this often helps to make a realistic prognosis.

Case example

A 44-year-old married man came to the attention of a junior hospital psychiatrist after taking an overdose in the context of marital breakdown. He described depressed mood, anhedonia, and continuing suicidal ideation. Although he made a fairly rapid improvement sufficient to return to work, his symptoms only partially resolved. The psychiatrist tried a number of antidepressants and some cognitive therapy to little avail, and, determined to explore all treatment options, he was thinking of suggesting ECT or referral for dynamic psychotherapy.

His consultant suggested discussing the patient with his GP, who turned out to know him well. The GP felt that, although the patient had benefited from treatment to get over the acute episode of distress, he had been 'back to normal' for some time. The patient had 'always had rather a gloomy outlook, just like the rest of his family'.

The patient was eventually discharged back to the care of the GP with a diagnosis of dysthymic personality.

Endogenous and *reactive* depression is another rather outdated distinction based on whether or not a precipitating life stress predating the depressive episode can be identified. Most depressive episodes are at least in part 'reactive'; therefore, resolving the external stress and/or helping the patient cope with it more constructively should certainly be part of management. But it is important to consider biological treatments if symptoms of severe depression are present, however understandable the cause. For example, drug treatment can be helpful for some patients with depressive illness following life events such as bereavement (see Chapter 6), or in medically ill patients (see Chapter 11), including those with terminal disease. It is impossible to predict which patients will respond to drug treatment.

The term 'psychotic depression', which is self-explanatory, is sometimes used, but the matching term 'neurotic depression' has largely been dropped because of the pejorative overtones of the word 'neurotic'.

Seasonal affective disorder (SAD) is a condition in which depressed mood accompanied by lethargy, excessive sleep, increased appetite, and irritability recurs each winter. It was believed to respond exclusively to light treatment; however, recent studies indicate it can be just as effectively managed with standard methods of treatment, such as medication. It is probably not distinct from depression, and should be managed in the usual way. The best way of increasing light exposure is probably daily walks.

Masked depression describes presentation with somatic symptoms when the patient denies depressed mood and may even appear cheerful and smiling. Self-evidently, this would be an unusual clinical situation requiring careful assessment; the term 'masked depression' is not unanimously accepted or commonly used, however.

Diagnosis of depressive illness

Most episodes of depression are brief and mild, and are dealt with by the patient's own resources, or by talking with a relative or friend. Of those patients who do present for help, the vast majority are dealt with in primary care. The diagnosis of depressive illness in clinical settings will have some regard to the official classifications set out above. However, clinical training and experience also comes into play. Mild reactions to difficulties experienced in life may not in practice be diagnosed as clinical depression. The clinician should look for features such as biological symptoms of depression, anhedonia, and guilt before entertaining the diagnosis. Depressed mood which seems unduly severe or prolonged in relation to its apparent precipitant, the presence of somatic symptoms, and prominent guilt, pessimism, anhedonia, suicidal thinking, and low self-esteem, all suggest depressive illness.

Rating scales for depression

Standardized rating scales exist to permit quantitative measurement of the severity of depressed mood. Their main use is in research work, as in comparing response to different treatments. They may be used clinically as screening instruments to help detect depression in high-risk populations, such as patients attending general hospitals. However, they are not in themselves diagnostic, and are not validated for medico-legal use.

Observer-rating scales include the Hamilton. Self-rating scales include the Beck, Zung, and HAD (Hospital Anxiety and Depression) scales, although the last is, strictly speaking, a screening instrument rather than a measurement tool.

Clinical features of mania

Mania causes much less diagnostic difficulty than depression. (In that respect, it resembles severe or melancholic depression, where there is seldom much doubt about the diagnosis, and where the international classifications are largely in agreement.)

Manic symptoms can be considered the opposite of depressive ones. Mood may swing rapidly between cheerfulness, irritability, or aggression. Energy is increased, with overactivity, disinhibition, distractibility, reduced need for food and sleep, increased sexual interest, and financial extravagance. This behaviour may have disastrous consequences for the patient and for others, leading to debts, relationship problems, or legal difficulties.

Thought and speech are copious (*pressure of speech*), often with rapid, loose connections between one topic and the next (*flight of ideas*), rhymes, and puns. Sometimes, the connections between the thoughts can be disrupted. Thought content is usually grandiose or paranoid. Delusions and hallucinations, also with a grandiose or paranoid content, may develop.

Hypomania is a term for mild episodes without delusions or hallucinations.

Manic stupor is a rare form in which activity is greatly reduced despite elated mood and grandiose thought content.

Transient periods of depression, sometimes lasting only minutes at a time, occur during many if not most manic illnesses. If the periods of depression are more prominent, the illness may be called a *mixed affective state.*

Differential diagnosis of mood disorders

Medical conditions

Depression can be an integral part of the symptomatology of some medical conditions, including neurological disorders such as Parkinson's disease, dementia, multiple sclerosis, and anaemia; endocrine disorders such as hypothyroidism; virus infections such as influenza; and deficiencies of vitamins such as B_{12} and folate.

Manic symptoms may be due to organic brain lesions, especially in the frontal lobe; toxic confusional states; and endocrine disorders such as thyrotoxicosis or Cushing's syndrome.

Drug reactions

Drugs that may precipitate depression include antihypertensives, especially reserpine and methyldopa; corticosteroids and possibly sex hormones; L-dopa; digitalis; certain cytotoxics; certain antimalarials; sulphonamides; and antipsychotics. Cholesterol-lowering drugs are also implicated.

Drugs that may precipitate mania include corticosteroids, antidepressants, L-dopa, LSD, and amphetamines.

Psychiatric conditions

Depressed mood often accompanies other psychiatric disorders. In elderly patients, distinguishing between depressive illness and dementia is a common dilemma, although sometimes they are present together. Both depressive and manic symptoms may occur in combination with symptoms of schizophrenia: schizo-affective disorder. Agitated depression and mixed depressive/anxiety neurosis are easily mistaken for pure anxiety states. Antisocial personality disorder may be confused with mania.

Substance misuse commonly coexists with mood disorders. Depression of mood can be secondary to alcoholism, due to the depressing effects of alcohol on the brain. Equally, patients with depression not infrequently attempt to self-medicate with alcohol; this is counterproductive, however, because the euphoriant effects of alcohol only last an hour or two, and are followed by a superadded lowering of the mood. Manic patients commonly abuse substances. Hence, all psychiatric assessments must include a record of the patient's pattern of substance use.

Treatment of depressive illness

Most depressive episodes present in general practice, and quickly resolve with primary care treatment. It is likely that this represents a combination of the natural tendency of such conditions to resolve spontaneously, together with the positive effects of a sympathetic interview, diagnosis, explanation, and reassurance.

The prescription of medication or the use of counselling is also likely be helpful, although in both cases the non-specific effects of treatment ('placebo effects') are likely to be just as, if not more, important than the specific clinical effectiveness of the particular treatment employed.

Only a small percentage of such cases are referred to specialists; a figure of 10 per cent would probably be on the high side. The majority of these are managed as outpatients; some of the more severe cases will be allocated help from the community mental health team, such as a community psychiatric nurse and/or attendance at a day centre.

Hospital admission may be required for patients who are suicidal, or refusing food and drink. Compulsory admission under the Mental Health Act 1983 may be required.

A few cases will need to have ECT (see Chapter 24). ECT is a widely feared treatment, although it is very effective in emergency cases when the patient has stopped eating and drinking properly, and is in danger of death through dehydration. However, modern treatments seem to be increasingly effective, and I prescribe ECT only about once a year or less in my practice. It is now, in effect, either an emergency treatment or a treatment of last resort.

Medication and psychological treatment are thus the main specific therapeutic options. However, usually no individual treatment is 100 per cent effective; a good recovery in a more severe case will often involve two or three therapeutic modalities, such as medication and psychological treatment, each contributing a partial amount, but adding up in combination to an effective treatment package.

NICE guideline

This effectively advocates a 'stepped care' approach (http://www.nice.org.uk/page.aspx?o=236667). It advocates *screening*, although it is disputed that this would meet standard UK criteria for the introduction of screening programmes (Gilbody *et al.*, 2006). *Watchful waiting*, that is, review in 2 weeks, is advocated for mild cases, and seems sensible. *Guided self-help* and *short-term psychological treatment* for mild and moderate cases are probably less realistic, however, due to lack of availability of same in primary care.

Prescription of a specific serotonin reuptake inhibitor (SSRI) is the next step advocated, and this aroused some controversy, even though it was essentially preaching to the choir, as SSRIs and later drugs have effectively taken over in primary care. Few GPs would now start with a tricyclic, let alone monoamine oxidase inhibitors (MAOIs). For *initial presentation of severe depression, treatment-resistant depression, or recurrent depression*, a combination of CBT and medication is suggested, but this again seems a counsel of perfection, in view of the limited availability of CBT.

The guideline contains disappointingly little on the community mental health team. The help of such professionals is, in practice, more available than psychological treatment; it is probably also more suitable for rehabilitation of chronic patients, who may need help with practical matters such as benefits and return to work.

Regarding *ECT*, NICE suggests that it should be 'used only to achieve rapid and short-term improvement of severe symptoms after an adequate trial of other treatment options has proven ineffective, and/or when the condition is considered to be potentially life-threatening, in individuals with a severe depressive illness', advice that seems reasonable.

However, NICE opposes maintenance ECT, the practice of giving a periodical application, say, once a month, to try to prevent recurrence in chronic severe depressive illness. This practice, although rare in adult psychiatry, is not uncommon in elderly psychiatry, where the frail older patient may experience fewer side-effects from ECT than from medication. This particular recommendation of NICE has therefore caused controversy.

Medication

Antidepressant medication is probably the most frequently used treatment. The main types of antidepressants are tricyclic antidepressants, SSRIs, and MAOIs. They are discussed in more detail in Chapter 23.

SSRIs are widely used in general practice. However, they are probably weaker drugs in more severe depressive states; hence, by the time patients have been referred to secondary care, they have probably already failed to improve on SSRIs. There is no logic in switching from one drug to another in the same category, as the similarities between them far outweigh the differences.

Therefore, there is a strong case for the use of the previous generation of antidepressant drugs, such as the tricyclics (e.g. amitriptyline) in secondary care. The tricyclics may have more side-effects, but are probably more powerful in more severe cases.

The key point with medication is that it must be continued. The standard advice is for patients to continue with the medication until they are fully recovered, and then for a further 6 months. At this stage, if the patient has remained well, the possibility of a dose reduction can be considered.

Unfortunately, many patients stop medication as soon as they feel a bit better; this is often followed by a quick return of symptoms, and the patient may then come to feel that the condition is incurable, and that the medication is ineffective. However, the truth is the exact opposite: the drug probably is effective, and the condition probably is responsive to the drug; the symptoms would therefore probably not have recurred if the patient had carried on with the medication.

- *Tricyclic antidepressants* such as amitriptyline and imipramine have long been regarded by psychiatrists as the standard first-line treatment for depressive illness; they are probably the most effective drugs for severe depression. They are effective in about 70 per cent of depressed patients.

- *SSRIs* such as fluoxetine and paroxetine are now considered by many GPs to be the treatment of first choice, because they are safer in overdose than tricyclics and may have fewer side-effects. Others consider that SSRIs, which are more expensive, should be reserved for patients who cannot take tricyclics or have failed to respond to them.

- *MAOIs* such as phenelzine and moclobemide are less often prescribed but are sometimes dramatically effective when other drugs have failed.

- *Lithium and other mood stabilizers* are mainly used in the prevention of recurrent affective disorder, but may also useful in an established depressive episode as adjunctive treatment to one of the antidepressants listed above.

A therapeutic trial of an antidepressant drug is often required when diagnostic doubt exists. Frequent changes of drug are to be avoided, and compliance needs checking. If an effective drug is found, it should be continued at least 6 months after recovery to reduce the risk of relapse, and then gradually tapered off if the patient remains well.

Case example

A GP telephoned the psychiatrist who was responsible for her sector, and who did monthly clinics in her surgery, to discuss a 47-year-old woman who had been depressed for several months. Having benefited from a 'recent course of amitriptyline', she had now relapsed, with a full depressive syndrome, including low mood and biological symptoms such as loss of appetite and insomnia. The GP requested advice on 'a change of antidepressant and/or admission'.

On further discussion, it became clear that the patient had derived clear though partial benefit from amitriptyline 50 mg nocte; not appreciating the need for continuing medication, she had stopped the tablets when she began to feel better. The psychiatrist suggested that the patient had had the right treatment, but not enough of it for long enough, and advised restarting amitriptyline, and working up to a dose of 150 mg nocte. She offered to see the patient if needed, particularly if the GP was worried about suicide risk.

The GP was happy with this plan and, 3 weeks later, reported that the patient had restarted amitriptyline, but had been unable to go beyond 75 mg because of side-effects. Nevertheless, she was very much better. The psychiatrist strongly advised continuing medication until the patient was fully well and for 6 months thereafter, before cautiously considering reduction, and once again offered to see the patient for further education and advice about depression and its management.

Electroconvulsive therapy (ECT) (see Chapter 24)

As previously indicated, ECT has a place in emergency treatment, and when other treatments have failed. It is currently infrequently used, but tends to have good results in the more severe cases in which it is utilized. ECT is effective in about 80 per cent of patients with severe depression, notably in psychotic cases with delusions or hallucinations. Mild depression seldom responds well to ECT. Prescribing an antidepressant alongside ECT is usually recommended. Benzodiazepines, used for insomnia or anxiety, should be stopped before ECT is started, as their anticonvulsant properties will interfere with the effectiveness of ECT in producing a convulsion.

Psychological methods (see Chapter 22)

A continuing supportive relationship with a trusted professional forms a valuable part of the treatment of all depressed patients.

Occupational therapy can also be most helpful in encouraging the patient to resume the full range of daily activities.

Cognitive therapy, designed to modify habitual negative thinking patterns which contribute to depressed mood, is as effective as drug treatment in moderate or mild depression. *Interpersonal therapy*, focused on relationships with others, is also useful.

Psychodynamic psychotherapy may perhaps be indicated for long-term problems. However, during severe depression, a purely psychotherapeutic approach is not appropriate because it will not correct delusions or hallucinations, and may increase patients' feelings of guilt and unworthiness.

Social casework may be helpful if the patient's family relationships or life circumstances are disturbed, whether as cause or result of the illness.

Resistant depression

This term covers patients with significant depressive illness who do not seem to respond to standard treatment, or respond only partially. Recovery, or at any rate improvement, is possible with continued treatment in most cases. Probably, combinations of medication, such as antidepressants with a small dose of a major tranquillizer or a mood stabilizer will need to be tried. The following points need to be considered:

• Reassess the diagnosis, excluding underlying physical pathology.

• Are social/family problems perpetuating the illness?

- Could cognitive therapy help habitual negative thinking patterns?

- Has the patient actually taken the medication?

- Have adequate doses have been given for long enough?

- Consider change of antidepressant class (tricyclic/MAOI/SSRI).

- Consider adding an 'adjuvant' such as lithium or an alternative mood stabilizer.

- Other 'adjuvant' drugs such as a small dose of an antipsychotic drug can be considered.

- Thyroid treatment can be tried, even if the patient is not hypothyroid; for example, liothyronine is used.

- Combination antidepressant treatment (tricyclic plus SSRI) is not infrequently tried. The use of combinations of tricyclic and MAOI is now very unusual, and requires specialist supervision.

Treatment of mania

Hospital admission may be desirable to prevent the adverse consequences of extravagance or disinhibited behaviour. Compulsory admission under the Mental Health Act 1983 may be required, since many manic patients have no insight into their illness. Neuroleptic drugs (see Chapter 23) are the first-line treatment; for example, olanzepine 5 mg b.d. Lithium is an effective adjunct to neuroleptics, but does not act so quickly and would not be used alone for treatment of a manic episode except for mild cases.

Prophylaxis of affective disorder

Prophylaxis in the form of long-term medication should be considered for patients whose lives are significantly disrupted by recurrent illness; say, two or three episodes within 5 years.

For bipolar patients, *lithium* is an effective prophylactic that prevents or at least ameliorates further episodes in 70–80 per cent of cases. *Carbamazepine*, an anticonvulsant drug, is an alternative to lithium, and the two drugs may be given in combination if neither has been successful on its own. Other drugs, including other anticonvulsants such as *valproate* and *lamotrigine*, may also be used.

For unipolar patients, lithium is sometimes effective, but antidepressant drugs are probably the best prophylaxis.

Psychological and social measures are also important. Interpersonal and cognitive-behavioural psychotherapies have preventive value. Many patients value the information and peer support available through voluntary organizations such as the Manic Depressive Fellowship.

Prognosis

From 70 to 90 per cent of episodes of affective illness recover within a few months even without treatment. The rest become chronic and may last for years. Prognosis is better if treatment begins early during the episode. Even if their first episode has recovered, 70–80 per cent of patients will suffer one or more further attacks at some stage in their lives. Some patients become ill at regular intervals, or at the same time each year, often spring or autumn. Bipolar patients may alternate between depressed and manic phases, or either type may be more frequent. The course for an individual patient is unpredictable.

References

Gilbody, S., Sheldon, T. and Wessely, S. (2006). Should we screen for depression? *BMJ* **332**, 1027–1030.

Kendler, K. S., Thornton, L. M. and Gardner, C. O. (2001). Genetic risk, number of previous depressive episodes, and stressful life events in predicting onset of major depression. *Am J Psychiatry* **158**, 582–586.

Üstün, T. B., Ayuso-Mateos, J. L., Chatterji, S. *et al.* (2004). Global burden of depressive disorders in the year 2000. *Br J Psychiatry* **184**, 386–392.

6 Anxiety and stress-related disorders

Anxiety and stress-related disorders can be considered as an exaggerated response to stress. In contrast to psychosis, such patients are free from delusions and hallucinations, and usually retain insight. These disorders include the following range of common, related, and overlapping conditions:

- *generalized anxiety states*: continuous, unfocused, 'free-floating' anxiety

- *panic disorder*: episodes of acute, severe anxiety

- *specific phobias*: anxiety related to specific objects (e.g. spiders) or situations (e.g. agoraphobia, social phobia)

- *obsessive-compulsive disorder*: anxiety related to obsessional thoughts or compulsive ritual behaviours

- *reactions to stress*: including adjustment reactions and post-traumatic stress disorder (PTSD).

Anxiety is a feature of them all. Patients with a mixture of symptoms from several categories were sometimes said to have *general neurotic syndrome*, although the term is not in clinical use today.

Hughes' Outline of Modern Psychiatry, Fifth Edition. David Gill.
© 2007 John Wiley & Sons, Ltd   ISBN 9780470033920

Boundaries of anxiety disorder

The above conditions overlap as follows:

- with each other
- with depression
- with normality.

In other words, the symptoms of an anxiety disorder are not qualitatively different from normality, unlike a psychotic disorder, where the definitive symptoms, such as delusions and hallucinations, are not seen in people in good mental health. After all, everyone worries, to a greater or lesser extent. The difference is that the person with an anxiety disorder worries to a pathological extent.

Anxiety and depression also coexist. Some anxiety symptoms will be present in every person with depression. Some patients with mild anxiety do not have low mood, but they are in a minority: most patients with diagnosable anxiety disorders have some coexisting mood symptoms.

Anxiety could to some extent be viewed as an early, mild form of depression. In this model, anxiety is prominent in the early stages, but, as the condition develops, low mood becomes more pronounced, and eventually comes to dominate the clinical picture. Accordingly, the diagnosis would then be one of a depressive illness.

Hierarchy of diagnosis

Thus, just as a diagnosis of psychosis 'trumps' a diagnosis of neurosis (anxiety, depression, and other non-psychotic conditions), so a diagnosis of depression is usually held to trump a diagnosis of anxiety. Hence, it would not be usual to diagnose, say, a generalized anxiety disorder, as well as a depressive illness. However, patients are sometimes diagnosed with more than one anxiety disorder; for example, generalized anxiety disorder and a phobic anxiety disorder.

Frequency

Community surveys suggest that 10–15 per cent of the population are significantly affected by anxiety symptoms at any one time, and about 25 per cent will suffer at some stage in their lifetime. However, an exact prevalence is impossible to determine because neurotic symptoms are not qualitatively different from normal experience, and prevalence will depend on the cut-offs in the criteria used.

In medical settings, anxiety is even more common than in the general community. In primary care, anxiety states frequently coexist with mild forms of depression, and it has been questioned whether there is any real distinction between the two. Anxiety, again often mixed with depression, is a significant problem for at least 25 per cent of patients in general hospital wards and clinics.

Epidemiology

Age

Anxiety neuroses usually start in early adult life. Symptoms may continue into middle or old age, but a first episode in later life should raise suspicion of major depressive illness or organic disease.

Sex

Anxiety neuroses are more common in women than men.

Causes

Genetics

Up to 20 per cent of patients' first-degree relatives are affected, usually by the same type of neurosis, but the familial tendency can be partly explained by the influence of home environment in early life.

Physiological and biochemical factors

These factors may mediate some of the effects of other aetiological influences; however, they are not of clinical utility at present.

- Overactivity of the sympathetic nervous system and increased secretion of adrenaline/noradrenaline (NA) are closely related to the physical manifestations of anxiety. ACTH and cortisol are also raised.

- Disordered activity of the limbic system of the brain, probably involving the inhibitory neurotransmitter gamma-amino-butyric acid (GABA); most anxiolytic drugs enhance GABA transmission. It is possible that the effects of GABA are brought about via influencing the 5-HT and NA systems.

- 5-HT release is increased in anxiety; 5-HT systems in the brainstem have been studied closely; reduction of receptor subtypes such as 5-HT1A has been postulated as linked to anxiety.

- NA release is increased in anxiety.

- Variation of symptoms with current physical status; for example, female patients usually describe an exacerbation in the premenstrual phase.

Personality

Almost everybody may undergo a neurotic reaction if under a sufficient degree of stress, but those of sensitive or insecure personality have a lower threshold for developing neurotic symptoms. There is therefore an overlap between anxiety disorder and personality disorder; the main distinguishing feature is the specific starting point in time of an anxiety disorder, whereas a personality disorder is permanently present. Chronic neurotic symptoms can come to be seen as an anxious (so-called 'avoidant') personality disorder or a dependent personality disorder.

Sometimes, a neurotic disorder is clearly an exaggeration of aspects of the patient's personality; for example, obsessive-compulsive disorder often develops in those with obsessional characters.

Events and social stress

Most acute episodes appear to be precipitated by an adverse life experience. Long-term psychosocial problems such as marital difficulties often appear to contribute in chronic cases, although the direction of cause and effect may be uncertain. The role of an event in the generation of post-traumatic stress disorder (PTSD) is discussed below.

Clinical features

One or more of a wide range of mental and/or physical symptoms may be the presenting complaint.

Mental symptoms

- apprehension/worry, either general ('free-floating') or focused

- poor concentration

- irritability

- insomnia, usually of the 'initial' type where the patient cannot get off to sleep but lies awake worrying.

Physical symptoms

- cardiovascular symptoms such as tachycardia or palpitations

- respiratory symptoms such as dyspnoea or chest pain

- gastrointestinal symptoms such as dry mouth, nausea, anorexia, dysphagia or diarrhoea

- muscle tension, including tension headache

- fatigue

- dizziness

- sweating

- tremor

- frequency of micturition

- flushing of the face and chest.

These physical symptoms can be explained by overactivity of the sympathetic nervous system, muscle tension, and/or over-breathing. In many medical settings, both patient and doctor place more emphasis on the physical aspects than the mental ones, resulting in diagnostic confusion and unhelpful or even harmful treatment (see Chapter 9).

Patients are oversensitive to minor environmental changes, and difficulties in personal relationships are often associated.

Differential diagnosis

- *Personality disorder*: personality disorder is a more persistent condition than neurosis, and tends to present with disturbance of behaviour and social adjustment, whereas neurosis presents with symptoms. The distinction between 'neurotic illness' and 'neurotic personality' is clear-cut in some patients – for example if an anxiety state develops in a previously well-adjusted subject following a stressful event – but in other cases they coexist, as when a habitually nervous, dependent subject has an episode of particularly intense distress.

- *Other psychiatric illnesses* such as major depression or psychosis. If delusions or hallucinations are present, the main diagnosis must be a psychotic disorder, although the patient may have neurotic symptoms too.

- *Medical illness*, including systemic disorders such as thyrotoxicosis, and brain disorders such as temporal lobe epilepsy.

- *Substance misuse*: alcohol, caffeine (in tea, coffee, or cola drinks), or other drugs.

- *Stress reactions* of normal degree: anxiety is to be expected in certain situations and, if not excessive, may actually improve ability to cope (the Yerkes–Dodson curve – performance improves with initial increases in stress, but beyond a certain point, further increases result in performance declining).

Treatment

General principles of psychological treatment and of medication treatment are discussed in Chapters 22 and 23 respectively. I will now discuss how these are applied in the specific case of anxiety disorders.

Simple explanation and advice are helpful to most patients, and may themselves be sufficient in milder transient episodes. Explanation, particularly regarding the causes of physical symptoms, is important. Simple lifestyle advice regarding exercise and diet, and avoidance of excess alcohol, caffeine, and smoking may be relevant.

Self-help through reading, sometimes dignified with the term 'bibliotherapy', can be useful as well, and Helen Kennerley's *Overcoming Anxiety* (2006) is widely recommended.

Medication

Use of medication is the most available treatment if the patient consults his GP.

Anxiolytic drugs

Anxiolytic drugs such as *benzodiazepine* are best taken only when symptoms actually occur, or shortly before the patient has to face an anxiety-provoking situation. Regular medication encourages tolerance and dependence, and for this reason benzodiazepines are recommended for short-term use only. Unfortunately, because of fears of addiction, these drugs may now be in danger of being underused. In patients with stable personality, with a likely short-term situation such as acute distress following bereavement to deal with, they can be a safe and effective treatment.

For the small minority of chronic severe sufferers who have tried and failed with other treatments, long-term benzodiazepine treatment may be the least problematic therapeutic option.

Antidepressants

Sedative *tricyclics* such as trimipramine are often given in anxiety disorders. Their full benefit may take several weeks in depression, but their useful hypnotic and anxiolytic properties are immediate and dose-related. For example, trimipramine 25 mg nocte regularly plus 25 mg mane p.r.n. will help sleep and make available a safe antianxiety treatment for daytime use in a patient with mild anxiety symptoms. Antidepressants are effective in panic disorder. MAOIs should be tried if other antidepressant classes are ineffective.

SSRIs are widely used in general practice; some patients probably benefit. However, in some patients, they can exacerbate anxiety, with troublesome agitation and gastrointestinal upset; the problem is so significant that some have recommended 'covering' a newly started SSRI with a second drug such as the notably sedative *trazodone* or a benzodiazepine. Unfortunately, it is not possible to predict which patients will experience these adverse effects.

I rarely if ever prescribe SSRIs for anxiety; cheaper and, in my hands, more effective drugs – tricyclics – are to be preferred. Trazodone, trimipramine, or, among the newer drugs, mirtazepine, have predictable and dose-related anxiolytic effects, and are much more suitable.

Beta-blockers

Beta-blockers such as propranolol can help to control the physical symptoms of anxiety, such as palpitations; they are useful in mild anxiety states in some patients, especially in primary care. They are seldom effective in severe anxiety states, as they have little effect on the psychic aspects of anxiety.

Buspirone

Buspirone is popular in the USA, but less so in the UK; in practice, its efficacy seems weak.

Antihistamines

Antihistamines such as promethazine have useful sedative and hence anxiolytic properties. It is worth remembering that these drugs were the drug class from which the original antipsychotics were developed; they have always been pre-scribed as sedatives to some extent, as in children, and in anaesthetic premedica-tion. They are now recommended as an alternative to the over-prescribing of benzodiazepines.

Antipsychotic drugs in low dose

Small amounts of chlorpromazine or, more recently, olanzepine are widely used; they carry their own risks, such as extrapyramidal side-effects, weight gain, and so forth, although these are very small in the small doses usually indicated for anxiety.

Psychological treatment

The ordinary forms of counselling – the sort widely available, sometimes in GP surgeries – are popular with patients. However, there is little evidence of effec-tiveness; the evidence base is for structured forms of psychological treatment such as behaviour therapy and cognitive-behavioural therapy (CBT).

For example, take the treatment of a specific phobia, such as that of water, using CBT principles. Components of treatment would include the following:

- assessment interview

- leading to the building up of a trusting therapeutic relationship

- the patient is encouraged to set practical goals, such as resuming swimming
- patient develops anxiety hierarchy
- plan of graded exposure
- regular review sessions, achievements recognized, blocks assessed and dealt with.

By anxiety hierarchy is meant a series of situations in which the person is exposed to the feared stimulus in a gradually increasing manner. In this case, it might include

- thinking about a swimming pool
- looking at a picture of a swimming pool
- walking past the swimming pool and similar actions
- working up gradually to jumping into the swimming pool.

As will readily be surmised, the approach is common sense and practical, and it can to some extent be systematized; therefore, computerized versions have been developed, both for anxiety and for depression. NICE has recently opined (http://www.nice.org.uk/page.aspx?o=TA097) that there is evidence of effectiveness of these computerized versions, and that they should be considered for clinical use. However, it seems unlikely that they will completely replace the need for skilled therapists. It seems more likely to me that they will form a component of therapy – for example, for use if the patient has to wait for treatment – but that there will still be a need for the therapist to see the patient.

Social management

Environmental problems causing continued stress can sometimes be modified through social casework. Many common stresses, such as an unhappy marriage, job dissatisfaction, and poverty, cannot be directly remedied, but the patient can often be helped to deal with them more constructively.

Prognosis

Some patients have a single brief episode that resolves completely (with or without treatment), some have recurrent episodes, and others are chronically incapacitated. Patients who develop an acute neurotic illness following a tempo-rary stress, but who had a sound premorbid personality, usually do better than those with long-standing symptoms, chronic stress, or neurotic personality traits.

Chronic neurosis can give rise to severe handicap, and is associated with raised mortality from suicide and accidents, and from neurological, respiratory, and cardiovascular disease. However, some patients improve when they reach later life.

Features of individual types of neurosis will now be described.

Case example

A young man in his late 20s described increasing fear and panic surround-ing his high-pressure sales job. He was very successful at this, depending in large extent, on his gregarious and popular personality. However, after the development of financial problems from his excessive spending, and relationship difficulties, he went off work, and developed gradually increas-ing anxiety about going outside the house.

His GP gave him an SSRI, which made him worse, causing agitation and vomiting. He was then referred to community mental health services, and responded to trimipramine, and to the development of a supportive rela-tionship with his community psychiatric nurse, who employed CBT in helping him rebuild his confidence. He also helped him come to an arrange-ment with his creditors.

Through liaison with his line manager and his human resources depart-ment, he was successfully rehabilitated via a graduated return-to-work programme.

Generalized anxiety disorder (anxiety state)

The prevalence of pure generalized anxiety disorder is about 3 per cent of the population, and a further 8 per cent have mixed anxiety and depressive disorder. Physical and/or mental symptoms of anxiety, as listed above, are present most of the time in the absence of real danger, and are 'free-floating' rather than focused on any particular stimulus.

Most acute episodes seen in primary care are precipitated by obvious stressors, and respond to supportive interviews designed to help the patient express and clarify feelings, and address any practical problems. Patients often ask for 'counselling', although the unlimited demand means that this may not always be available. In fact, 'watchful waiting' may be the best option, as most such episodes have a strong tendency to resolve naturally.

If a specific treatment were required, the GP would have a choice of the medications outlined above: a beta-blocker, an antihistamine, or a sedative antidepressant such as small doses of trimipramine or trazodone. SSRIs can make things worse. Benzodiazepines should be avoided in most cases.

Panic disorder

This diagnosis, made more frequently in the USA than the UK, has only been part of psychiatric classification for the past 20 years or so, and its status remains controversial. It remains unclear whether there is a separate population of patients who just get panic attacks, and who do not have predominant diagnoses of either anxiety or depression. In clinical practice, patients often seem to have a mixture of varying anxiety and depression symptoms over the years.

The condition is described as a chronic one, which usually begins in young adult life.

Panic attacks are intermittent episodes of acute anxiety with marked physical symptoms: shortness of breath, dizziness or faintness, palpitations or tachycardia, trembling or shaking, choking, nausea, depersonalization or derealization, numbness or tingling, flushes or chills, and chest pain. The patient may be terrified of dying or losing control. The attack may be misdiagnosed as a medical emergency such as a heart attack or epileptic fit.

First attacks often occur without apparent reason, but, later, return to the situation in which previous episodes took place can precipitate further attacks and set up a pattern of avoidant behaviour (see agoraphobia below).

CBT, benzodiazepines, and antidepressant drugs are effective treatments.

Agoraphobia

Agoraphobia literally means 'fear of the marketplace'. Patients are afraid to visit shops or use public transport, especially if alone, and some are afraid to leave home at all. Panic attacks may occur in the feared situation, and some cases are secondary to panic disorder. Many patients are young women of dependent personality, whose partners may be overprotective and often have neurotic symptoms themselves. Behaviour therapy involving regular exposure to the feared situation is the best treatment. Medication may also help.

Social phobia

Social phobias involve anxiety about being with other people, sometimes in a general sense, sometimes only in formal settings such as parties or restaurants. Mild cases are very common, and merge into the normal personality variant of shyness. Behaviour therapy is the treatment of choice. SSRIs have also been heavily promoted for this indication, but I think that they are best avoided in anxiety states.

Simple phobias (specific phobias, monophobias)

Simple phobias are common in both childhood and adult life; only the more severe cases tend to come to the attention of psychiatrists or psychologists. Anxiety is focused on a single phobic stimulus such as spiders, cats, air travel, or vomiting, although almost anything can form the nucleus of a phobia. Sometimes the condition has an obvious explanation, as in the case of a young woman bitten by a dog who became preoccupied with fear of dogs and altered her whole lifestyle to avoid possible contact with them; a 'maladaptive learned response'. Other phobias have no identifiable cause. Behaviour therapy is the treatment of choice, and consists of gradually increasing exposure to the feared phobic stimulus.

Obsessive-compulsive disorders

Patients feel a strong *obsession* to ruminate on a thought topic, and/or *compulsion* to carry out some practical action. Patients know that these symptoms come from within the self; in other words, that these are their own thoughts and actions. (Hence, they are quite distinct from the experiences of thought insertion or delusions of control sometimes seen in schizophrenia.) They also know that the thoughts or actions are irrational, and that they are contrary to their own beliefs and well-being; they are sometimes described as 'ego dystonic'. They realize that the thoughts and actions are inappropriate and should be under personal control, but attempts to resist them cause increased anxiety and are usually not successful. Common types of obsessional thinking include the following:

- fears of harming others (very rarely put into practice) or contracting a serious disease

- sexual or blasphemous thoughts which are abhorrent to the patient

- ruminations on insoluble problems in mathematics or philosophy.

Common types of compulsive rituals include:

- checking, for example, that the door is locked or lights switched off

- washing, often carried out in order to allay fears of contamination or harm

- cleaning, for the same reason.

Patients may spend so much time on their rituals that normal daily activities are neglected. Compulsive hand washers often develop skin rashes. The illness is particularly distressing because the patients are so well aware that their symptoms are irrational.

Community surveys indicate that obsessive-compulsive disorder is present in 2–3 per cent of the general population and, in contrast to other neurotic disorders, is equally common in men and women.

Similar symptoms may occur as a sequel to organic brain disease, and schizophrenic phenomena such as thought interference, passivity experiences, and delusions may also cause diagnostic confusion. However, in organic disease and schizophrenic cases, insight and resistance are usually absent.

Behaviour therapy with exposure and response prevention, and antidepressants, especially those such as clomipramine and SSRIs, which act on the 5-HT system, are effective treatments.

Post-traumatic stress disorder (PTSD)

Psychiatry has always recognized that mental disorders can follow traumatic events. The names have tended to change over the years, including 'shell shock', 'war neurosis', or 'battle fatigue'. However, it was only in 1980 that DSM–III described PTSD; it appears in ICD also, and the diagnosis has evolved significantly since its introduction.

PTSD is described in survivors of major traumatic experiences of a kind outside the normal range of human experience. Such experiences include large-scale disasters, whether natural or man-made, which cause multiple deaths and injuries (for example, transport accidents and earthquakes); wartime combat; or individual trauma such as rape or domestic fire. The DSM sets out definitions of the various aspects necessary for a diagnosis of PTSD.

The traumatic event (DSM definition) must involve 'direct personal experience of an event that involves actual or threatened death or serious injury, or other threat to one's physical integrity; or witnessing an event that involves death, injury, or a threat to the physical integrity of another person; or learning about unexpected or violent death, serious harm, or threat of death or injury experienced by a family member or other close associate' (criterion A1).

The person's immediate response (criterion A2) must have involved 'intense fear, helplessness, or horror'.

There are three cardinal groups of symptoms:

- *re-experiencing* the traumatic event (nightmares and flashbacks): criterion B

- *avoidance* of trauma-associated circumstances (cf. phobic anxiety): criterion C

- *increased* arousal (cf. generalized anxiety): criterion D.

There may be general feelings of detachment, loss of interest, inability to feel emotion, and 'survivor guilt'.

Finally, the symptoms must be present for more than 1 month (criterion E), and the disturbance must cause clinically significant distress or impairment in social, occupational, or other important areas of functioning (criterion F).

PTSD: examples of stressors sufficient to qualify for criterion A

- violent physical assault

- sexual assault or abuse

- combat

- serious accidents

- natural or man-made disasters

- diagnosis of a life-threatening illness.

Prevalence

How common is PTSD? Community surveys show that exposure to traumatic events is the rule rather than the exception, having happened to up to 90 per cent of subjects at some time. PTSD is much less common, being found in less than 10 per cent in the same surveys. This apparent discrepancy is because:

- Not all those exposed to a traumatic event develop PTSD.

- PTSD tends to resolve naturally in many cases.

As would be expected, rates of PTSD after accidents are somewhat higher, and figures of approximately 20 per cent at 3 months and 15 per cent at 1 year have been suggested among road traffic accident victims who attend hospital. Those who appear to have felt entirely out of control during the traumatic incident appear most at risk. The disorder may persist for years, with relapses at anniversaries. Many cases are complicated by alcohol misuse.

Types of trauma

A single traumatic event such as a fire has been termed 'type I trauma'. By contrast, repeated, prolonged trauma, such as child abuse, has been denoted type II trauma. It has been suggested that these result in different reactions in the patient and in their family and friends. In type I trauma, the event will be clearly remembered and acknowledged and the patient will receive support from family and friends.

By contrast, type II trauma is said to be poorly remembered, and to be associated with more severe symptoms. This is a controversial area, involving the disputed 'recovered memories', as Brandon *et al.* (1998): 'When memories are "recovered" after long periods of amnesia, particularly when extraordinary means were used to secure the recovery of memory, there is a high probability that the memories are false, i.e. of incidents that had not occurred.'

What about the 'post' in PTSD? Since the concept was formulated, it has become clear that the delay between trauma and onset of symptoms – to which the 'post' in PTSD refers – only occurs in a minority of patients (e.g. 10–20 per cent). The vast majority develop symptoms straightaway.

Prevention of PTSD

'The road to hell is paved with good intentions' might be our watchword here, at least in respect of well-meaning efforts to prevent PTSD. Efforts to encourage – or even require – those who have been exposed to trauma to talk things over with a counsellor or other adviser, either individually or in a group, come under the heading of *debriefing*. To many, both in the mental health professions and in the wider community, it would seem natural and obvious that such an endeavour would be helpful. After all, 'it's good to talk'. Unfortunately, the evidence shows that this can actually be harmful, increasing rates of PTSD at follow-up – the exact opposite of what it was designed to do.

It seems that most people actually do better on their own than if they are directed down a mental health route; informal support mechanisms, whether going to the pub with workmates or having a good cry with loved ones, seem more healthy. Accordingly, the NICE PTSD guideline (http://www.nice.org.uk/page.aspx?o=CG026NICEguidelineword) advises against routine use of debriefing.

Treatment of PTSD

'All PTSD sufferers should be offered a course of trauma-focused psychological treatment (trauma-focused cognitive behavioural therapy or eye movement desensitization and reprocessing),' recommends the NICE PTSD guideline (http://www.nice.org.uk/page.aspx?o=CG026NICEguidelineword). As regards CBT, this is a laudable sentiment, but it is wishful thinking: there are just not enough therapists.

The mainstay of treatment is psychotherapy in which patients are encouraged to express their memories and feelings about the disaster in an individual or group setting. Antidepressant drugs may also help.

As regards EMDR (which stands for 'eye movement desensitization and reprocessing'), this controversial treatment is also regarded by NICE as an evidence-based treatment, in spite of the fact that no one has a clear idea of how it might work.

PTSD: controversies

It will be apparent that the definition of a traumatic event has been widened in successive editions of the DSM; almost any accident could be described as a 'threat to one's physical integrity', and 'witnessing an event' is surely qualitatively different from being involved. This has led to people having received compensation for harassment in the workplace on the basis of PTSD, when the initial definition of PTSD related to serious physical trauma.

As indicated above, there are doubts about the 'post' in PTSD. The very name 'PTSD' may be misleading, in that it assumes that the trauma is causative, while not mentioning the importance of vulnerability. Further, the clinician has to make a judgement about the severity of trauma when he was not there and is not in any case an expert on it. Critics have suggested that these inherent flaws in the concept of PTSD should lead to its removal from the international classifications of psychiatry. However, it seems likely to be with us for some time yet.

Adjustment disorders

Adjustment disorders are maladaptive reactions to psychosocial stress, lasting no more than about 6 months. Common symptoms include anxiety, depression, insomnia, behavioural changes, and physical complaints. These symptoms appear in excess of the 'normal' reaction to the stressor concerned, and produce some impairment of occupational and social function. Counselling or social casework is usually considered more appropriate than drugs, although some patients do benefit from antidepressants or anxiolytics.

Bereavement

Grief following major bereavement has been described as having four classic phases:

- shock, numbness, disbelief

- protest, searching, pain

- despair

- acceptance.

This model is a crude guide to a gradual process, which may take well over a year to complete. Similar reactions are found after other loss events such as death of a pet, break-up of a relationship, loss of a job, or mutilating surgery.

An abnormal grief reaction may be diagnosed if grieving is unduly prolonged, if grief cannot be expressed, or if there is denial that death has occurred. Bereavement may precipitate psychiatric illness, usually depression, or suicide in vulnerable people. Abnormal grief reactions are more common if the deceased was young, if the death was sudden or violent, or if the bereaved person's relationship with the deceased was complicated by guilt or ambivalence.

Psychotherapy is often appropriate for abnormal grief reactions; for example, the technique of 'guided mourning' to help the patient acknowledge and grieve the death.

If severe depression develops after bereavement, treatment should be prescribed in the usual way.

References

Brandon, S., Boakes, J., Glaser, D. and Green, R. (1998). Recovered memories of childhood sexual abuse. Implications for clinical practice. *Br J Psychiatry* **172**, 296–307.

Kennerley, H. (2006). *Overcoming Anxiety*. London: Constable & Robinson.

7 Personality disorders

Definition

Personality disorders involve deeply ingrained maladaptive patterns of behaviour that cause harm to the subject and/or other people. These disorders are generally recognizable by the time of adolescence, and continue through most or all of adult life.

The older term 'psychopathy' may be used for any personality disorder, but is usually reserved for the 'antisocial' type.

Great caution must be exercised before the diagnosis is given, as it can have adverse implications, and can lead to the patient's being rejected from services as untreatable.

Indeed, it has been observed, only half-jokingly, that the only people who do not have a personality disorder are those without a personality. This makes the important point that all of us have personality traits that could be maladaptive or counterproductive in certain circumstances.

Classification

It is first necessary to discuss how 'normal' personality may be classified. There are two general approaches, the ideographic and the nomothetic.

Ideographic theory views each person as a unique individual, with aspects of personality that are not possessed by anyone else. The structure of the personality

Hughes' Outline of Modern Psychiatry, Fifth Edition. David Gill.
© 2007 John Wiley & Sons, Ltd   ISBN 9780470033920

may be different between individuals, even though similar traits may be present; the relative importance of such traits may also differ. This approach gives great weight to detailed appreciation of the individual history in case studies.

Nomothetic theory, by contrast, sees each person as possessing greater or lesser amounts of a number of personality traits, these traits being present to a greater or lesser extent in all members of the population. In other words, each personality, according to nomothetic theory, is made up of a unique selection from a sort of *à la carte* menu of personality traits, each of which is assumed to have the same meaning or effect in each person.

The nomothetic model has been predominant in recent years, as it is obviously suitable for a quantitative approach using self-report personality questionnaires, structured interviews, and factor analysis of the results thereof. For example, it has been suggested that a five-factor model (neuroticism, extroversion, openness, agreeableness, and conscientiousness) can account for much of the observed personality characteristics of different individuals, and that there may be a strong genetic aspect to such traits (Yamagata *et al.*, 2006).

Although the evidence base for a nomothetic approach to understanding personality may continue to grow, it is counter-intuitive to think that it will ever be able to account for the infinite variety of individual personality.

Use of personality measures such as the MMPI (Minnesota Multiphasic Personality Inventory) is claimed to give quantitative measures of aspects of personality. However, their use remains uncommon in UK clinical practice in psychiatry.

The various types of personality disorder, as described below, overlap with each other, many individuals having traits characteristic of more than one type. Hence, if a patient satisfies criteria for more than one type, it does not necessarily mean that he has 'two personality disorders', in the sense of two separate conditions that are additive. The disorders are therefore not necessarily 'twice as severe' – it is more likely that they just do not fit neatly into the written classifications.

DSM versus ICD

There is much common ground between the two classifications in how they deal with personality disorder, but also a small number of significant differences. Probably the most significant difference is that DSM–IV includes *schizotypal personality disorder*; this does not appear in ICD.

Schizotypal personality disorder is said to be characterized by 'ideas of reference . . . magical thinking . . . unusual perceptual experiences, including bodily illusions . . . odd thinking and speech . . . suspiciousness or paranoid ideation'. It has been suggested that the category may serve to contain the excess of cases of schizophrenia diagnosed by US psychiatrists in previous years as compared with those from the UK and other countries (WHO, 1973).

(*F21 schizotypal disorder* does appear in the ICD–10; the list of clinical features is very similar, but it is included within the same block as schizophrenia. Confusingly, ICD indicates that its 'evolution and course are usually those of a personality disorder'. In any event, the diagnosis of schizotypal disorder is not frequently made in UK clinical practice; most clinicians would regard it as a mild or prodromal form of schizophrenia, and would advise standard management of that condition, including medication.)

By contrast, the DSM concept of *borderline personality disorder* (see below) has achieved clinical currency in the UK, even though it does not appear in ICD–10.

The DSM also includes *narcissistic personality disorder,* which overlaps with histrionic personality disorder, on the one hand, and with antisocial personality disorder, on the other hand. It is not separately coded in ICD–10.

The final main difference is that DSM groups the personality disorders into three clusters:

- *Cluster A: odd eccentric,* including paranoid, schizoid, and schizotypal personality disorder

- *Cluster B: dramatic-emotional-erratic,* including antisocial, borderline, histrionic and narcissistic personality disorder

- *Cluster C: anxious-fearful,* including avoidant, dependent, and obsessional compulsive personality disorder.

There is no comparable grouping in ICD–10, and this concept is not, in my experience, in widespread use in clinical practice.

Types of personality disorder

The types of personality disorder described in ICD–10 will now be delineated. As will be appreciated, they do overlap.

- *Paranoid personality disorder F60.0*: in this condition, subjects appear touchy and oversensitive; they are suspicious of the motives of others and prone to the development of overvalued ideas, including ideas of reference (see Chapter 8). They may be excessively self-reliant and self-isolatory, and often quarrel with neighbours or officialdom. The symptoms fall short of satisfying criteria for psychosis. However, some do go on to develop a psychiatric illness with paranoid symptoms, typically paranoid psychosis or schizophrenia.

- *Schizoid personality disorder F60.1*: these subjects tend to be shy, reserved, introspective, emotionally cold, and shunning close relationships. They are often eccentric 'with preference for fantasy, solitary activities, and introspection'. A small proportion develop schizophrenia.

- *Dissocial (antisocial, sociopathic, psychopathic) personality disorder F60.2*: subjects show repeated antisocial behaviour, not modified by experience or punishment. This type will be discussed in more detail below. There is an excess of males over females with this diagnosis.

- *Emotionally unstable personality disorder F60.3*: subjects are emotionally unstable, and prone to outbursts of excessive anger or distress. The US equivalent is *borderline personality disorder*, and this term has come to be more frequently used. The essential concepts are the same, however. The patient may engage in repeated acts of deliberate self-harm, such as cutting or overdoses, or otherwise sabotage his or her own interests, as when they are on the point of getting a new job or starting a new relationship. There is an excess of females over males with this diagnosis.

- *Histrionic personality disorder F60.4*: These patients are prone to overdramatization and transient emotional displays, particularly regarding relationships. They are described as self-centred and emotionally shallow, and with little concern for the feelings of others. This disorder was formerly known as *hysterical personality disorder.*

- *Anankastic (obsessive-compulsive) personality disorder F60.5*: these subjects tend to be cautious, painstaking, and perfectionist and may show stubbornness and lack flexibility. They may do well in occupations requiring extreme attention to detail; conversely, they may be handicapped in forming intimate relationships, with all the give-and-take that this entails. Under stress, they may develop a neurotic reaction, characterized by depression or full-blown obsessive-compulsive disorder.

- *Anxious (avoidant) personality disorder F60.6*: as evident from the name, subjects are affected by chronic feelings of worry, apprehension, and low-grade anxiety symptoms generally. They may avoid social interaction, being generally shy, and often compare themselves adversely with others, leading to low self-esteem. Under stress, these patients can develop a range of anxiety or depressive conditions.

- *Dependent personality disorder F60.7*: subjects are characterized by 'pervasive passive reliance on other people to make one's major and minor life decisions, great fear of abandonment, feelings of helplessness and incompetence, passive compliance with the wishes of elders and others, and a weak response to the demands of daily life. Lack of vigour may show itself in the intellectual or emotional spheres; there is often a tendency to transfer responsibility to others.' A typical instance would be an individual who has normal intelligence, but who fails to separate from the family, and lives a retired life at the parental home, perhaps not working, and often not presenting until the death of the parents.

Under '*Other specific personality disorders F60.8*', ICD gives the following headings: eccentric, 'haltlose' (mixture of frontal lobe, antisocial, and histrionic personality traits), immature, narcissistic, passive-aggressive, and psychoneurotic, but supplies no further information about their characteristics.

In clinical practice, it is more important to make a clear diagnosis of personality disorder, based on the temporal and other characteristics, and then to describe the difficulties presented by the patient. The types of personality disorder in the classifications are really only a guide, and the majority of patients have features from more than one type of personality disorder, as described.

Multiple personality is a rare condition of dubious validity: it seems to develop in vulnerable individuals, called forth by the interest and attention that the concept may excite in the treating professionals.

Sexual deviations (see Chapter 19) may be considered as variants of personality.

Epidemiology

A recent review (National Institute for Mental Health, 2003) indicates that the prevalence of personality disorder in the community is 10–13 per cent, although, obviously, this depends on the definition used. Some forms (e.g. antisocial personality disorder) are more common in men, with others (e.g. borderline personality disorder) more common in women. Antisocial personality disorder has a prevalence of about 2–3 per cent in the community, but this is as high as 75 per cent in prison populations.

Differential diagnosis

'Normal' personality

There is no fixed dividing line between the normal and the disordered personality. Many of the personality traits mentioned above are disadvantageous only if present to extremes. Mild degrees may carry benefits in the right setting; for example, an anankastic personality may do well as a librarian, and a histrionic personality in the entertainment world. Personality disorder should be diagnosed only if the personality traits consistently impair well-being, personal relationships, or work, or lead to dependence on drugs or alcohol.

Learning disability

The other main permanent feature of an individual's mental make-up is his level of intelligence. The DSM helpfully codes both personality disorder and learning disability on the same Axis II. It used to be customary to do psychological testing of intelligence for many psychiatric patients, but this is now unusual unless there is a definite indication. Hence it is important to remember that mild degrees of learning disability can easily be missed.

A common situation in clinical practice would be a patient with low normal intelligence (IQ just over 70), but with the intelligence level making it much harder for the patient to cope with personality and/or mental health problems.

Psychiatric illness

Personality disorders are relatively permanent conditions, whereas psychiatric illnesses involve a potentially reversible change from the patient's usual function. In other words, *it is the time course which is crucial.* Personality disorder, unlike mental illness, has no identifiable beginning. The distinction between personality disorder and psychiatric illness can be difficult, however, for the following reasons:

- The same patient may have both.

- Personality disorders may only be obvious during times of stress.

- Patients are often unable to describe the difference between their current symptoms and their usual personalities.

An account from an informant and long-term observation are essential in trying to resolve the issue.

Organic brain disease

Organic brain disease often causes personality change. The effects of head injury, for example (such as poor impulse control, behavioural disturbance, etc.), can be hard to distinguish from personality disorder.

Treatment

By definition, personality disorders involve persistent characteristics that cannot easily or quickly be eradicated. However, it is wrong to assume that all these patients are untreatable: it may well be possible to contain or even modify undesirable personality traits and their ill-effects.

The principles of treatment include the following:

- consistent care, perhaps including:
  - identified key worker or therapist
  - written contract

- realistic goals – possibly, at first, harm minimization only

- assessment of risk to self and/or others

- proportionate response to manage risk

- sometimes, multiagency working (e.g. probation, substance misuse).

An important recent report, *Personality disorder: No longer a diagnosis of exclusion* (National Institute for Mental Health, 2003) sets out guidance for treating such patients within existing mental health services.

Case example

A woman in her mid-20s had always privately engaged in self-injurious behaviour. After her divorce, she took overdoses and cut herself much more frequently, at least once a week. Repeated assessments failed to indicate any mental illness. Antidepressant medication had been tried without improvement; admission to acute psychiatric wards seemed to be associated with a worsening of her behaviour. She was admitted to a therapeutic community where self-harm was against the rules and would lead to discharge. Although she was apparently reluctant to address her psychological problems in the daily group sessions, her behaviour became much less troublesome during the year of her membership. Problems did return after she left, but remained at a comparatively low level. The cost of the treatment was less than that of the care she would have otherwise required.

Psychotherapy aiming for greater insight and improved behaviour patterns benefits some cases. However, many patients cannot tolerate in-depth individual work.

Group psychotherapy offers an alternative in which patients can learn from each other. This is the mainstay of *therapeutic community* treatment, in which the residents are responsible for setting and maintaining the rules (often referred to as 'the boundaries'; for example, a typical rule is that patients must not self-harm – distress must instead be dealt with by talking to others).

Dialectical behaviour therapy is a fairly new type of treatment for borderline personality disorder (Palmer, 2002). It combines elements of CBT with 'dialectical thinking' and 'mindfulness'.

Nidotherapy (derived from Latin *nidus*, 'nest') is another novel word, at least, and is based on the idea of changing the patient's environment in an effort to produce therapeutic progress (Tyrer and Bajaj, 2005).

Drug treatment is sometimes helpful, in which case it usually needs to be continued on a long-term basis. Antidepressants, low-dose antipsychotics (sometimes given in depot form), and mood stabilizers (lithium or carbamazepine) have been successfully used in some cases. Drugs with a high potential for dependence, such as benzodiazepines, are best avoided in these patients.

Prognosis

Long-term follow-up studies indicate a wide range of outcomes. Some patients improve considerably over time, whereas in others the features of disorder become even more deeply ingrained, and the risk of suicide is raised.

Sociopathic (dissocial) personality disorder

The Mental Health Act 1983 (using the older term *psychopathic disorder*) gives this definition: 'A persistent disorder or disability of mind (whether or not including significant impairment of intelligence) which results in abnormally aggressive or seriously irresponsible conduct on the part of the person concerned.'

Causes

• *Genetic predisposition* is suggested by adoption studies.

• *Brain damage*, usually dating from early life, is present in some cases, and the EEG may show an immature pattern. Temporal lobe lesions may be especially implicated.

• A *disturbed upbringing* is often described, suggesting that the condition may partly result from lack of guidance in childhood regarding acceptable behaviour.

Clinical features

Sociopaths, most of whom are male, consistently behave in ways that are unacceptable to their culture and damaging to themselves, but seem unable to learn from experience. They seek immediate pleasures without considering the long-term consequences, and are unable to make lasting relationships with others, although some possess great superficial charm and are skilled in casual contacts. Subjects often report frequent changes of job, frequent moves of residence, and multiple sexual partners, and live under stress of their own making. They often become depressed at such times and/or experience transient delusions or hallucinations. Drug or alcohol misuse and criminal behaviour are frequent. 'Inadequate', 'aggressive', and 'creative' types have been described. Many prison inmates have sociopathic traits.

Differential diagnosis

- *psychiatric illness*, especially hypomania and schizophrenia
- *organic brain disease*, especially frontal and temporal lobe lesions
- *drug-induced states*, especially by amphetamines or LSD.

Treatment

There is no firm evidence that psychiatric treatment is helpful, but the Mental Health Act 1983 permits compulsory admission if it is considered likely that treatment will 'alleviate or prevent deterioration of the condition'. Many psychopaths have been admitted to hospital under the Act in the past, although there is increasing reluctance to do this unless there is clear treatability.

The most effective management is thought to be psychotherapy in a group composed of other sociopaths. The key point is to encourage the patient to take responsibility for his own conduct. Therapeutic communities for this purpose include those at the Henderson Hospital, Broadmoor Hospital, and Grendon Underwood Prison. Individual psychotherapy is seldom successful, as patients are often manipulative and unreliable in attendance.

Lithium and/or long-acting depot antipsychotics are sometimes tried to control aggression and mood swings. However, use of this medication must be very cautious. As well as elevated risk of overdose, dependence, or abuse, medication may affect the patient's understanding of his condition. If the doctor is prescribing antipsychotics, the patient may see himself as mentally ill, and think that he does not have responsibility for his conduct. He might seek to blame the doctor for inadequate treatment if he committed a criminal offence, for example. In general, the role of medication is limited.

Prognosis

Flagrant antisocial behaviour usually diminishes with age, but problems with relationships continue. About 5 per cent of patients commit suicide (see also Chapter 21 on forensic psychiatry).

References

National Institute for Mental Health in England (2003). *Personality Disorder: No Longer a Diagnosis of Exclusion.* http://www.dh.gov.uk/assetRoot/04/05/42/30/04054230.pdf.

Palmer, R. L. (2002). Dialectical behaviour therapy for borderline personality disorder. *Adv Psychiatr Treat* **8**, 10–16.

Tyrer, P. and Bajaj, P. (2005). Nidotherapy: making the environment do the therapeutic work. *Adv Psychiatr Treat* **11**, 232–238.

WHO (1973). *Report of the International Pilot Study of Schizophrenia.* Geneva: WHO.

Yamagata, S., Suzuki, A., Ando, J. *et al.* (2006). Is the genetic structure of human personality universal? A cross-cultural twin study from North America, Europe, and Asia. *J Pers Soc Psychol* **90**, 987–998.

8 Paranoid states

Definition

Paranoid states involve distorted attitudes and beliefs, often concerning persecution. For practical purposes, the important distinction is whether the beliefs are *delusions* or *overvalued ideas* (for the difference, see Glossary).

Predisposing factors

- *Paranoid personality characteristics*: paranoid personalities (see Chapter 7) are abnormally sensitive and conscious of their own rights, tend to see other people's behaviour as hostile, and are prone to develop ideas of reference. Overvalued ideas have often been present throughout adult life and have influenced the patient's choice of lifestyle; for example, the patient lives alone with minimal social contacts. The personality disorder may not present medically, but it colours the presentation of a superimposed mental illness. For example, a paranoid person who becomes depressed might not trust doctors or might suspect that medication is poisonous.

- *Deafness*, and other forms of sensory deprivation.

- *Social isolation*.

- *Cultural isolation; for example, that due to migration.*

Hughes' Outline of Modern Psychiatry, Fifth Edition. David Gill.
© 2007 John Wiley & Sons, Ltd   ISBN 9780470033920

Differential diagnosis of paranoid states

Paranoid symptoms are found in many of the common psychiatric conditions described elsewhere in this book, including *schizophrenia, affective disorders* (depressive illness and mania), *drug and alcohol misuse*, and the *dementias*. The following list describes some other syndromes in which paranoid symptoms are a main feature:

• *Persistent delusional disorder* (older terms include *paranoid psychosis, paraphrenia,* and *paranoia*): delusions are present, but, in contrast to paranoid schizophrenia, there are usually no hallucinations, the rest of the personality is preserved, and onset is in later life. The majority of patients have a paranoid premorbid personality, and interviews with informants may be essential to determine whether the symptoms are new (an illness has developed), or whether they have always been present (personality) and have come to light for other reasons.

• *Acute paranoid reaction*: a transient condition provoked by stress.

• *Induced delusional disorder (folie à deux)*: a rare condition in which the same persecutory delusions are shared by two people, or sometimes several people, who live in close contact and are often genetically related. The 'principal', who initiates the delusions, suffers from schizophrenia or other mental illness. The 'associate', who reproduces the delusions often has a dependent personality and low intelligence, and usually gives up the delusions if separated from the principal.

• *Morbid jealousy (pathological jealousy, Othello syndrome)*: patients, usually men, are deluded that their sexual partners are unfaithful. Morbid jealousy is often part of another syndrome: paranoid schizophrenia, depressive illness, organic brain syndrome, or alcoholism. Many patients have sexual dysfunction and/or poor personality adjustment. A small percentage may show homicidal behaviour, and lesser degrees of violence are even more common, so morbid jealousy is an important condition despite being rare. A formal risk assessment must be made in such cases, and an appropriate care plan put in place. Referral to forensic psychiatric services may have to be considered. Antipsychotic drugs may be effective. Separation from the partner may have to be advised depending on the risks as evaluated.

Management

Establishing a trusting relationship with the patient, though not always easy, is of prime importance in the treatment of paranoid states.

Objective information about the social setting and cultural background must be sought. Some 'paranoid delusions' are based on genuine persecution, and some 'religious delusions' could be viewed as spiritual experiences rather than as a manifestation of mental illness.

A psychotherapeutic approach is often suitable for milder cases, but if delusions are present, an antipsychotic drug is indicated. Small doses of the strongest antipsychotic drugs such as haloperidol are probably the treatment of choice. Some patients are reluctant to take medication because they suspect it is poisoned, or insist they are not ill. Compulsory detention and treatment under the Mental Health Act 1983 may be necessary if there is disturbed or violent behaviour, or a risk thereof.

Culture-bound syndromes

These conditions, confined to particular cultures, are conveniently mentioned here, although it may not be strictly correct to class all of them as 'paranoid states'. Examples are as follows:

- *amok*: an acute confusional state in Malaysian men, leading to murder and/or suicide

- *latah*: echolalia and echopraxia in Malaysian women

- *koro*: panic caused by fear that the penis is disappearing, in young Chinese men

- *dhat*: complaints of losing semen in the urine, in young Indian men.

These rare syndromes are of academic interest to the UK psychiatrist, rather than practical importance.

Further reading

Enoch, M. D. and Ball, H. N. (2001). *Uncommon Psychiatric Syndromes* (4th edn). London: Arnold.

9 Physical symptoms and psychiatric disorder

Introduction

In the West, we naturally think of illness as either physical or mental. In most circumstances, this works fine: a person with a broken leg is cared for in the orthopaedic ward, and a person with an acute psychotic episode is seen by psychiatric services.

In other circumstances, this physical/mental distinction is less helpful. For example, the condition of a patient who has symptoms such as pain when no physical disease can be found is sometimes referred to as *somatization*, on the basis of a presumption that the symptoms can represent a manifestation of underlying psychological distress. *Medically unexplained symptoms* is a more neutral alternative term.

Another instance of the physical/mental distinction being less helpful is when a patient has both a physical disorder, say, cancer, and a symptom such as depression of mood. The doctrine of *mind–body dualism* (usually attributed to Descartes) can lead here to fruitless debate as to whether the depression is psychiatric in origin or an effect of the cancer, when what is really required is not

Hughes' Outline of Modern Psychiatry, Fifth Edition. David Gill.
© 2007 John Wiley & Sons, Ltd   ISBN 9780470033920

discussion, but a cooperative practical effort of physician and psychiatrist to assist the patient.

In this chapter, I therefore attempt to describe the different ways physical symptoms may present in psychiatric practice, with some suggestions as to management. The chapter should be read in conjunction with Chapter 11 on *liaison psychiatry*, which covers related matters, including service provision.

Assessing physical symptoms in psychiatric practice

The assessment depends in part upon the setting. In some cases, for example, the patient on antipsychotic medication who complains of a shakiness of the hands, the most likely diagnosis (*extrapyramidal side-effects of medication*) will be obvious. Another common instance of side-effects of medication is the patient on tricyclic antidepressants, who complains of a dry mouth.

However, it is always important to remember that the emergence of a physical symptom could represent the first sign of an *underlying physical disorder*. This is particularly pertinent in new referrals, for example, to the outpatient clinic. Usually, it is the responsibility of the referring GP or other doctor to exclude physical disease. However, the psychiatrist must check that appropriate investigations have been done, and continue to remain on the alert and review the matter during the course of treatment. Otherwise, sooner or later, he will find himself in the unenviable position of having tried unsuccessfully to treat someone for, say, depressive illness, with low mood and lack of energy, when the underlying problem turned out to be anaemia or some other physical condition.

Somatic (physical, bodily, biological, or vegetative) complaints form part of the symptom pattern in all the common primary psychiatric disorders. Psychiatric conditions in which somatic complaints are particularly important include:

- *Depressive illness* (see Chapter 5): this is often associated with anorexia, weight loss, constipation, tiredness, and pain. Because of their pessimistic and hopeless cognitions, depressed patients may attribute these symptoms to physical disease of a serious and/or stigmatized kind, such as cancer or AIDS. Those with psychotic depression may develop full-blown delusions of having incurable illness.

- *Anxiety states* (see Chapter 6): autonomic overarousal, heightened muscle tension, and over-breathing can produce a wide range of bodily symptoms. Anxious patients may attribute these symptoms to serious physical disease; for example, they fear a heart attack if they experience palpitations.

- *Schizophrenia* and *delusional disorders* (see Chapter 4): somatic delusions and hallucinations may occur in schizophrenia and are sometimes bizarre; for example, the belief that the internal organs are upside down. Rare related conditions are characterized by fixed somatic delusions; for example, patients with *monosymptomatic hypochondriacal psychosis* might believe that their skin is infested with parasites or their bodies emit a foul smell.

Somatic presentations may arise because emotional problems carry a stigma in the patient's family or cultural setting, and/or because patients genuinely perceive the bodily symptoms to be predominant.

Many psychiatrically ill patients, perhaps especially those from ethnic minorities, first present to their doctors with somatic complaints. These patients are often referred to medical or surgical outpatient clinics because the psychological background is unrecognized. This can result in a long series of unhelpful and expensive hospital investigations and treatments.

Sometimes somatic symptoms have a demonstrable physiological basis, and sometimes they seem to result from misinterpretation of ordinary bodily sensations. Such misinterpretation may be based on past experience of physical disease in other people or in the patient himself.

The psychiatrist performs a service both to the patient and to medical colleagues if he is able to diagnose and treat such somatic presentations of the major mental illnesses.

Unexplained physical symptoms

Introduction

Under this heading, I will now discuss the group of related problems in which the patient continues to have physical symptoms and/or seek medical care when examination and investigation indicate that no causative physical disease can be identified. Thus, a physical symptom such as back pain can be clearly due to a physical pathology such as a prolapsed intervertebral disc. If the patient presenting with pain had no identifiable pathology after appropriate examination and investigation, the traditional approach was to tell the patient he had nothing wrong with him and discharge him.

In recent years, the obvious limitations of such an approach have become clear. Many patients without objective physical pathology do have health problems and are suffering; some unexplained symptoms reflect underlying mental disorder, such as depression or anxiety. In most, elements of psychosocial difficulty can be identified, and this was the part of the basis for the development of *liaison psychiatry services.*

Rather more controversially, the symptoms themselves can be taken as the basis of a 'functional' diagnosis, such as chronic pain syndrome, chronic fatigue syndrome, and others. These syndromes may be advocated by doctors of various disciplines, often with the support of patient groups, who sometimes vehemently deny any role for psychological factors in their genesis.

Classification and terminology

This group of conditions includes *somatoform disorders, hypochondriasis, factitious disorders, malingering,* and so-called 'functional' disorders such as *irritable bowel syndrome.* They are grouped together here partly for convenience; they may not be all related to each other, and the status of some fairly recently introduced concepts, such as *somatoform disorders,* is controversial. Others, such as *Munchausen's syndrome by proxy,* have attracted intense media interest, and may not best be seen as mental disorders.

Terminology for these disorders is complex, and varies substantially between ICD and DSM. In the ICD, most are listed in the chapter *Neurotic, stress-related and somatoform disorders (codes F40–F48).* However, this is widely seen as something of a 'ragbag', containing a variety of conditions which had to be put somewhere, but which, as previously indicated, may not fundamentally have much in common.

The following summary is based on UK clinical practice. The syndromes may be primary, or secondary to another mental disorder, in which case diagnosis and management would be guided by that of the underlying condition.

Hypochondriasis (ICD F45.2 hypochondriacal disorder)

Hypochondriasis involves an unwarranted fear or belief that one has one or more serious physical diseases (in contrast to somatization, in which the patient tends to concentrate on the symptoms themselves). The fears and beliefs persist despite negative medical tests, but are not of delusional intensity. The syndrome is equally common in both sexes, usually starts in young adult life, and follows a chronic course; indeed, in many cases, it is often best regarded as a type of anxious personality trait. It is compatible with a normal level of psychosocial functioning.

Dysmorphophobia (subtype of ICD F45.2 hypochondriacal disorder)

Dysmorphophobia patients are preoccupied with a defect of appearance, such as a misshapen nose, which other people consider trivial. They often seek plastic surgery and in some cases this is helpful, but other patients remain dissatisfied even after repeated surgical revisions. In contrast with *monosymptomatic hypochondriacal psychosis*, the beliefs of dysmorphophobia are not of delusional intensity.

Chronic pain (ICD F45.4 persistent somatoform pain disorder)

This syndrome involves persistent severe pain that cannot be explained by a physical disorder. An example would be a patient who has had an operation for back pain, but still has severe pain, or a patient who has been in a minor road traffic accident and sustained whiplash injuries, but is still complaining of incapacitating neck pain years later.

This can be a controversial category. In some cases, there are obvious psychological factors at play, but many of these patients vehemently deny any mental health aspect of their problems. Frequently, they are seen in *pain clinics*, often run by anaesthetists, where a variety of physical treatments (injections, TENS machines, medications, etc.) will be tried. A *biopsychosocial model* of pain is usually acknowledged, with a role for rehabilitation along cognitive-behavioural lines. Psychiatrists and psychologists sometimes have sessional commitments to such clinics. Dramatic improvements seem unusual in pain clinic patients.

It important to ensure that patients have appropriate antidepressant medication treatment as part of the management; tricyclics in proper doses have useful analgesic and anxiolytic properties, even if there is not a typical depressive syndrome present.

Particularly controversial aspects of chronic pain include the disputed syndrome of 'fibromyalgia', and individual cases where there are medico-legal or insurance claim dimensions.

Somatization disorder (Briquet's syndrome ICD F45.0)

In this disorder, patients repeatedly consult their doctors about a variety of physical symptoms, in different body systems, for which no organic cause can be found. Patients often have very thick notes, with repeated consultation of a number of specialties. The disorder is a chronic one that fluctuates over a period of several years, usually beginning in early adult life, and affecting women more often than men. Most patients have severe social or interpersonal problems, and there may be coexisting depression, anxiety, and personality disorder. History of adverse upbringing, including deprivation or abuse or both, is usual. Management is extremely difficult. Harm minimization through liaison with the patient's GP to try to avoid excessive referrals and invasive and possibly harmful procedures may be the most realistic option.

Conversion and dissociative disorders (ICD F44, formerly called hysteria)

Conversion disorder is the current term for syndromes in which there is loss of physical function, such as paralysis of a limb, blindness, or fits, that cannot be explained by physical disease. The condition is regarded as not intentionally produced, thereby distinguishing it from *factitious disorder* (see below). It tends to develop acutely in stressful circumstances. Such symptoms appear to express an emotional conflict or need, and may bear some symbolic relationship to the nature of the stress. For example, one student developed a paralysed right hand the day before a written examination. The symptoms often appear to bring advantages for the patient: a 'primary gain' of keeping psychological stress at bay, and a 'secondary gain' of attracting sympathy and support or avoiding unwelcome obligations.

Most cases seen today tend to resolve quickly, although they may recur under repeated stress. Florid cases, with severe features such as chronicity and unconcern about the symptoms ('la belle indifférence'), are rare in modern Western society. Civilian cases tend to occur in women, but male cases are encountered in military settings during wartime. Epidemic forms occur.

Dissociative disorder refers to a similar presentation; however, the loss is not of physical function but of mental, such as psychogenic amnesia. *Fugue* is a classic manifestation, in which the patient travels away from his home area, and turns up far away with no memory of himself or how he got there. Liaison with police, who will check missing persons alerts, is often necessary. Obvious stressors (e.g. legal, family, or financial) in the background are often discovered. Gradual recovery is usual.

Factitious disorder (Munchausen's syndrome)

This is listed in ICD as *F68.1 Intentional production or feigning of symptoms or disabilities, either physical or psychological [factitious disorder].* (This is in a different chapter, namely, *Disorders of adult personality and behaviour (F60–F69).*)

Patients contrive repeated hospital admissions by fabricating acute physical symptoms such as bleeding or acute abdominal pain. They usually give a dramatic history, sometimes under a false name. They may submit to unpleasant investigations, or even to surgery, before suddenly discharging themselves when detection is imminent and travelling to another hospital to repeat a similar performance. Some patients go so far as to inject themselves with noxious material in order to produce fever, or to pick at a surgical wound to prevent its healing. Alternative terms quoted in the ICD include *hospital hopper syndrome* and *peregrinating patient.* The patient appears to crave the attention and succour derived from hospital care; it is not done for external gain, which is the main distinguishing feature from *malingering* (see below).

Munchausen's syndrome by proxy (MSBP) (not listed in ICD)

This was a term coined to describe the behaviour of parents, usually mothers, who intentionally produce illness in their child, who is then presented for medical attention. The term and its paediatrician originator, Meadow, subsequently became controversial. The syndrome may have seen overdiagnosed, resulting in possible wrongful removal of non-abused children from their parents and even criminal convictions. The more neutral term *fabricated or induced illness (FII)* is now preferred by paediatricians.

It is probable that MSBP does not denote a unique psychiatric syndrome in the parent. It is better to regard it as criminal behaviour, rather than a psychiatric matter; it should be investigated by the police, and social services should undertake a risk assessment in respect of the children according to standard child protection procedures. Psychiatric evaluation of the parent on standard lines will be appropriate; a variety of disorders may be present, including personality disorder.

Chronic fatigue syndrome (ICD neurasthenia F48.0)

The term chronic fatigue syndrome may be applied to a patient whose persistent tiredness lacks a physical pathology to account for it. The diagnosis of neurasthenia was popular in the late nineteenth century, and its symptoms included fatigue after minimal effort, loss of interest, irritability, poor concentration, and sleep disturbance.

Similar syndromes have attracted great interest in recent years under new names such as *chronic fatigue syndrome*, *post-viral syndrome*, and *myalgic encephalomyelitis* (ME). There is an association with chronic pain and 'fibromyalgia', on the one hand, and with psychiatric disturbance including anxiety and depression, on the other hand. However, there is no agreed physical basis for these conditions; for example, no objective inflammation or other pathology ('-itis') of the muscles or brain has been found to justify the use of the term *encephalomyelitis*.

Some cases follow infection with the Epstein–Barr virus (which causes infectious mononucleosis or glandular fever) or other viral illnesses such as influenza, hepatitis, brucellosis, or encephalitis. In other cases, no such infection can be identified, leading to controversy about whether chronic fatigue is primarily 'organic' or 'functional' in origin. Many cases probably represent the combination of the after-effects of a viral infection with a psychogenic reaction to stress in a person with obsessional and perfectionist personality traits.

Some patients present after many years of overwork, in jobs where they may have been overpromoted on the basis of their diligence, but beyond their intrinsic capabilities. Their inability to maintain this after a minor health problem is probably best not seen in medical terms.

Many patients have depressive symptoms, but it is not clear whether these are part of the syndrome itself, or a secondary reaction to it. Whatever the aetiology, psychosocial factors appear to be of prime importance in maintaining persistent symptoms and disability. Some patients, convinced that they are suffering from continuing viral illness, insist on continuing to rest, and this causes loss of fitness and eventually makes fatigue worse. Others are willing to engage in a programme of gradually increasing activity, although they are often reluctant to consider that their problems may have a psychological dimension.

Cognitive-behavioural treatment and graded exercise have been shown to be effective in randomized trials. Other proposed treatments such as 'pacing', based on prolonged rest periods, are not supported by this level of evidence, although they are popular with some patient groups (Reid *et al.*, 2006).

Somatoform autonomic dysfunction (ICD F45.3)

Somatoform autonomic dysfunction is a little-used ICD category covering 'cardiac neurosis . . . and psychogenic forms of . . . irritable bowel syndrome' among many other examples given. Symptoms are said to include

> objective signs of autonomic arousal, such as palpitations, sweating, flushing, tremor, and expression of fear and distress about the possibility of a physical disorder. Second, there are subjective complaints of a nonspecific or changing nature such as fleeting aches and pains, sensations of burning, heaviness, tightness, and feelings of being bloated or distended, which are referred by the patient to a specific organ or system.

Management

Excluding organic disease

A small minority of 'somatizing' patients referred to psychiatrists have a genuine physical illness that has been missed. The initial evaluation should therefore always include making sure, preferably by personal discussion with the referring doctor, that appropriate physical assessments have been done. Some psychiatrists favour carrying out a physical examination themselves. If no evidence of organic disease is found, the patient should be firmly reassured at the outset, but repeated reassurance is unhelpful. Following this, the psychiatrist often contracts with the patient that any requests for more sophisticated tests and second opinions should be addressed to the referring doctor, as patients may otherwise use this as a means of avoiding underlying psychological issues.

General approach

Somatizing patients need tactful handling. Some are reluctant to consider a psychological aspect of their condition, are on bad terms with their doctors (the term 'heartsink patient' has been applied to chronic somatizers in general practice), and become angry if psychiatric referral is broached. Others welcome an opportunity to discuss the psychosocial background to their symptoms. If several health-care professionals are involved, it is important for them to cooperate with each other, to ensure a consistent policy.

A key point is that most of these disorders are to be coped with over long periods, rather than cured. The vast majority will be cared for by the primary health-care team. A GP who has known a patient for many years will often be able to identify lifelong hypochondriacal tendencies, and so contain an increase in symptoms and consultations at times of stress without needless interventions.

Case example

A 27-year-old woman had been looked after by one GP throughout her life. Her parents had separated, her father being an alcoholic, and there was some suggestion that she had been sexually abused by her stepfather. She herself tended to form abusive relationships with a succession of violent males, her main outlet being frequent consultations with her doctor with bitter complaints of symptoms in a variety of body systems. Although the GP viewed her as one of her 'heartsink' patients, and never felt that she was achieving much progress, she managed to contain her with only infrequent symptomatic treatments and simple investigations.

While her usual GP was on holiday she consulted a locum, complaining of pelvic pain and in great distress. She was referred to the local gynaecologist. At the hospital, where she saw a succession of junior doctors, various medications were tried to no effect, and eventually a hysterectomy was performed. The patient then complained that her pain had actually got worse. A psychiatric referral followed, and a diagnosis of somatization disorder was made, but the patient refused to engage in any form of psychological treatment and spoke of suing the gynaecologist.

Underlying psychiatric disorders

Underlying psychiatric disorders must be treated. For example, somatic delusions in psychotic depression often disappear after successful treatment of the depressive illness.

Specific psychological interventions

It is important to explain the symptoms to the patient, not belittling them as trivial or unreal, but introducing the idea of mind–body interactions, for example, by explaining the physiology of anxiety, or by pointing out time links between psychological stress and onset of symptoms. Giving positive suggestions that improvement is likely to occur with time is probably helpful. Specific therapy with a cognitive-behavioural approach (see Chapter 22) may enable patients to view their symptoms in a more logical way, and gain greater control over them. In other cases, a psychodynamic approach to the conflicts underlying the physical complaint is helpful.

Psychotropic drugs

Antidepressant drugs are sometimes effective for somatic complaints including pain, even if the patient is not overtly depressed, and neuroleptic drugs such as trifluoperazine or pimozide may control somatic delusions and hallucinations.

Case example

A man of 48 was made redundant from an unskilled factory job, and could not find further work. He started to suffer severe headaches, and consulted his GP several times. The GP's impression of a depressive component was vehemently rejected by the patient, and there seemed no alternative to neurology referral. While waiting for outpatient consultation, the patient's pain became incapacitating over a weekend and he was admitted as an emergency. During a 2-week admission, he had extensive investigations, all of which were normal, and continued to refuse the ward staff's efforts to encourage him to talk about his apparent emotional problems. He was discharged with a diagnosis of 'tension headache, depressed' on amitriptyline 50 mg nocte, in the belief that this drug was purely an analgesic. He continued to suffer headaches, and to decline more intensive psychiatric input. In follow-up, he never regained full physical or psychological health, although it was clear that he was rather better when taking amitriptyline than when not.

Malingering and exaggeration

Malingering (*ICD Z76.5, malingerer [conscious simulation]: person feigning illness with obvious motivation*) is listed in the ICD not as a mental disorder, but in the little-used chapter, *Factors influencing health status and contact with health services Z00–Z99.*

Malingering can be defined as the deliberate feigning or exaggeration of illness for external gain. It includes the following:

1. Pure malingering: complete fabrication of symptoms; this is probably rare

2. Partial malingering: exaggerating real symptoms or falsely saying that past symptoms are continuing

3. False attribution: falsely saying that real symptoms are due, for example, to a compensatable accident

DSM–IV lists malingering under 'additional conditions which may be a focus of clinical attention'; that is, not as a mental disorder in itself. It advises that 'malingering should be strongly suspected in any combination of the following:

- medico-legal context

- discrepancy between complaints and objective findings

- uncooperative in examination/treatment

- antisocial personality disorder.'

This sets a fairly low threshold for suspecting malingering, but the DSM gives no further guidance as to how the question should be addressed.

Malingering may occur in an effort to avoid detention or military service; these forms may include apparent drowsiness, together with unusual symptoms such as 'seeing little green men' or coprophagia. (Presumably, the individual considers that these necessarily indicate mental illness.) This group of features, together with so-called approximate answers (for example, question: how many legs has a dog? Answer: three) and apparent mental confusion, were sometimes referred to as the 'Ganser syndrome'. However, there is no unifying pathology underlying the term, which has fallen into desuetude.

Malingering or, more commonly, exaggeration also occurs in civil settings. There are documented examples in the literature of malingered PTSD and chronic pain. There is evidence that it may affect substantial numbers of evaluations (e.g. 40 per cent) (Richman *et al.*, 2006) where a financial outcome depends on the result, such as disability benefit payments or compensation for personal injury. It is assessed by clinical examination, and examination of medical records, looking in particular for consistency and plausibility, or their absence (Gill, 2006). Symptom validity testing (Richman *et al.*, 2006) is a comparatively new technique that may help to elucidate some of these difficult cases.

References

Gill, D. (2006). Faking it London: *Solicitors Journal.* Expert Witness Update.

Reid, S. *et al* (2006). Chronic fatigue syndrome. *Clinical Evidence* (15th edn), pp. 1530–1541. London: BMJ Books. http://www.clinicalevidence.com/ceweb/conditions/msd/1101/1101. jsp.

Richman, J., Green, P., Gervais, R. *et al.* (2006). Objective tests of symptom exaggeration in independent medical examinations. *J Occup Environ Med* **48**, 303–311.

Further reading

Sharpe, M. *et al.* (2006). Bodily symptoms: new approaches to classification. *J Psychosom Res* **60**, 353–356.

10 Organic brain syndromes

Delirium and *dementia* are the two main types of organic brain syndrome, with *focal lesions* also to be considered. The term *organic brain syndrome* means a general disturbance of brain function due to a physical disorder. The characteristic feature is a reduction in intellectual functioning (as tested in mental state examination of orientation, concentration, and memory).

If the disturbance comes on suddenly, as in the context of a very high fever, there will be acute organic brain syndrome, most often referred to as *delirium* or *acute confusional state*, with *reduced conscious level* — drowsiness — as the cardinal feature. If, however, the disturbance comes on gradually, as in *dementia* due to Alzheimer's disease, the reduction in intellectual functioning will occur in clear consciousness; that is, there is no drowsiness (at least, until the terminal stages). (Dementia could, by extension, be referred to as 'chronic organic brain syndrome', but the phrase is seldom used.)

Localized lesions give rise to *focal impairments*, such as stroke. This tends to be more the province of neurology. But some types are relevant to psychiatry, and can be considered as psychiatric focal lesions. Examples include Korsakov's psychosis, in which the main abnormality is memory defect; this is due to isolated damage to mesial temporal lobe structures, such as the mammillary bodies. Frontal lobe syndrome (disinhibition, etc.) due to frontal lobe tumour is another example.

Hughes' Outline of Modern Psychiatry, Fifth Edition. David Gill.
© 2007 John Wiley & Sons, Ltd   ISBN 9780470033920

Organic brain syndromes are conditions in which psychiatric symptoms result primarily from a biological disorder affecting brain function. This underlying biological disorder may involve structural cerebral pathology and/or metabolic disturbance. The patient's psychological reaction to the illness (see Chapter 11) is also important in organic cases.

DSM–IV does not include the term 'organic brain syndromes' because it is thought to encourage a misleading separation between 'organic' and 'functional' states. DSM–IV uses the concept of 'secondary' disorders instead, but it means essentially the same thing as 'organic' for practical purposes.

Causes

Cerebral conditions

- degenerative; for example, senile and presenile dementias, Parkinson's disease

- space-occupying lesions; for example, primary brain tumour, cerebral metastasis, subdural haematoma

- infections; for example, bacterial or viral meningitis or encephalitis, including HIV, syphilis, and TB

- head injury

- epilepsy

- vascular; for example, arteriosclerosis, stroke, hypertensive encephalopathy, collagen disease

- miscellaneous; for example, multiple sclerosis, normal pressure hydrocephalus.

Systemic conditions

- infections; for example, septicaemia, pneumonia

- metabolic disturbances; for example, renal or hepatic failure, diabetes, electrolyte imbalance, remote effects of carcinoma, porphyria

- endocrine disorders; for example, thyrotoxicosis, hypothyroidism, Cushing's syndrome

- poisons; for example, alcohol or drug intoxication or withdrawal, carbon monoxide, heavy metals

- cardiac or respiratory conditions causing cerebral anoxia

- vitamin B deficiency.

Clinical features

Organic cerebral disorders in which the whole brain is affected usually present with cognitive impairment and/or clouding of consciousness, which may be accompanied by neurological symptoms or signs. The classical picture in acute cases is called *delirium* and in chronic cases *dementia*. Localized lesions give rise to *focal impairments*. Delirium, dementia, and focal syndromes are described below.

Less typical presentations include mood change, lability of mood, paranoid ideation, and changes in behaviour or personality. Organic cases may present with neurotic or psychotic symptoms resembling those found in 'functional' disorders, but often showing atypical features such as fluctuating symptomatology, visual hallucinations, vague or transient paranoid delusions, or first onset of neurotic symptoms in middle or old age. Cognitive testing may reveal unsuspected defects.

The symptom pattern depends more on the time course of the illness, and the part of the brain involved, than on the type of underlying pathology. Therefore, for example, a confusional state due to fever generally resembles, in its psychiatric aspects, confusion due to, say, renal failure.

Clinical features may also be modified by the patient's premorbid personality, premorbid vulnerability to psychiatric disorder, past life experience, current medication, and social circumstances.

Delirium

Definition

Delirium (acute brain syndrome, acute confusional state) is clouding of consciousness – that is, reduced awareness of the environment – accompanied by abnormalities of cognition, perception, thought, and mood, from an organic cause. The alcohol withdrawal syndrome (delirium tremens) is a common example, but delirium may be due to any acute condition affecting the brain.

Clinical features

The cardinal feature is a reduced level of consciousness, although mild degrees of this can be easy to miss in clinical practice. The patient is confused and disoriented, often restless, overactive, and fearful, but sometimes underactive and withdrawn. Inattention, including reduced ability to focus, sustain, or shift attention, is common. Illusions; hallucinations of visual, auditory, or tactile type; and changeable paranoid delusions may be present.

Severity fluctuates, usually being worse at night, because when there is less light, the environment is more likely to be misinterpreted, curtains appearing as threatening monsters, for example.

Management

The first priority is diagnosis and treatment of the medical cause, such as occult infection, acute intoxication (e.g. opiates), withdrawal of alcohol or benzodiazepines, or adverse reaction to medication, polypharmacy being a common cause in the elderly.

These patients will often present in the general hospital, and are frequently on a medical 'take'. Probably the commonest type would be 'acute-on-chronic'; that is, a person with a – perhaps unrecognized – background of mild cognitive impairment who becomes acutely confused in association with an intercurrent medical problem such as chest infection – or even something as mild as constipation.

Nursing care, best carried out by one or two familiar people, is important. It includes attention to fluid intake and bladder and bowel function, provision of quiet, warm, well-lit surroundings without too many strange people around, protection against such hazards as unsupervised smoking in bed, and clear explanations before doing any practical procedures.

Drug treatment, preferably with an antipsychotic started at low dose and increased as necessary, may be required to reduce disturbance or distress. Haloperidol in doses as low as 0.5 mg can be effective in the elderly; younger, fitter patients may require higher doses. Most cases are treated in general medical wards without involving psychiatrists.

Prognosis

Outcome depends on the cause. Young, fit patients with a clear cause – say, infection – will usually make a complete recovery if the cause resolves. In older patients, the outlook varies between complete recovery, partial recovery with residual cognitive problems, and death. For general hospital inpatients, development of full-blown delirium is a predictor of increased mortality or, for those who survive, a prolonged hospital stay and/or possible need for long-term care or placement in a nursing or residential home.

Many cases of dementia, as indicated above, first present as a confusional state. There will be improvement with the resolution of the medical problem that precipitated the confusion, but then the underlying cognitive problems become apparent.

Dementia

Definition

Dementia is an acquired global impairment of intellect and memory, often accompanied by changes in personality, mood, and behaviour, from an organic cause. Dementia is usually progressive and irreversible, although some cases have treatable causes, which are important to recognize.

Causes

In clinical practice, the three most common types of dementia are as follows:

- Alzheimer's disease (AD)
- vascular (multi-infarct, arteriosclerotic) dementia (VaD)
- dementia with Lewy bodies (LBD).

AD accounts for 60–70 per cent of dementia cases; the three common types probably together account for over 90 per cent of cases in clinical practice. Most clinical cases would probably have contributions from more than one of the pathologies indicated, if the cellular pathology were examined under the microscope (although brain biopsy *in vivo* is rarely done in dementia because it will not in most cases change management).

Dementia can also be classified according to neuropathological and other research information. Such classifications vary but would include dementia of AD type, Lewy body dementia (LBD), Pick's disease, Huntington's disease, and the prion diseases.

A general account of dementia is given below, followed by a description of some individual conditions.

Clinical features

Onset is usually gradual, unless the dementia is the sequel of a delirious illness. Memory loss is usually the first symptom. This involves recent rather than remote memories, and results in disorientation. Other intellectual functions also deteriorate. In the early stages, the patient may be aware of the memory problems, but, if so, will tend to make light of them or otherwise confabulate so as to minimize the problem in most cases. Most established patients do not complain very much about their memory.

Self-care (appearance) may decline. Affective changes are common, and may consist of lability of mood, sustained depression, or, more rarely, euphoria. Exaggeration of previous personality traits and coarsening of personality accompanied by socially unacceptable behaviour may occur.

Insight may be present in the early stages. Strong emotion, including aggression (sometimes referred to as 'catastrophic reaction'), can understandably occur when patients realize their memory is in severe decline; thus, cognitive testing must always be done sensitively, lest the patients be unduly distressed by realization of their intellectual decline. However, complaints of memory problems volunteered by the patient are seldom a prominent part of the clinical picture.

Insight is usually absent in the later stages. Except in terminal cases, consciousness is unimpaired.

If patients are in their own familiar environment, with friends or family around, they may go undiagnosed, as they may continue to cope with surprising degress of cognitive impairment. But when support disappears – for example, due to illness of a neighbour who regularly checked on them, or when an acute medical problem presents – then the patient may decompensate and the dementia become apparent.

'Sundowning' is often seen, that is, a worsening in confusion in the afternoon and evening; its cause is not clearly known, but may relate to tiredness or to vasospasm. It may be helped by simple nursing measure such as change in rest, exercise, or toileting routines.

'Cortical' and 'subcortical' types of dementia may be distinguished. Cortical dementia includes disturbance of 'higher functions', such as dysphasia, agnosia, and apraxia. In subcortical dementia, these functions are preserved, but the patient is forgetful, slow, and apathetic and may show marked emotional lability with sudden outbursts of laughter or rage.

Diagnosis

Diagnosis is made on clinical grounds from the history and mental state examination including simple cognitive testing.

In taking the history, if there is a suspicion of dementia, it will be appropriate to do cognitive testing early in the interview. This will give guidance as to whether the patient can give a proper history or not (so as not to spend too much time, and annoy the patient, by inappropriately persisting in trying to take a history that must ultimately be incoherent).

Disorientation may be unsuspected by the examiner unless tested; short-term memory (as assessed by name and address test or three-object recall) will usually be abnormal.

Formal psychometric tests can be used to confirm the diagnosis and specify the type of defects present, and repeated at intervals to monitor progress. The Mini-Mental State (Folstein et al., 1975) is widely used in UK clinical practice.

Investigation

All patients require a full medical history and physical examination. Treatable causes (such as brain tumour, subdural haematoma, normal pressure hydrocephalus, infections, hypothyroidism, or vitamin B_{12} deficiency) may be revealed by investigations such as blood count and ESR, urea and electrolytes, liver function tests, thyroid function tests, B_{12} and folate, calcium and phosphate, serological tests for syphilis, HIV antibody testing (with informed consent), chest radiography, EEG, and brain scan.

Potentially treatable factors can be identified in many dementia patients, but good results from treatment are obtained in few. Expensive or invasive investigations are only indicated if their results would alter management, and are seldom justified in patients whose dementia is very severe or whose general physical state is very poor.

Differential diagnosis

Depression is the main condition liable to be confused with dementia, especially in the elderly. *Depressive pseudodementia*, as the name implies, refers to states of depressive illness where the presentation mimics dementia. It can usually be distinguished from dementia by the history of comparatively recent and quick onset, almost always in a patient with a history of previous episodes of depressive illness. Mental state examination may show pronounced features of low mood, and psychological testing may produce better results than in true dementia. In doubtful cases, a therapeutic trial of antidepressant drugs or ECT should be undertaken. In some patients, the two disorders co-exist, indeed depression is thought to be a risk factor for the development of dementia.

Management

The cause of the dementia should be corrected if possible. Acetylcholinesterase inhibitors are licensed for use in AD; see details below.

For the majority of cases, specific treatment produces limited benefit. The aim of management is therefore to keep patients functioning at their optimum level by maintenance of good physical health and provision of a suitable environment. It is usually best for patients to remain in their own homes with help from community services (see Chapters 20 and 25); indeed, the vast majority of patients with dementia do reside in the community. Much of the care necessary is provided by relatives and friends. The burden on them can be lessened by arranging respite care every so often, and by offering prompt emergency help in the event of an intercurrent illness or a social crisis.

Admission to hospital or nursing home may worsen confusion and distress, although it may be inevitable in the later stages. Long-term inpatient hospital care for dementia is now almost extinct in the NHS. It is now in England mainly provided through private nursing and residential homes, for which the patient has to pay until almost all his money is gone. This includes his home, which otherwise he might have wished to pass on to his children. In other parts of the UK, this care is provided free by the state.

Prognosis

In the minority of patients with a treatable cause, progression of the dementia can be arrested, and there may even be partial recovery, but most cases gradually deteriorate. The effect of acetylcholinesterase inhibitors, if any, is to delay decline, by putting back the time when the patient will no longer be able to be cared for at home. Acute confusional episodes due to other pathology, such as chest or urinary infections, strokes, faecal impaction, or inappropriate medication may be superimposed.

Drug treatment of behavioural and psychotic symptoms of dementia (BPSD) may be necessary, but it carries risks; atypical antipsychotics such as olanzepine and risperidone are contraindicated because of the risk of stroke.

Specific types of dementia will now be described.

Senile dementia of Alzheimer type (SDAT)

Epidemiology

SDAT accounts for over half of all cases of dementia in old age. It is present in 5 per cent of people over age 65 and 20 per cent of people over 80. Women are affected nearly twice as often as men, probably mainly reflecting women's longer lifespan.

AD is also the commonest of the primary 'presenile' dementias, with onset earlier in life, say, between the ages of 40 and 60.

Cause

Genetic predisposition exists and a link with allele e4 of apolipoprotein E is established. About 20–30 per cent of the population has at least one copy of e4; about 50 per cent of AD patients have at least one copy of e4. However, most cases are probably polygenic and multifactorial.

Most cases of early-onset AD arise sporadically, but others are inherited, usually in polygenic fashion, although in a few families there is a dominant gene. Mutations in the amyloid precursor protein (APP) gene on chromosome 21 have been found in a few affected families. APP is implicated in the formation of senile plaques, one of the key neuropathological findings in AD. The role of APP ties in with the well-known increased rate of AD in trisomy 21 (Down's syndrome) patients.

Genetic testing is seldom done in clinical practice unless the AD is strongly familial.

Neuropathology

Shrinkage of the brain causes enlargement of the ventricles and sulci, as revealed by CT or MRI brain scanning Microscopically, there are three characteristic changes: neuronal loss, senile plaques, and neurofibrillary tangles. Neurons are decreased both in number and size, and astrocytes proliferate. Senile plaques, which have argyrophilic cores containing an amyloid-like substance, develop in the grey matter. Nerve fibres form tangles called Alzheimer's neurofibrillary degeneration. Lewy bodies (see below) may also be present.

Neurochemistry and neurophysiology

Post-mortem brain studies show a deficiency of the enzyme choline acetyltransferase, which is concerned in the synthesis of acetylcholine, and defective cholinergic transmission is considered the likely basis of the symptoms. Cerebral blood flow and oxygen consumption are reduced. The EEG usually shows theta or delta waves, with alpha rhythm slow or absent. Brain scans show cerebral atrophy, selectively affecting the medial temporal lobe in early cases.

Symptoms

Onset is gradual over a year or more. Loss of recent memory is usually the first symptom, and is followed by deterioration in other mental functions, emotional lability or sustained depression, and personality change. Delusions and hallucinations, fits, and neurological signs may occur in advanced cases. Insight is usually absent, and the patient comes to medical attention because relatives or neighbours notice failing memory, confusion, poor hygiene, and self-neglect. Diagnosis is made on clinical grounds, as there is no laboratory test for AD, although tests may be required to exclude other causes of dementia.

In early-onset dementia, rapid progression was said to be usual, but there is doubt as to whether deterioration is really quicker, on average, than in later-onset cases. Marked neurological abnormalities are common.

Treatment

The acetylcholinesterase inhibitors *donepezil*, *galantamine*, and *rivastigmine* are now licensed for use in AD. Their use was sanctioned by NICE in 2001 (http://www.nice.org.uk/page.aspx?o=14487), but with the following conditions:

• MMSE > 12

• prescription to be initiated in specialist clinics, most services now running a 'memory clinic' for this purpose

- treatment normally to continue only if MMSE > 12, and judged to be of overall clinical benefit.

It is unusual for such conditions to be attached to drug licences; this reflects the high cost of the drugs, and the continuing doubts about their effectiveness. Trial data indicate improvements, or at least slower declines, in measures of cognitive function, which are claimed to delay the requirement for the patient to enter institutional care. However, clinical experience is that dramatic responses are unusual. The overall impact of the drugs in clinical practice has been modest.

Memantine is an NMDA-receptor antagonist that affects glutamate transmission; it is licensed for treating moderate to severe AD; however, its cost-effectiveness has been doubted (http://www.nice.org.uk/page.aspx?o=322952).

NICE recently reviewed the effectiveness of all these drugs in relation to their cost; the manufacturers – not surprisingly, considering the potential size of the market – have entered appeals, as have other groups; this debate can be followed at the NICE website. At the time of writing, NICE has just – controversially – withdrawn approval for the NHS use of these drugs in early dementia in England, although they remain available in Scotland.

Prognosis

Dementia shortens life. Pneumonia is a frequent terminal event. Death 5 years after the onset of dementia would be a typical course, but much depends on overall health and the quality of care.

Vascular dementia

Vascular dementia (VaD) is common; it frequently co-exists with AD.

Epidemiology

VaD usually starts between the ages of 60 and 70 but sometimes earlier. Men are affected slightly more often than women.

Pathology

The cause is focal infarction of the brain due to haemorrhage, thrombosis, or embolism, usually associated with cerebral arteriosclerosis. There may be a single cerebral vascular accident, multiple small infarcts, or small vessel disease causing white matter damage. Most patients have hypertension, focal neurological signs, and evidence of arteriosclerosis in other organs.

Symptoms

Loss of memory, intellectual deterioration, and mood changes occur. Insight and personality are retained longer than in AD, and the continued insight may contribute to the depression that is often present. Deterioration is stepwise rather than gradual, as repeated small strokes or episodes of hypertensive encephalopathy occur and leave residual damage.

Prevention and treatment

Some cases might be prevented by control of hypertension in its early stages, and by attention to potential sources of emboli in the brain. Some improvement in the established condition may be achieved by treatment of very high blood pressure levels, cessation of smoking, and regular low-dose aspirin.

Prognosis

Average survival time is about 5 years; the usual causes of death are ischaemic heart disease and stroke.

Lewy body dementia

Definition and neuropathology

Comparatively recently, in fact since the last edition of this book, Lewy body dementia (LBD) has been recognized as a distinct condition. This is a type of dementia in which Parkinsonian features are prominent. Conscious level and cognitive function tend to fluctuate; and visual illusions or hallucinations may occur, as may frank psychotic symptoms.

It has been recognized that Parkinson's disease can sometimes proceed to dementia. Patients with LBD seem to be on a continuum between pure Parkinsonism, on the one hand, and dementia on the other hand.

Lewy bodies are oval structures that are in fact eosinophilic inclusion bodies within degenerating dopamine-bearing cells in the substantia nigra and related areas; they are the neuropathological basis of Parkinson's disease. The presence of such Lewy bodies (which are morphologically similar but distinct) in other areas of the brain appears at least partly to underlie the clinical syndrome of LBD.

Epidemiology

It is not yet clear what proportion of dementia cases overall should be classified as LBD. Clearly, this would depend on how a case should be defined. It has, however, been suggested that it is the second commonest cause of dementia after AD.

Clinical features

LBD is marked by fluctuating cognitive performance and conscious level, Parkinsonism (in the majority of cases), and psychiatric symptoms including visual hallucinations.

Treatment

Treatment is inherently difficult. Drugs used to help Parkinsonian features tend to exacerbate any psychotic symptoms present. Parkinsonian treatment should be reviewed and reduced if possible, beginning probably with any anticholinergics.

Conversely, antipsychotic drugs, if employed for psychotic symptoms – whether inherent or due to side-effects of anti-Parkinson drugs – will make Parkinsonian symptoms worse. Patients are often very sensitive to neuroleptics, both typical and atypical, and they should be avoided if at all possible. A difficult balance has to be struck.

Pick's disease

Pick's disease is regarded as one of the frontotemporal lobe dementias; although it is a rare cause of dementia overall, it may account for up to 5–10 per cent of early-onset cases. Some cases are familial, probably caused by a dominant gene. Onset is between the ages of 50 and 60, and women are affected twice as often as men. Cerebral atrophy occurs, with loss of neurons and gliosis, most marked in the frontal and temporal lobes. Characteristic Pick bodies (cortical inclusions) are seen.

Symptoms of frontal lobe damage occur first (character change, disinhibition, poor judgement, etc.), followed by language problems if the temporal lobes are affected. Day-to-day memory may be relatively spared in the early stages, but impairment of memory and intellect gradually develops later. Dysphasia, apraxia, agnosia, and extrapyramidal symptoms are sometimes present. Death occurs 2–10 years after the onset.

Huntington's disease (Huntington's chorea)

Huntington's disease is a rare form of inherited presenile dementia. Its molecular genetics and the clinical implications thereof have been extensively studied.

Epidemiology

Five per 100 000 of the population are affected, with marked regional variation. Men and women are equally at risk.

Cause

The cause is an abnormality in the IT-15 gene, located on the short arm of chromosome 4, which encodes the protein huntingtin. This results in an autosomal dominant inheritance pattern with about 90 per cent penetrance. The number of repeat sequences of the abnormal DNA triplicate (CAG) – leading to excessive glutamine in the protein – has some relationship to the age of onset and severity of the clinical disorder. However, the role of the protein in brain function is still unclear in spite of enormous research effort.

Half the children of an affected parent develop the condition, and because the age of onset is usually in midlife, many patients have already had children themselves by the time symptoms begin. 'Anticipation' is also seen; that is, age of onset decreases in succeeding generations. Occasionally, patients have no family history, and such cases may be explained by spontaneous mutation or doubtful parentage.

Neuropathology and neurophysiology

Generalized atrophy of the brain is most severe in the frontal lobes, caudate nuclei, and putamen. Low-energy metabolism in the caudate nucleus, identified by PET scan, is characteristic and could be used as a presymptomatic test. Deficiency of GABA and excess dopamine have been demonstrated at post-mortem.

Clinical features

Onset may be at any age, but is most often in midlife (mean age 49). The juvenile form, starting in adolescence, accounts for 10 per cent of cases. Choreiform movements and dementia are the most characteristic symptoms, but there may be any type of psychiatric abnormality – for example, neurotic, depressive, or schizophrenic symptoms or psychopathic personality features – and great variation in the clinical course.

Treatment

Choreiform movements can be modified with phenothiazines or tetrabenazine. Any psychiatric symptoms present should be treated with appropriate drugs.

Diagnosis

Presymptomatic testing by genetic probes is now available through departments of medical genetics. The test may be carried out on an adult individual or an unborn child. Testing raises ethical issues, since there is no means of preventing or treating the disorder in those carrying the gene, and tests should be carried out only in the context of thorough family counselling. In practice, only a minority of at-risk individuals choose to be tested.

Prognosis

The average survival time is about 15 years.

Transmissible spongiform encephalopathies (prion dementias)

These are rare forms of dementia, caused by accumulation of abnormal prion proteins in the brain. Prion stands for proteinaceous infectious particle, a unique form of infective agent, as it contains no genetic material. Prions are now accepted as the cause of a group of transmissible spongiform encephalopathies including scrapie (in sheep), chronic wasting disease (in deer), and bovine spongiform encephalopathy (BSE) ('mad cow disease').

Human examples of these disorders include *Creutzfeld–Jacob Disease* (CJD) and *kuru* (formerly found in Papua New Guinea cannibals; this epidemic peaked in the 1960s and is now more or less extinct, due to the decline of cannibalism). Sporadic CJD has always rarely occurred. Iatrogenic CJD cases involved transmission of the condition by use of pituitary tissue ('harvested' to obtain growth hormone) from brains post-mortem that turned out to be CJD infected. New variant (nvCJD) cases are those linked to BSE. Although at the height of the health scare regarding BSE, huge numbers of cases were predicted, as of August 2006, only 156 had been identified (http://www.cjd.ed.ac.uk/figures.htm).

BSE was described in British cattle in the 1980s and was probably due to use of scrapie-infected sheep products in cattle feed (the temperature at which such products should be treated to render them safe had been reduced by the government for reasons of economy). Other countries such as France had similar epidemics, which were not as well publicized.

Gerstmann–Sträussler–Scheinker syndrome and fatal familial insomnia are other rare human examples.

Causes

In some families, these dementias appear to be due to an inherited prion gene mutation, which follows an autosomal dominant pattern. Other cases are infective, due to an abnormal prion protein acquired in various ways. The disorders can be transmitted to experimental animals, and human cases have followed neurosurgery, corneal grafting, or administration of cadaveric growth hormone.

Neuropathological features

Prion protein, a modified cell membrane protein, accumulates within the CNS. There is neuronal loss, astrocytic hyperplasia, and spongiform vacuolation in grey matter, with amyloid plaques.

Clinical features

Dementia, accompanied by myoclonus or ataxia, usually starts in middle life. EEG changes are characteristic, and diagnosis can be confirmed by finding a prion gene mutation in a blood sample. These diseases are always fatal, within a few months typically.

NvCJD is said to differ clinically from 'classical' CJD, in that the symptoms are often initially psychiatric, and progression is slower.

HIV dementia

Cognitive impairment is associated with HIV infection and AIDS. However, it is difficult to generalize about the prevalence of dementia, as the outlook for the condition varies greatly between countries where there is good health care and those where access to AIDS drugs is limited and the outlook much poorer. Regarding the UK, the predictions at the start of the epidemic of very large numbers of HIV-dementia cases have fortunately proved wide of the mark.

Nevertheless, substantial numbers of patients in the late stages of this illness do develop a frank dementing syndrome due to invasion of the brain by the HIV virus. Typical features include forgetfulness, slowness, and apathy, accompanied by motor weakness, with multiple neurological abnormalities in the later stages.

Cerebral atrophy is shown on brain scan. Treatment with antiviral agents may bring about worthwhile clinical improvement.

Differential diagnosis in the HIV-positive patient includes other cerebral infections such as toxoplasmosis, herpes simplex, and those caused by cryptococcus and cytomegalus; cerebral lymphoma; and depressive illness. Specific treatments are available for several of these conditions; therefore, it is desirable to reach an accurate diagnosis.

Prevention of dementia

Purandare *et al.* (2005) suggest that 'The prevalence of dementia would be reduced by 50 per cent if risk reduction strategies were successful in delaying its onset by 5 years', and three strategies have been put forward:

- treatment of vascular risk factors

- neuroprotection, through vitamins, antioxidants, and anti-inflammatory agents

- building up neuronal reserves, through increased activity.

Focal brain damage

Amnesic syndrome

The most common type of amnesic syndrome is Wernicke–Korsakov syndrome, which is fundamentally due to thiamine depletion, almost always in the context of alcohol misuse. 'Wernicke' refers to the acute encephalopathic presentation (confusion and neurological signs, usually in a known alcoholic – parenteral thiamine treatment is mandatory), and 'Korsakov' to the chronic memory defect state. The brain structures involved, necessary for the laying down of new memories, have been described as the circuit of Papez (Sperling, 2001): the hippocampus and nearby areas in the mesial temporal lobe, fornix, mammillary bodies, and thalamus.

Causes

The causes of this syndrome are as follows:

- *thiamine deficiency*, usually secondary to *alcoholism*, and occasionally secondary to other causes of nutritional deficiency

- *carbon monoxide* poisoning

- *vascular* lesions

- the aftermath of *hypoxia* (such as may follow anaesthetic accidents, or attempted suicide by hanging) or *hypoglycaemia*

- *encephalitis.*

Clinical features

The memory of recent events is grossly impaired, but immediate recall and long-term memory are both preserved, as are other intellectual functions. Many patients confabulate; that is, they conceal their memory defect by elaborate falsification.

Treatment

Thiamine may be helpful if thiamine deficiency is present. Memory aids may enable some patients to function adequately, but many need constant supervision. Alcohol should be avoided, but therapy for this is inherently difficult due to the memory problems.

Frontal lobe lesions

The frontal lobes are the seat of the higher mental functions, particularly the carrying out of complex mental operations, the 'executive functions'. *Personality change* is often the first sign of a frontal lobe lesion. Behaviour becomes disinhibited, tactless, or ill-judged; mood is inappropriately euphoric; drive and concentration are diminished, although there is no formal intellectual impairment; and insight is lacking.

Neurological signs include a grasp reflex, anosmia, optic atrophy, and incontinence. If the lesion involves the motor cortex, there may be epileptic fits or contralateral spastic paresis.

Broca's area, in the inferior frontal lobe, is involved in language production; lesions here result in expressive dysphasia but relatively unimpaired comprehension.

Temporal lobe lesions

Personality change may take the form of increased aggression and emotional lability, or resemble that seen with frontal lobe lesions.

Temporal lobe epilepsy may develop. This condition, even more than other types of epilepsy, has important psychiatric aspects. It is associated with neurotic disorder, mood disorder, schizophrenia, and high suicide rate.

Intellectual deficits can be verbal or non-verbal depending which side is involved. Memory defects occur with bilateral lesions.

Neurological impairments include contralateral homonymous upper quadrant visual field defect, contralateral limb weakness or sensory loss, and language difficulties in the case of dominant hemisphere lesions.

Wernicke's area, is required for comprehension; damage here produces reduced understanding, but speech output is fluent, albeit inaccurate.

Psychiatric symptoms of schizophrenic or affective type may occur.

References

Folstein, M. F., Folstein, S. E. and McHugh, P. R. (1975). Mini-Mental State: a practical method for grading the state of patients for the clinician. *J Psychiatr Res* **12**, 189–198. http://www.medicaleducation.co.uk/resources/Miniment.pdf.

Purandare, N., Welsh, S., Hutchinson, S. *et al.* (2005). Preventing dementia. *Adv Psychiatr Treat* **11**, 176–183.

Sperling, R. (2001). The volumes of memory. *J Neurol Neurosurg Psychiatry* **71**, 5–6.

Further reading

Lishman, W. A. (1997). *Organic Psychiatry: Psychological Consequences of Cerebral Disorder* (3rd edn). Oxford: Blackwell Scientific.

11 Liaison psychiatry

Liaison psychiatry refers to the branch of psychiatry involving assessment and treatment in the general hospital of referred patients, for example in casualty or following deliberate self harm.

Psychiatric disorders, including anxiety, depression, and/or organic brain syndromes, are present in up to 50 per cent of any population of medical or surgical patients. Some disorders are mild and transient, but 10–20 per cent of patients are severely affected. The majority of patients identified by research surveys are not receiving psychiatric treatment, and apparently have not been recognized by medical or nursing staff.

This psychiatric 'co-morbidity' adds to patients' suffering, and, because it tends to be associated with poor response to medical treatments and extended hospital stays, it adds to health-care costs.

The association between psychiatric and physical conditions may be explained in several ways:

- *Pre-existing psychiatric illness* or *personality disorder* may have played a role in causing the physical disorder, or hindering recovery and response to treatment (see below).

- *The stress of the physical illness* (see below) may precipitate psychiatric disorder.

- *An organic brain syndrome* (see Chapter 10) has developed secondary to the physical illness or its treatment.

Hughes' Outline of Modern Psychiatry, Fifth Edition. David Gill.
© 2007 John Wiley & Sons, Ltd   ISBN 9780470033920

- There is *somatic presentation* of a primary psychiatric condition (see Chapter 9).

- *Medically unexplained symptoms*, rather than objective medical or surgical pathology, dominate the clinical picture.

The links between medical and psychiatric illness are reflected in the raised suicide rate of some, but not all, medical conditions: high-risk disorders include HIV/AIDS; cancer, especially of the head and neck; Huntington's disease; multiple sclerosis; peptic ulcer; renal failure; spinal cord injury; and systemic lupus erythematosus (SLE). Primarily neurological conditions such as epilepsy are even more likely to be associated with psychiatric problems.

Psychological influences on the course of physical disease

The question of whether psychological factors are directly linked to the development or prognosis of physical disease is controversial, and difficult to study. Classing certain illnesses as 'psychosomatic' is no longer accepted, but psychological factors can certainly make an indirect contribution by their effects on lifestyle. Links include the following:

- *Behavioural factors*: patients with psychiatric illness or abnormal personalities are especially prone to:
  - voluntary behaviour that endangers health, such as heavy smoking and drinking, and reckless driving
  - poor compliance with medical management of disease; for example, delay in reporting new symptoms and failure to take tablets or follow lifestyle advice.
  - all psychiatric disorders carry a raised mortality, with about 80 per cent of the excess being due to physical illness and about 20 per cent to accidents or suicide.

- *Personality and attitudes*: some research studies suggest that people who tend to repress their emotions, especially anger, have an increased risk of developing cancer. Other research suggests that patients with established cancer tend to live longer if they adopt a 'fighting spirit' stance against their illness than if their response is a 'helpless-hopeless' one. The validity of these associations remains disputed; there are difficulties in establishing the direction of cause and effect in studies of this kind, and behavioural factors such as degree of treatment compliance might account for any links which are found.

- *Life events* and *social stress*: mortality and morbidity increase after major adverse life events such as bereavement. This may reflect changes in behaviour, such as self-neglect or deliberate self-harm, or it might have a direct physiological basis, such as hormonal or immunological change.

The stresses of physical illness

Any physical illness and/or its treatment can give rise to multiple losses and threats, such as the following:

- *unpleasant physical symptoms* such as pain, breathlessness, or nausea

- *body-image problems*, as in weight loss or gain, or surgical removal of a body part

- *biological influences on cognition and mood* due to brain disease, metabolic disturbance, or drugs such as steroids

- *enforced restrictions on lifestyle*, causing boredom or loss of self-esteem as well as practical and financial problems

- *interpersonal problems*, involving changed family dynamics and sexual relationships

- *concern and uncertainty* about future prognosis; some patients are also troubled by existential and spiritual issues in relation to, for example, the reasons for their illness or the prospect of death and dying

- *a sense of stigma*, attached most strongly nowadays to HIV/AIDS but also to many other physical disorders, such as epilepsy and skin disease.

Adjustment and coping

Many patients show emotional adjustment reactions following the first presentation of a physical illness or its subsequent progression. Anxiety is common in the early stages, when symptoms have been noticed but no firm diagnosis made. If investigations confirm that a serious, progressive medical condition is present, some patients are actually relieved to know what they have to face. Others, not having suspected their diagnosis previously, go through a period of 'denial' in which they do not seem to appreciate the gravity of the situation, and/or experience acute distress or anger. This is followed by depression or sadness before the final stage of acceptance can be reached. The pattern and the time course of the adjustment process varies markedly, depending on many factors: the nature of the physical illness, the patient's personality and social circumstances, and relationships with health-care staff.

The majority of patients with serious physical disease adjust successfully, through a variety of 'coping styles'. In general, those who take positive action toward understanding and mastery of their illness tend to adapt better than those whose reaction is passive or helpless. Sometimes the illness brings psychological benefits such as closer family relationships, keener appreciation of life, and a sense of greater maturity. A minority of patients show persistent 'maladaptive' reactions, which may include anxiety, depression, anger, or denial. These always impair quality of life, and may cause poor cooperation with, and response to, medical treatments.

Even patients who remain well after initial treatment for a serious disease such as cancer may have their lives permanently overshadowed by fear of recurrence and death, and become hypochondriacal about minor bodily symptoms. When incurable progressive disease is a reality, many physical, psychological, social, and spiritual issues arise, and the palliative care (hospice) movement is concerned with optimizing all these aspects of care for patients with advanced cancer and other serious illnesses.

Clinical depression in medically ill patients

Depression is common in this situation, but there are no agreed diagnostic criteria. Two main difficulties arise:

* distinguishing pathological mood disorder from appropriate sadness and adjustment

* determining the cause of somatic symptoms, such as anorexia, loss of energy, and sleep disturbance, which could be due to either mood disorder or the physical illness, or both.

If depressed mood is severe and/or prolonged more than a few weeks after the patient receives bad news about his or her condition, depressive illness (clinical depression) should be suspected. Detection of clinical depression is important because good relief of symptoms can often be achieved with antidepressant drugs.

Key symptoms suggesting clinical depression in the physically ill include guilt, perceiving the illness as a punishment, hopelessness, loss of interest, loss of pleasure (anhedonia), inability to feel warmth toward family and friends, or suicidal ideation. Depression sometimes presents with exacerbation of physical symptoms, such as difficult-to-control pain.

Management and prevention

General approach

Patients often perceive deficiencies in their relationship and communication with health-care professionals. Time to express concerns to a sympathetic listener, ask questions about the physical illness and its treatment, and receive honest answers may be all the treatment required for milder cases. Better provision of information to medical and surgical patients may help prevent psychiatric problems.

Recognizing organic brain syndromes (see Chapter 10)

Psychological disturbances secondary to biological factors may be reversible, but are often missed.

Psychological therapies (see Chapter 22)

Cognitive-behavioural approaches are effective and widely used. Brief psychodynamic therapy is indicated for a few with more complex or deep-seated problems. Interventions have been used preventively to enhance psychological adjustment in the majority, and prevent psychiatric morbidity in the few. These include monitoring by nurse-counsellors, and supportive/educational group discussions for those with a particular physical condition, either with a professional therapist or on a self-help basis. There is some evidence that such measures reduce psychiatric symptoms, and improve quality of life; however, not all patients want them.

Psychotropic drugs (see Chapter 23)

Antidepressants are especially useful (Gill and Hatcher, 1999). Even for patients who have good cause to be depressed, these drugs can help improve mood and relieve associated symptoms such as insomnia and pain. Antipsychotic drugs are used to control agitation or behaviour disturbance in patients with organic brain syndromes.

ECT (see Chapter 24)

ECT is occasionally indicated for relief of severe depression, and is safe in physically ill patients provided they are fit for anaesthetics and do not have raised intracranial pressure.

Liaison psychiatric services

Liaison psychiatrists work with medical and surgical staff, and may have their own multidisciplinary teams of clinical psychologists, social workers, and specialized psychiatric nurses. Their role includes the following:

- *Assessing and treating referred patients.* A report by the Royal College of Physicians and the Royal College of Psychiatrists classified clinical problems into the following groups:
  - organic disease with associated psychiatric disorder
  - cerebral complications of organic disease
  - bodily symptoms not due to organic disease (medically unexplained symptoms)
  - abuse of alcohol and drugs
  - deliberate self-harm (DSH)
  - sexual or relationship problems; eating disorders.

- *Educating general hospital staff* about recognizing psychiatric disorder and the principles of its management.

- *Implementing screening programmes* for detection of psychiatric disorder; for example, asking all patients to complete the Hospital Anxiety and Depression (HAD) Scale and interviewing the high scorers.

- *Research* into relationships between medical and psychiatric illness.

- *Staff support*: helping to address work-related problems and stress.

Space does not permit individual medical conditions to be considered here. Many psychiatric studies have been carried out on disorders such as HIV/AIDS, cancer, cardiac disease, diabetes, epilepsy, Parkinson's disease, renal failure, skin diseases, and stroke. Each condition has some unique features but similar general principles apply to them all.

Reference

Gill, D. and Hatcher, S. (1999). A systematic review of the treatment of depression with anti-depressant drugs in patients who also have a physical illness. *J Psychosom Res* **47**, 131–143.

Further reading

The Psychological Care of Medical Patients (2003). Royal College of Physicians/Royal College of Psychiatrists.

12 Drug misuse

Definitions

Drug misuse implies the use of drugs outside social, medical, or legal norms. It is widespread among young people in the UK. Although statistically it is strongly linked with violent and criminal behaviour, there are large numbers of 'weekend' or 'recreational' drug users who do not come in conflict with the law and who would claim that their drug taking is no more abnormal than drinking alcohol.

Relevant terms include the following:

- *Addiction*: dependence on drugs with consequent detriment to social, physical, or economic function.

- *Dependence*: psychological dependence is a strong desire to take a certain drug to produce pleasure or relieve distress, and physical dependence is indicated by the development of bodily symptoms if the drug is withdrawn.

- *Tolerance*: physical adaptation to a drug, leading to a need for increasing dosage to achieve the same effect. Tolerance often precedes development of physical dependence.

Hughes' Outline of Modern Psychiatry, Fifth Edition. David Gill.
© 2007 John Wiley & Sons, Ltd   ISBN 9780470033920

Epidemiology

Age

Illegal drug taking largely occurs in adolescents and young adults; up to 50 per cent of teenagers experiment with illegal drugs, but most have stopped using by their 20s. The most commonly used drug is cannabis. There was apparently a rise in prevalence of illicit drug use in the early 1990s, in association with the emergence of dance culture. The rise has persisted.

Although older people occasionally continue with illegal drugs, even up to their 50s or 60s, a much greater problem in middle and old age is the misuse of alcohol and of prescribed medication.

Sex

Illegal drug taking is more common in men than women. Misuse of prescribed drugs may be more common in women.

Causes

Patients who develop serious problems with illicit drugs often have psychological and social contributory factors such as socio-economic deprivation, disordered personality, disturbed family background, membership of social groups in which drug taking is prevalent, and ready availability of drugs.

Prescription drug misuse often comes from misguided medical prescribing for chronic neurotic or painful symptoms, which actually are rooted in the patient's personality.

A small minority of health professionals become addicted to narcotics and other substances (including anaesthetic gases and veterinary preparations) that they obtain at work.

Psychiatric and physical complications

A history of drug misuse is often found nowadays in young male patients presenting with serious mental illnesses such as schizophrenia and schizo-affective disorders. Such patients may be especially prone to violent behaviour. In some, the drug misuse appears to have triggered the psychosis; others have used the drugs as self-medication for their psychotic symptoms.

A typical case would be a young person with a chronic psychotic illness, precipitated and maintained by cannabis use. It may strike the patient as unfair that he should be advised against this drug, which his friends can perhaps take without apparent ill effect. However, cannabis is undeniably a potent exacerbating factor in psychosis.

The government has also confused the issue recently, downgrading the legal classification of cannabis, and issuing unclear guidance as to how the police should deal with a person possessing it. In fact, it remains illegal and harmful, especially to psychiatric patients.

Medical complications, sometimes fatal, often arise from the intravenous injections of opiates and other drugs. They include infections (abscesses, phlebitis, septicaemia, hepatitis, endocarditis, pneumonia, and HIV) and arterial occlusions leading to gangrene of limbs. Drug misuse in pregnancy may be teratogenic, and lead to complications with the pregnancy or birth. Poor diet and poor hygiene in drug misusers lead to various impairments of health.

Legal aspects

Chemicals with the potential for misuse can be classified according to their legal status:

- *legal and freely available:* alcohol (see Chapter 13), tobacco, caffeine, and solvents

- *sanctioned for medical use on prescription:* hypnotics, minor tranquillizers, opiates, anabolic steroids, and anticholinergics, especially procyclidine

- *illegal:* for example, cannabis and cocaine.

The Misuse of Drugs Act 1971 governs the production, distribution, prescribing, and possession of certain drugs. The drugs controlled under this Act are divided into classes A, B, and C, with class A drugs being most dangerous and carrying the most severe penalties for misuse. The Act also distinguishes Schedules 1 through 5, which govern the rules for possession, storage, prescription, and keeping of records. Further details are given in the *British National Formulary* (BNF).

The legal status of a drug may not be an accurate reflection of its dangerousness. Alcohol (see Chapter 13) and tobacco, which are legal and even socially encouraged in many settings, are possibly more threatening to life and health from a strictly chemical point of view than some of the illegal substances considered in this chapter.

Much of the harm of illegal drugs probably comes from the fact that they are illegal; if they were legalized and made commercially available, they could be taxed and regulated in the same way as legal substances such as alcohol. There is a strong civil liberties argument for this course of action. It is also illogical for some types of mood-altering substances to be legal and others illegal. However, it seems unlikely that there will be the political will to tackle these anomalies in the immediate future.

Pharmacology

Drugs which invite misuse fall into the following groups:

- *opiates*

- *depressants and tranquillizers*, such as alcohol, barbiturates, chlormethiazole, and benzodiazepines

- *stimulants*, such as cocaine, amphetamines, caffeine, and khat

- *hallucinogens* (psychedelics and psychotomimetics), such as LSD, mescaline, phencyclidine, psilocybin, and psilocin (magic mushrooms).

Other drugs include nicotine, cannabis, volatile inhalants, and various so called 'designer drugs' such as ketamine and GHB. Many drug misusers take a mixture of drugs, the choice depending on availability, price, and fashion as well as pharmacology.

Prevention

Efforts to reduce supply are the province of police and customs.

Much effort and expense have been devoted to educational presentations to schoolchildren, given by drug advisory bodies or specialized police officers; such programmes are designed to prevent drug misuse but could have the opposite effect on some individuals. They have not been demonstrated to be effective.

Secondary prevention (harm minimization) has benefits; see below.

Treatment

While drug misuse can be seen as an illness requiring treatment, it is just as valid to regard it as a behaviour chosen by individuals, treatment for which will succeed only with the subject's motivation and cooperation. The Mental Health Act 1983 specifically excludes compulsory detention or treatment for drug addiction per se, although the Act does apply to mental disorders caused by substance misuse. It was recently suggested that a new Mental Health Act in England and Wales would permit compulsory treatment of addictions per se, but this has caused great controversy, and the proposals are not yet clear at the time of writing.

Because of the large amount of drug-related crime, Drug Treatment and Testing Orders (DTTOs) have been introduced as community sentences. A DTTO is essentially a probation order with a condition of treatment. The person has to agree, and they receive help to move away from drugs and crime. It is obviously a sensible idea, but its effectiveness is unclear.

The long-term aim of treatment may be either *complete abstinence* from drugs or *controlled drug use*. Patients might be treated in dedicated inpatient settings, attend special outpatient clinics for controlled drug supplies, or consult community drug misuse teams staffed by specialized nurses and social workers with input from a consultant psychiatrist.

Abstinence

If physical dependence is present, and the patient elects to withdraw, initial treatment can be carried out in hospital or, more frequently now, in the community. This may include detoxification. Withdrawal symptoms can be minimized by gradually reducing the dose of the drug, and perhaps substituting another, less harmful drug that has cross-tolerance with the original.

Relapse prevention

Of psychological approaches to preventing relapse, the most promising is the cognitive model, which looks at situations and cues predisposing to resumption of drug use. A minority of addicts receive long-term rehabilitation treatment in residential units, which are often run on therapeutic community lines and require members to abstain from drugs completely.

Controlled drug use

Many users do not wish to give up drugs, and the treatment aim is therefore 'harm reduction'. Advice includes instruction on safer injection techniques, giving out clean needles to reduce needle sharing, and encouraging change from injected to oral drugs. Some teams adopt an 'assertive outreach' approach to drug users who lack the initiative to seek regular help for themselves.

Physical complications often need attention, and many addicts have social difficulties or personality problems for which extensive and prolonged help may be given, to uncertain effect. There are no accurate statistics on outcome of treatment, and results must be considered in relation to the natural history of drug misuse as a behaviour of adolescence and young adulthood that tends to die away in later life.

Treatment services vary greatly around the country. Informal, advice-based services are common, and may be run by a charity, a local authority, or health services; community drug teams are often part of mental health services. Some GPs (http://www.smmgp.org.uk/index.php) have developed a special interest in the area.

Opiates

Opiates include morphine, heroin, methadone, pethidine, buprenorphine, and dipipanone. Opium and morphine are derived from the opium poppy; the others can be synthesized chemically.

Legal status and availability

Strong opiates are class A drugs, but some weaker ones are available over the counter as codeine preparations or in cough syrup. Most addicts obtain their supplies on the black market, but a few cases of addiction are iatrogenic due to inappropriate prescribing.

Administration

Administration used to be mostly intravenous, but since the awareness of HIV, it is more frequently by smoking ('chasing the dragon').

Psychological and social effects

Intravenous injection may produce either intense pleasure or malaise. Chronic opiate use leads to apathy, moodiness, and clouding of consciousness. Addicts' social circumstances deteriorate, and the need to obtain the drug dominates their lives.

Physical effects

Nausea, constipation, and constricted pupils are seen in the acute stages. Large doses cause respiratory depression and death; for example, this occurs by injection of a stronger than usual supply, or resumption after release from prison of a previous high dose when tolerance has worn off. Chronic use produces a characteristic greyish skin colour, weight loss that can be extreme, and flat affect.

Intravenous use may cause medical complications as above. Use in pregnancy is associated with obstetric complications: abrupt opiate withdrawal can cause intrauterine death, and opiate use at term causes respiratory depression and withdrawal symptoms in the baby. Management of the pregnant opiate user should include gradual withdrawal in the second trimester if possible, with close cooperation between all the professionals concerned.

Tolerance and dependence

Greatly increased tolerance and physical dependence develop within a few weeks of starting regular use. Endorphin neurotransmitters are probably involved. There is a severe withdrawal syndrome of craving, sleepiness, rhinorrhoea, lacrimation, abdominal colic, and diarrhoea.

Detection

Opiates can be detected by blood and urine tests.

Treatment

There is a legal requirement for all doctors to notify the Home Office Drugs Branch, Queen Anne's Gate, London SW1H 9AT, of opiate addicts with whom they come in contact.

Overdose should be managed as a medical emergency; treatment may include the opiate antagonist *naloxone* to reverse respiratory depression. Other management depends on whether patients wish to become *abstinent* or not. If they do wish to get off, they will be helped either by gradually reducing the dose or by detoxification. For those who elect to withdraw, *clonidine* or *lofexidine* may be given. The antagonist *naltrexone* can be used for help in relapse prevention, but its effectiveness is unclear.

Most users prefer, at least initially, to stay on opiates, so *harm reduction* programmes are the mainstay. *Methadone maintenance* is key; the patient is prescribed a legal supply of opiate in oral (liquid) form. This is designed to satisfy cravings and reduce the need to purchase illegal supplies, with associated crime in order to finance this. Oral administration can be observed if there is concern that the patient may be selling his supply (this is usual in other countries, although less frequent in the UK). Oral administration is also the safest route of ingestion.

If the patient can be stabilized on methadone, and develop a good relationship with the clinic, his lifestyle and health may improve, and he may eventually consider gradual reduction in dose and abstinence. There is evidence (Mattick *et al.*, 2006) that methadone as part of a maintenance programme 'can reduce the use of heroin in dependent people, and keep them in treatment programs'.

Buprenorphine sublingual is an alternative to methadone. Maintenance prescriptions of *diamorphine* or *dipipanone* also have their proponents, but they are in a minority. Maintenance prescriptions can only be issued by doctors with a special licence, working from a treatment centre, and it is advisable for the prescriptions to be dispensed from a designated pharmacy. (Any doctor may prescribe diamorphine for relief of severe pain.)

For those who continue to inject, many chemists provide sterile needles free of charge under the 'harm-reduction' policies designed to restrict spread of HIV and other infections.

Prognosis

Some opiate addicts give up their habit either spontaneously or with medical help. The prognosis is not inevitably one of remorseless progression to needle sharing and death. Mortality is increased several-fold, of the order of 2 per cent per annum; the most frequent causes of death are respiratory depression from drug overdose, infections, and suicide. Often, patients who reduce opiate use move toward misuse of other substances, notably alcohol.

Amphetamines (Speed)

Legal status and availability

Injectable amphetamines are class A, and oral amphetamines class B drugs. They used to be widely prescribed for depression (in the 1950s and 1960s) and for obesity (until quite recently). They are stimulants, and are thus related to cocaine (see below). They are now only licensed for treatment of attention deficit hyperactivity disorder (ADHD) in children and adolescents as part of a comprehensive treatment programme, and for narcolepsy or obstructive sleep apnoea syndrome. Inappropriate private prescription by 'slimming clinics' still occurs occasionally, and patients sometimes get supplies over the Internet. Easy chemical synthesis also makes for continued widespread availability.

Administration

Administration is oral, intravenous, or inhaled.

Psychological effects

Amphetamines are stimulants; they cause euphoria, increased activity, insomnia, and anorexia. *Amphetamine psychosis* is characterized by visual or auditory hallucinations and paranoid delusions similar to those of paranoid schizophrenia. (As amphetamines act by stimulation of CNS dopamine systems, this effect is a main plank of the 'dopamine hypothesis' of schizophrenia.) Amphetamine psychosis nearly always recovers if the drug is withdrawn.

Physical effects

Amphetamines stimulate sympathetic nervous system activity.

Tolerance and dependence

Psychological dependence and tolerance occur but probably not physical dependence. Depressed mood, low energy, and increased sleep may follow withdrawal.

Detection

Amphetamines can be detected by blood and urine tests.

Treatment

Various medications have been tried, but none is generally accepted as helpful. Individual support or group therapy, concentrating – in the absence of physical dependency – on relapse prevention is more important.

Cocaine and crack

Cocaine is derived from the coca shrub grown in South America. Crack is cocaine that has been separated from its hydrochloride salt.

Legal status and availability

Cocaine is a class A drug not used in medical practice except in ENT and related surgery (to control bleeding by its vasoconstrictive actions – hence its necrotizing effects on the nasal septum in misusers).

Administration

Cocaine is inhaled as snuff or injected. Crack can be smoked to produce a rapid effect.

Psychological effects

The psychological effects are similar to those of amphetamine. *Cocaine psychosis* resembles amphetamine psychosis but also includes the tactile hallucination of a sensation of insects crawling on the skin (formication).

Physical effects

Cocaine may cause cardiac arrhythmia. Repeated inhalation may cause perforation of the nasal septum.

Tolerance and dependence

Psychological dependence occurs only with ordinary cocaine, but crack is considered to be more addictive and tolerance rapidly develops – there may be physical dependence, but this is controversial.

Detection

Cocaine can be detected by blood and urine tests.

Treatment

Addicts should be notified to the Home Office. Maintenance prescriptions can only be issued by doctors with a special licence. Because of the lack of a physical withdrawal syndrome, no specific treatment of withdrawal is indicated. Most users stop – and many do, or at any rate drift in and out of using – without medical attention.

Cannabis (Indian Hemp, Hashish, Pot)

Cannabis is the name given to products of the plant *Cannabis sativa*, which include hashish and marijuana. 'Skunk' is an especially potent form. The psychoactive ingredient is *tetrahydrocannabinol* (THC). *Cannabis sativa* grows wild in many countries including Britain. THC can also be chemically synthesized.

Legal status and availability

Cannabis is a class C drug, but freely available from unofficial sources and probably used by at least 10 per cent of young people in this country. Legalizing cannabis has been suggested, but this would have adverse consequences for psychiatric patients because of its propensity to cause and worsen psychosis.

Administration

Cannabis is usually mixed with tobacco and smoked, but can also be taken orally or intravenously.

Psychological and social effects

Cannabis usually produces sedation, but it can exaggerate an unpleasant pre-existing mood state of anger, depression, or anxiety. Psychotic symptoms, including perceptual distortions, visual hallucinations, and confusion, can occur. The use of cannabis is often implicated in worsening the clinical course of schizophrenia, precipitating onset or relapse and retarding recovery. Sustained long-term use is believed to cause an 'amotivational syndrome' of apathy and cognitive defect, partially reversible if the drug is stopped.

Physical effects

Cannabis has many physiological effects, including cardiovascular ones, which may be dangerous in people with heart disease. Cannabis taken in pregnancy is thought to be teratogenic. Chronic effects include those of the associated tobacco smoking. Cannabis has analgesic and other properties, which have been the subject of randomised trials. For example, it has been tried in multiple sclerosis, but so far has not been considered to be an improvement on existing treatments (Robson, 2001).

Tolerance and dependence

Psychological dependence is common. Physical dependence probably does not occur.

Detection

Cannabis can be detected in body fluids for up to 2 weeks after consumption.

Prognosis

Occasional cannabis use may be harmless in some people, despite the concern about psychotic illness described above. However, cannabis predisposes indirectly to use of more dangerous drugs through encouraging contact with other drug users.

Lysergic ACID diethylamide (LSD, ACID)

LSD is a synthetic compound. It is a hallucinogen. Such drugs became well known in the 1950s, when the author Aldous Huxley foolishly publicized his subjective impressions of taking mescaline. This contributed to their use and abuse by the impressionable, and they were made illegal in the late 1960s. They were even used in abortive therapeutic experiments on psychiatric patients, some of whom later claimed that they had been harmed thereby.

Legal status and availability

LSD is a class A drug, easily synthesized by amateur chemists.

Administration

Administration is oral. LSD is often sold soaked into blotting paper.

Psychological effects

The psychological effects include perceptual distortion, reactivation of distant memories, extreme depression or ecstasy ('bad trips' or 'good trips'), and acute psychotic experiences. Death can result, for example, from delusions of being able to fly from high places. 'Flashbacks' of LSD-induced experiences may continue for years after the last dose.

Physical effects

The physical effects are those of sympathetic nervous system overactivity.

Detection

LSD cannot be detected by laboratory tests.

Tolerance and dependence

Tolerance and dependence do not occur.

MDMA (Ecstasy)

MDMA (3,4, methylenedioxyamphetamine) is a class A drug that alters perceptual and emotional experience, giving enhanced appreciation of colour and sound, and increased empathy with others. The drug also has stimulant properties. It is popular at pop festivals and 'rave' parties, but may cause sudden death in such settings through cardiac arrhythmia, dehydration, and hyperthermia. The acute intoxication may resemble neuroleptic malignant syndrome or serotonin syndrome. It may precipitate or cause psychosis. Long-term use may have neurotoxic effects. Tolerance may develop.

Glues and solvents

Fumes from products based on toluene and acetone have been increasingly used for their psychological effects in recent years. Such products include glues and solvents for domestic or industrial use. They are freely available and popular among children, particularly male adolescents.

Administration

Administration is by inhalation from paper, bottle, or bag (glue-sniffing).

Psychological effects

The psychological effects are euphoria and perceptual disturbance, progressing to stupor. Long-term neuropsychological damage may occur.

Physical effects

These substances are toxic to the liver, kidney, heart, and brain, and inhalation may cause accidental death. Chronic use causes a characteristic acneiform rash around the mouth and nose.

Tolerance and dependence

Psychological dependence is common, but tolerance and physical dependence probably do not occur.

Treatment

Abstinence is the goal here.

Tobacco

Nicotine is the constituent of tobacco that causes psychological effects and dependence, whereas carbon monoxide and tar cause most of the physical ill effects. Cigarette smoking is more harmful than other forms of tobacco consumption. About one-third of the population smoke, and rates are rising among young women. Smoking is widespread among patients and nurses in psychiatric hospitals.

Psychological effects

Nicotine is both a central nervous system stimulant and an anxiolytic.

Physical effects

The acute effects are those of sympathetic nervous system overactivity. Chronic effects include raised susceptibility to lung cancer and many other cancers, cardiovascular disease, chronic bronchitis, and, during pregnancy, stillbirth and abortion.

Tolerance and dependence

Both psychological and physical dependence occur. There is a withdrawal syndrome consisting of anxiety, depression, irritability, insomnia, and craving.

Management

Nicotine chewing gum is a less toxic alternative that helps some smokers give up. Psychological methods, including hypnosis and group therapy, are sometimes effective. Measures to reduce smoking in the community include education, media campaigns, banning tobacco advertisements, and increasing the price of cigarettes. There are moves to ban smoking in public places in the UK, a move that has already happened in Ireland and some other countries. Although it may seem an attack on civil liberty, the rights of non-smokers must also be respected, and a ban now seems inevitable at some stage. Psychiatric inpatients are very often heavy smokers, however, and it is unclear at present how their rights are to be safeguarded.

Caffeine

Caffeine, a xanthine alkaloid, is a constituent of coffee, tea, cocoa, and cola beverages. Most people in the UK consume several such drinks a day without apparent ill effects.

Psychological effects

Caffeine is a stimulant that increases well-being and reduces fatigue. Large doses cause anxiety and insomnia. 'Caffeinism' is an important differential diagnosis of anxiety disorders. Some psychiatric patients consume large amounts (say

10–20 cups of tea or coffee daily) in the mistaken belief that this helps to calm their nerves.

Physical effects

The physical effects include tachycardia, diuresis, and muscle tension.

Tolerance and dependence

Psychological, but not physical, dependence occurs.

Barbiturates

Legal status and availability

Barbiturates used to be widely prescribed as tranquillizers and hypnotics before their addictive potential became clear. Their prescription for this purpose is now almost extinct, although a very few older people may remain dependent. Barbiturates are still sometimes used for epilepsy. Black market barbiturates are less frequently used today.

Administration

Administration is oral or intravenous.

Psychological effects

The psychological effects are central nervous system (CNS) depression causing psychomotor impairment, drowsiness, or sleep.

Physical effects

Ataxia, nystagmus, slurred speech. Large doses may cause fatal respiratory depression. Cross-tolerance with alcohol and anaesthetics exists.

Tolerance and dependence

Tolerance and physical dependence develop rapidly. There is a withdrawal syndrome of anxiety, insomnia, tremor, fits, and delirium.

Detection

Barbiturates can be detected by blood and urine tests.

Benzodiazepines

Misuse has been an important problem: to some extent, they can be seen to have replaced the barbiturates as an over-prescribed sedative for the ups and downs of life, although with less serious side-effects (that is, lack of respiratory depression; this means they are safe in overdose). They act at receptors associated with gamma-aminobutyric acid (GABA) receptors.

The BNF (http://www.bnf.org/bnf/bnf/current/3139.htm) carries a sensible withdrawal schedule for patients who have become dependent. The patient is switched to an equivalent dose of diazepam (e.g. lorazepam 1 mg = diazepam 10 mg), and then about one-eighth of the daily dose is reduced per 2 weeks. Diazepam is chosen because it is long-acting.

References

Mattick, R. P., Breen, C., Kimber, J. and Davoli, M. (2006). Methadone maintenance therapy versus no opioid replacement therapy for opioid dependence. *Cochrane Database Syst Rev* Issue 2, CD002209.

Robson, P. (2001). Therapeutic aspects of cannabis and cannabinoids. *Br J Psychiatry* **178**, 107–115.

Resources

Department of Health guideline on treatment. http://www.dh.gov.uk/assetRoot/04/07/81/98/04078198.pdf.

Resources and information. http://www.drugscope.org.uk.

Society for the Study of Addiction. http://www.addiction-ssa.org.

13 Alcohol misuse

Moderate alcohol intake is, for many people, an acceptable and enjoyable part of life. However, those who drink to excess, or are particularly vulnerable to the unwanted effects of alcohol, may experience a wide range of medical and psychiatric problems.

Alcohol misuse may be defined in terms of:

- *quantity* of alcohol intake

- presence of *dependency*

- alcohol related *disability*, whether physical, mental or social.

There is no agreed definition of 'alcoholism'. Patients with obvious drink problems often seek to avoid the issue by diversion into discussion about whether they are or are not 'an alcoholic', but these are, by their very nature interminable, as the word means different things to different people. The words are used here as a useful shorthand only.

Safe limits of drinking

Quantities

The limits of 21 units per week for men and 14 for women suggested by the Royal College of Physicians have been widely influential. A 'unit' is one drink

Hughes' Outline of Modern Psychiatry, Fifth Edition. David Gill.
© 2007 John Wiley & Sons, Ltd   ISBN 9780470033920

(half a pint of ordinary strength beer, one glass of wine, or a single measure of spirits) and contains 8–10 g alcohol.

Pattern

'Binge drinking' can cause problems (accidents, especially head injury; acute alcoholic poisoning; and involvement in criminal activity such as assault and vandalism) over and above those found with the steady daily intake of equivalent amounts of alcohol. Hence, a person would certainly be drinking in an unsafe pattern if they drank only once per week, but consumed all their 'weekly allowance' on that single occasion.

Frequency

Up to 5 per cent of people in England and Wales have a serious drinking problem. About 25 per cent of men and 15 per cent of women drink more than the recommended limits given above. Alcohol misuse is often concealed. Its extent within a given population can be estimated by:

- *alcohol sales* per capita
- alcohol-related *hospital admissions*
- *drunkenness* convictions
- mortality from *cirrhosis of the liver*.

Epidemiology

Nationality

Wine-producing countries such as France and Italy have high rates of alcohol-related problems, especially cirrhosis. Northern European countries have lower rates of total consumption, so lower rates of cirrhosis, but higher rates of binge drinking with its attendant behavioural problems. Muslim and Jewish societies, with their religious constraints on drinking, have lower rates. Scotland and Ireland have higher rates than England and Wales.

Occupation

Groups at high risk include publicans, seamen, journalists, and doctors.

Age

Most cases present in middle age, but a growing number of young adults are seeking treatment, and concealed alcohol misuse is increasingly recognized as a problem in old age.

Sex

Men are more often affected than women, but the prevalence among women is increasing, with changing behavioural norms (the 'ladette' culture).

Causes

Genetics

There is evidence of a genetic component of alcoholism: a two–threefold increase in alcoholism in the relatives of alcoholics, especially male ones; a higher concordance between monozygotic than dizygotic twins; and a high rate in children of alcoholic parents who were adopted into non-alcoholic homes in infancy. Sociopathic personality disorder is over-represented among the male relatives of alcoholics, and depressive illness among female relatives.

Psychological factors

Psychosocial stress is often the precipitant for escalation of heavy drinking, alcohol being a temporary anxiolytic and euphoriant. Any psychiatric disorder may lead to self-medication with alcohol.

Social and cultural factors

Drinking problems are more common in settings where alcohol is cheap and easily available, and drinking is encouraged socially.

Economic

The greater the per capita consumption of alcohol in a society, the larger is the number of people with alcohol problems, and per capita consumption is inversely related to price. This means that a nation's alcohol taxation policy affects its rate of alcohol-related problems: a good historical example is the increase in alcohol problems in eighteenth-century England, after the government encouraged cheap home-produced gin to supplant French brandy. A current example is the association between the recent falls in the real price of alcohol in the UK and a rise in alcohol problems.

Effects of alcohol

Small quantities promote sociability and well-being, and may bring certain health benefits. People who take one or two drinks per day have been held to suffer less coronary heart disease and have a lower all-cause mortality rate than non-drinkers. However, the epidemiological evidence for this possibly attractive proposition remains conflicting. Higher consumption, whether on a long-term regular basis or in the form of acute drunkenness, can have many damaging effects.

Damage may result from direct toxicity of ethanol, or from associated phenomena including vitamin B deficiency, hypoglycaemia, dehydration, alcohol withdrawal, toxic congeners (other substances present in alcoholic drinks), and trauma sustained during intoxication.

Acute intoxication

Blood alcohol levels around 50 mg/100 ml cause increased well-being, reduced inhibitions, and reduced efficiency (seldom recognized by the subject). Heavier intoxication causes obvious cognitive impairment, ataxia, slurred speech, and vomiting, with subsequent amnesia.

Coma usually supervenes when blood alcohol reaches about 200–300 mg/100 ml. Coma in heavy drinkers may also result from head injury, drug overdose, a recent fit, hypothermia, or hypoglycaemia: this is a well-known clinical pitfall in casualty and in acute psychiatric presentations. The patient may well be a known alcoholic or obviously drunk: but may also have other disorders, such as an intracranial bleeding, that will be fatal if not picked up. Blood alcohol levels over 400 mg/100 ml may be fatal. Milder degrees of intoxication can lead to death indirectly through accidents or inhalation of vomit.

'Pathological intoxication' (*mania a potu*) is abnormal behaviour following only modest alcohol intake, usually described in brain-damaged people, although there is doubt as to the validity of this concept. It is sometimes used as the basis of a somewhat optimistic defence against criminal charges.

Neuropsychiatric complications

Delirium tremens (DTs), an indication of physical dependence, can be precipi-tated by abrupt withdrawal of alcohol in a heavy drinker, caused, for example, by the end of a drinking bout, efforts to give up drinking without professional advice, intercurrent illness, hospital admission, or arrest/imprisonment. Confu-sion, fever, visual or tactile hallucinations, and fits may occur. Delirium tremens is a medical emergency with an appreciable mortality, and should be treated by physicians. Treatment includes correction of any fluid or electrolyte imbalance, or hypoglycaemia, and a 5-day reducing course of a benzodiazepine, such as chlordiazepoxide, to counteract withdrawal symptoms by sedation and preven-tion of fits. These drugs have potential for dependence and abuse, and should not be continued after detoxification. Parenteral vitamins, thiamine being most important, are also given to prevent other neurological complications.

Wernicke's encephalopathy is an acute syndrome thought to result from defi-ciency of B₁ (thiamine). Haemorrhages occur in the mammillary bodies, thala-mus, and hypothalamus. Acute confusion is accompanied by nystagmus, diplopia, ataxia, and peripheral neuritis. The condition may be fatal unless promptly treated with thiamine.

Korsakov's syndrome, a more chronic disorder, is also believed to result from thiamine deficiency. It may be a sequel of delirium tremens or Wernicke's encephalopathy. Haemorrhage, necrosis, and gliosis are present in the mammil-lary bodies and hippocampus. A gross defect of short-term memory leads to disorientation, for which some patients attempt to compensate by confabulation. Peripheral neuropathy often co-exists.

Alcoholic dementia comprises global impairment of mental functioning, often accompanied by personality changes of the frontal lobe type. Brain scans show cerebral atrophy.

Epilepsy may be caused by direct toxicity of alcohol, especially if there is pre-existing brain damage, alcohol withdrawal, over-hydration, or hypoglycaemia.

Peripheral neuropathy results from thiamine deficiency, and affects motor, sensory, and autonomic nerves. Presenting symptoms include impotence or burning pain in the feet.

Other neurological complications include cerebellar degeneration, central pontine myelinosis, degeneration of the corpus callosum, retrobulbar neuritis, and subdural haematoma following falls.

Alcoholic hallucinosis often starts during a phase of abstinence. Auditory hallu-cinations, usually voices, develop in clear consciousness. If insight is lacking, the voices may form the basis of a delusional system. It may recover spontaneously after a few months, but other cases become chronic and require treatment.

Alcoholic paranoia is the development of paranoid delusions in the absence of hallucinations. Morbid jealousy (see Chapter 8) of the sexual partner is a frequent theme, in which case dangerousness (see Chapter 21) must be assessed because of the risk of assault or even homicide.

Alcoholic hallucinosis and alcoholic paranoia can be helped by antipsychotic drugs, but abstinence is crucial.

Physical complications

The mortality rate in alcoholics is about three times the general population rate.

Liver damage includes acute hepatitis, fatty infiltration, and cirrhosis. In men, cirrhosis seldom develops until heavy drinking has continued for at least 5 years, but women are more vulnerable. Cirrhosis has a high mortality rate even in those who become totally abstinent.

In pregnancy, heavy drinking may cause abortion, stillbirth, or the 'foetal alcohol syndrome', comprising microcephaly and other deformities, and learning disability.

Other physical consequences include peptic ulcer, pancreatitis, gastritis, cardiomyopathy, myopathy, gout, vitamin deficiencies, drug interactions (the effect of psychotropic drugs may be either enhanced or reduced), and raised susceptibility to infections, including tuberculosis and malignancies.

Accidents, including road accidents, and *accidental deaths* are common. *Suicide* is the cause of death in about 15 per cent of alcoholics, and 50 per cent of non-fatal self-poisonings are combined with alcohol.

Social consequences

- *Family disruption* occurs with marital breakdown and violence toward partners and children.

- *Working efficiency* is reduced, often leading to demotion or unemployment.

- *Crime*: many alcoholics steal to get money for drink, and intoxication may precipitate violence. About 50 per cent of violent crimes are committed when the offender is drunk, and about 50 per cent of men in prison have a drinking problem.

- *Drunken driving*: 80 mg/100 ml is the legal upper limit of blood alcohol for drivers in the UK.

Course of alcohol abuse

The traditional view, which may well apply to some of the most severely affected, is of a relentlessly progressive disorder. Alcohol problems commonly begin when social drinking becomes heavier for psychological reasons, such as living in a hard-drinking environment, or stressful work or family circumstances. This stage of psychological dependence is followed in some cases by development of physical dependence, manifested by loss of control over the amount consumed, and withdrawal symptoms (tremor, sweating, anxiety, and craving) if alcohol is unavailable for a few hours. Intake increases further to combat withdrawal symptoms. Alcohol tolerance increases initially, decreasing again when the condition becomes advanced. Drinking gains priority over other activities, and the various physical, psychiatric, and social problems ensue.

Other patterns include repeated relapses and remissions according to current circumstances and/or changes in mood. As with other kinds of substance misuse (see Chapter 12), some people drink heavily in early adulthood but 'grow out' of their habit later on. Many drinkers deny their problem, concealing the extent of their drinking and hiding bottles at home or at work. Heavy smoking, dependence on other drugs, and heavy gambling may be associated.

Vagrant (skid row) alcoholics are those without families, homes, or jobs, often handicapped by low intelligence or chronic mental illness, who live rough in city centres drinking cheap forms of alcohol.

Recognition

Patients with undetected drinking problems commonly present in primary care or hospital settings because of the physical or psychiatric complications of alcohol. Patients with, for example, depressive illness or peptic ulcer will not improve if treatment is directed to these diagnoses without attention to the underlying alcohol misuse. Ways of improving recognition include the following:

- *Taking a drinking history* as a routine part of medical or nursing assessment.

- *Screening questionnaires* such as CAGE:
  Have you ever felt you ought to Cut down on your drinking?
  Have people Annoyed you by criticizing your drinking?
  Have you ever felt Guilty about your drinking?
  Have you ever had a drink first thing in the morning (an 'Eye-opener') to steady your nerves or get rid of a hangover?

Two or more positive replies indicate a possible drinking problem, but must be followed up by direct enquiry. Brief counselling by trained nurses is effective in persuading general medical patients identified in this way to reduce their drinking.

- *Laboratory tests*: a raised blood level of liver enzymes, the most sensitive being gamma glutamyltranspeptidase (gamma GT) (over 40 iu/litre), and/or macrocytosis (mean corpuscular volume (MCV) over 96 fl) are suggestive of high alcohol intake. However, both tests may also give abnormal results in other illnesses unrelated to alcohol, so they are not in themselves diagnostic.

Treatment

Alcohol misuse cannot be regarded as a disease to be 'cured' by doctors. The responsibility for change in behaviour rests with the drinker, the professional's role being to facilitate this change. There is limited point in attempting to treat those who deny their problem, or do not want to overcome it. Some who are well motivated stop drinking of their own accord; others need professional help, but the strength of motivation is the most powerful predictor of treatment success.

Intervention is probably most effective at an early stage, but most alcohol misusers do not seek help until they are forced to do so and their condition is advanced. Once heavy drinking has become established and physical dependence is present, results of treatment are less favourable.

Total abstinence is the traditional goal, especially for those with physical dependence or physical complications. Controlled drinking is a realistic aim for some milder cases. Treatment methods include the following.

Detoxification

Detoxification by medical treatment, as outlined above for delirium tremens, is necessary to permit safe cessation of drinking in those who are chemically dependent (as evidenced by a physical withdrawal syndrome). It may be done safely at home or in a hostel if there is adequate supervision. A typical regime would be chlordiazepoxide 40–60 mg q.d.s., reducing gradually to zero over 5 days. Chlormethiazole (Hemineverin) was formerly the standard treatment, but is no longer recommended.

Psychological and social approaches

Systematic reviews indicate that most of the brief approaches that have been trialled are effective in reducing consumption, but that longer-term psychological treatments (including dynamic, behavioural, or supportive psychotherapy, individual or group, on an inpatient or outpatient basis) have little or no additional benefit. The trend is firmly toward inexpensive community treatments with input from health, social, and probation services. However, inpatient alcoholic units still exist, offering intensive group psychotherapy over several weeks or months. Long-term residence in a 'dry' hostel offers support for some severely damaged ex-drinkers.

Alcoholics Anonymous (AA) is a voluntary organization offering self-help group therapy at evening meetings, and it also runs groups for partners and children. The goal of lifetime total abstinence is central to AA's approach. Some people derive great benefit from AA, and continue frequent attendance at meetings for many years to make sure they remain 'dry'. For others, however, the AA approach, which has a quasi-religious aspect, is less attractive.

Motivational interviewing uses a model that can also be applied to other addictive behaviours, describing a 'cycle of change':

- precontemplation

- contemplation

- action

- maintenance/relapse.

Problem drinking is seen as being likely to recur, perhaps more than once, before the drinker gains control; returns to drinking are seen not as moral lapses but as learning experiences. This has the advantage of recognizing that multiple attempts are often necessary before a drink problem can be mastered.

Drugs

Disulfiram ('Antabuse' tablets or implant) blocks the action of acetaldehyde dehydrogenase, causing accumulation of acetaldehyde if alcohol is taken. Drinking therefore becomes both unpleasant and dangerous, with the risk of cardiac arrhythmia or extreme hypotension. Disulfiram can be helpful, but generally a patient with the willpower to take a tablet every day may have the willpower to remain abstinent without tablets. Because of the potential risk, disulfiram is mainly prescribed by specialists.

Many other drugs have been tried, including *lithium*, *fluoxetine*, and *naltrexone*; however, none of these have become established. Recently, *acamprosate* was introduced; it has been suggested as a useful adjunct to psychological treatments, but evidence is not yet conclusive.

Prognosis

It is very difficult to give a numerical overall prognosis, as the condition is not exclusively a medical one. Prognosis is poorer for those severely affected, especially with attendant physical health problems; loss of family, job, and home; or forensic problems. Prognosis will be better for younger, healthier patients without such complications, especially if they are identified earlier and engage well with treatment.

Prevention

There is evidence that a reduction in national per capita alcohol consumption, and hence a reduction in the number of people with alcohol-related problems, could be achieved by *increasing the price of alcohol*. Other measures which may be presumed to be helpful include *education* about the dangers of alcohol, increasing the availability of *non-alcoholic drinks* at business and social functions, *discouraging advertisements* for drink, and placing *restrictions on availability* in shops and catering establishments. However, some of these suggestions run counter to civil liberty arguments, and, perhaps more to the point, to powerful vested interests.

Reference

Ritson, B. (2005). Treatment for alcohol related problems. *BMJ* **330**, 139–141.

Further reading

Edwards, G., Marshall, E. J. and Cook, C. C. H. (2003). *The Treatment of Drinking Problems*. Cambridge: Cambridge University Press.

14 Deliberate self-harm

Fatal deliberate self-harm (*suicide, completed suicide*) and *non-fatal* deliberate self-harm (*DSH, parasuicide, attempted suicide*) are separate phenomena which overlap to some degree. Both medical and social factors are involved in their aetiology, prevention, and management.

Suicide

Definition

Suicide is an act of self-harm, undertaken with conscious self-destructive intent, with a fatal outcome.

Frequency

There are between 4000 and 5000 suicides in England and Wales per year; this is about 10 per 100 000 population, and around 1 per cent of all deaths. Official statistics have tended to underestimate the true rate because only cases with proven evidence of intent, such as a suicide note, were given suicide verdicts by

Hughes' Outline of Modern Psychiatry, Fifth Edition. David Gill.
© 2007 John Wiley & Sons, Ltd   ISBN 9780470033920

the coroner. Some deaths given 'accident' or 'undetermined' verdicts in the past were probably suicides. However, coroners may have become more ready to give suicide verdicts in recent years when the evidence points in that direction.

Methods

Methods that are most easily available are most likely to be used, and media publicity about a suicide is often followed by other deaths by the same method. Methods can be thought of as violent (hanging or jumping) and non-violent (drugs and other forms of poison). Males and mentally disordered persons tend toward violent methods; females toward non-violent.

Hanging/strangling/suffocation and gassing by car exhaust fumes (carbon monoxide) are now the most common methods taken overall, although poisoning (often by medicinal drugs) remains the commonest method in women. Other methods include drowning, shooting, cutting, jumping, and burning.

Epidemiology

- *Temporal trend:* the number of suicides in the UK and some other countries has declined somewhat in recent years (McClure, 2000), partly due to the detoxifying of the household gas supply (natural rather than coal gas) and motor vehicle exhaust fumes (introduction of catalytic converters) (McClure, 2000). Attempts have been made to relate this reduction to contemporaneous increases in antidepressant prescribing rates (e.g. Hall *et al.*, 2003), but this is impossible to prove.

- *Age:* the rate increases with age, but suicide in young men (age 15–24) has recently become more frequent.

- *Sex:* suicide is more than twice as common in men than women.

- *Marital status:* divorced people have the highest rates, followed by the widowed and single, and the married at the lowest.

- *Social class:* the highest rates are at both extremes of the social scale.

- *Occupation:* high-risk groups include doctors, veterinary surgeons, pharmacists, and farmers.

- *Residential circumstances:* inner-city areas with a mobile population have high rates. Psychiatric inpatients, those recently discharged from such hospitals, and prisoners are all at high risk.

- *Nationality*: there are large differences between the suicide rates of different countries. These are partly real, due, for example, to religious and cultural variation, but some apparent differences result from differing methods of ascertainment. High rates are found in Greenland, Hungary, Austria, Denmark, Japan, Germany, and Eastern Europe. Low rates are found in Eire, Italy, Spain, Greece, and the Netherlands.

- *National circumstances*: suicide rates fall in wartime. High suicide rates are found in association with economic depression, unemployment, and high divorce rates.

Causes

Psychiatric disorder

Psychiatric disorder is present immediately before death in up to 90 per cent of cases, as indicated by the 'psychological autopsy' technique of interviewing those who knew the dead person. Depressive illness, often inadequately treated, is the commonest diagnosis, especially in older people. Alcohol and drug misuse are also common, especially in the young. Personality disorder often coexists. 'Rational' suicide, by people without evidence of mental disorder, presumably in hopeless situations, seems to be rare in Western societies.

Follow-up of psychiatric patient populations indicates that in 5–15 per cent of subjects with mental illness, personality disorder, and/or drug or alcohol problems, suicide will be the cause of death. Risk of suicide is raised in all mental disorders, not just depression.

Other causes

- *stressful circumstances*, including life events such as bereavement, and long-term social difficulties such as unemployment

- *social isolation* in those who live alone and/or lack confiding relationships.

- *physical illness*: raised suicide rates are found in association with certain physical conditions, including epilepsy, other neurological disorders, peptic ulcer, renal failure on dialysis, and AIDS.

- *neurochemistry*: deficiency of 5-HT has been linked to suicidal behaviour in some studies.

The French sociologist Émile Durkheim, whose influential book *Le Suicide* was published in 1894, distinguished three types of suicide: 'anomic' related to a disorganized society, 'egoistic' among people isolated from their social group, and 'altruistic' for the benefit of others.

More recent research suggests that the psychological state of *hopelessness* is a key precursor of suicide.

Prevention

Some preventive strategies aim to improve the management of individuals at high risk; others to reduce factors associated with suicidality in society as a whole. Reduction of suicide rates, both for the general population and for psychiatric patients, is among the targets in the government's 'Health of the Nation' strategy.

A recent systematic review (Mann *et al.*, 2005) indicates that 'physician education in depression recognition and treatment and restricting access to lethal methods reduce suicide rates.' However, it is important to remember that not only depression but also all mental disorders (apart possibly from learning disability and dementia) carry an increased risk of suicide (Harris and Barraclough, 1997).

Medical care of the mentally ill

Many suicides have been in contact with GPs or psychiatrists shortly before death, suggesting that better medical management might have prevented the fatal act. Psychiatric patients who have voiced suicidal thoughts, have a past history of suicide attempts, or possess the socio-demographic factors listed above should be considered at high risk.

Prompt and energetic physical treatment of psychiatric illness should help prevent suicide in the mentally ill. High doses of psychotropic drugs may be required, but potentially suicidal patients should not be given large supplies, which might be used in overdose. ECT may be indicated for the suicidally depressed. In the long term, prophylactic medication and care may help to reduce suicide.

Suicidal patients who live with responsible relatives or friends can often be managed at home, but must have frequent follow-up reviews, and 24-hour access to professional help in case of emergency. Hospital admission, with close nursing observation, is indicated for the very severely ill and those without adequate home support.

In cases where more chronic psychiatric and social problems existed, a growing alienation from professional carers sometimes seems to have been a factor in the suicide. This can happen if staff themselves become hopeless or cynical in relation to an unrewarding case, and points to the importance of supportive care in suicide prevention.

Other strategies

- *counselling services*, such as the confidential telephone helpline for despairing and suicidal people run by the Samaritan organization.

- *restricting availability of methods*, such as catalytic converters for cars; controls on sale and possession of medicines, guns, and poisons. Restricting the amount of analgesics that can be bought without prescription, seems to have been associated with reduced suicide rates in the UK (Hawton *et al.*, 2004).

- *physical considerations* such as making psychiatric wards as safe as possible (for example, by removing potential ligature points, from which a patient might hang himself) and preventing public access to bridges or cliffs from which others have jumped to their death. Removal of a method can have a significant long-term effect, as it is not necessarily replaced by other methods; in the 1960s, changing the domestic gas supply from coal gas (containing carbon monoxide) to non-toxic natural gas was followed by a sustained reduction in total UK suicide rate.

- *educational programmes*; for example, efforts to improve the recognition and management of potentially suicidal patients in general practice, or to dissuade young people from suicidal behaviour.

The aftermath of suicide: effects on those involved

Bereavement counselling and practical help may be required in the immediate aftermath of the death, which will almost always be a very difficult time for relatives. In the longer term, the relatives of those who died by suicide are at high risk of psychiatric illness and social problems, and many take years to adjust, if they ever do, to a death which frequently seems like an act of aggression as well as of self-destruction. Sometimes, suicide can even seem to be an act with a violent aspect, perhaps directed toward those left behind, leaving the family almost as 'victims' of suicide. Others, however, might ultimately find their lives made easier if the dead person had been affected for many years by a severe and intractable personality disorder, mental illness, or drug/alcohol misuse.

Suicide can also exact a toll on others involved, such as train drivers, who can expect occasionally to be in the unenviable position of applying the brakes as they sight a person on the tracks ahead, knowing that it is physically impossible to stop in time. They even have their own slang expression ('one under') for these events. Mental health problems and medico-legal considerations are frequent.

The professionals involved in the care of a patient who has killed himself often react with distress and guilt, which is understandable but not always justified. A certain number of suicides are bound to occur in psychiatric practice, and it is not possible to predict exactly which patients are going to kill themselves, or when. After a suicide has taken place, review of the case may well suggest some way that management could have been improved; this should be used as a constructive opportunity to improve future standards of practice in the unit concerned, rather than a collective 'guilt trip' or, still worse, a search for a scapegoat.

Learning lessons

Some suicides, such as those resulting from an acute severe depressive illness which could almost certainly have been cured, are major tragedies. In other cases, such as those associated with chronic intractable mental or physical illness, the argument that it might have been preventable may be less strong.

The key initiative here is the National Confidential Inquiry into Suicide and Homicide by People with Mental Illness (Appleby *et al.*, 2006; Hunt *et al.*, 2006), which is a continuing national survey. Between 1996 and 2000, there were 4859 cases of suicide in England and Wales whose victims had been in recent contact with mental health services.

1100 (23 per cent) had been discharged from psychiatric in-patient care less than 3 months before death. Post-discharge suicide was most frequent in the first 2 weeks after leaving hospital; the highest number occurred on the first day. . . .

Deaths of young patients were characterized by jumping from a height or in front of a vehicle, schizophrenia, personality disorder, unemployment, and substance misuse. In older patients, drowning, depression, living alone, physical illness, recent bereavement and suicide pacts were more common. (Appleby *et al.*, 2006)

Hence, there should be a documented risk assessment before discharge from inpatient care, and follow-up of those on the enhanced tier of the Care Programme Approach within 7 days. All this should be straightforward in patients with a clear-cut mental illness such as schizophrenia. There is more difficulty in deciding what is appropriate for other patients who have contact with mental health services, such as 'young people with personality disorder, unemployment and substance misuse', none of which are readily treatable by medical means.

'Assisted' suicide

Recent proposals for legalizing 'medically assisted' suicide, as for those with terminal illness, have aroused much professional and public controversy, and seem unlikely to be accepted in the foreseeable future.

Non-fatal deliberate self-harm (Parasuicide, attempted suicide)

Definition and terminology

Non-fatal deliberate self-harm (DSH) is deliberate overdose or self-injury without a fatal outcome. Most such acts are not determined attempts at self-killing, and therefore the previous terms 'parasuicide' and 'attempted suicide' are less frequently employed. The term 'deliberate self-harm' (DSH) has become preferred, because it is neutral and gives a clearer description.

Accidental injuries and acts intended to cause pleasure are excluded from the definition of DSH. Factitious disorder involves a form of self-injury, such as self-injection with pus to produce fever. The intended outcome is to deceive health-care professionals into thinking that a person is unwell and needs care. However, in this case, the self-injury is clearly only a part of the picture, and thus factitious disorder is regarded as separate from DSH.

Frequency

Exact frequency is impossible to determine because milder cases may not be referred to hospital, or even present to health services at all. Community surveys indicate a lifetime prevalence of up to 5 per cent for DSH. A major epidemic occurred during the 1960s and 1970s, when self-poisoning became the commonest reason for a young person to be admitted to a medical ward. Rates have declined since then, although more than 140 000 people still present with DSH to hospital in England and Wales each year (Bennewith *et al.*, 2004).

Non-fatal DSH is at least 10 times more common than completed suicide, although there is some evidence that rates of DSH and suicide move in tandem.

Methods

About 90 per cent of DSH cases are self-poisonings, often by painkillers bought without prescription, such as paracetamol, and/or prescribed psychotropic drugs; they are often accompanied by alcohol. Others are by more violent methods, such as self-cutting or burning by cigarette ends.

Epidemiology

• *age*: highest in the late teens and early twenties

• *sex*: twice as common in women

• *social conditions*: highest rates are in social classes IV and V, and in inner-city areas with a high incidence of social problems.

Motives

Up to 10 per cent of episodes of DSH are serious suicide attempts that failed. In other cases, the reported motivation is to escape from an intolerable situation or state of mind, an appeal for help, or an attempt to influence another person. Some patients cannot explain their motivation. Motivation is frequently multiple, mixed, and complex and changeable. Patients often say that they wanted to die when they did the act, but that this coexisted with other motives and feelings, such as a need to get out of an impossible situation. By the time they are seen, the wish to die has usually passed and the patient is focused on other matters.

Causes

• *Life events and social difficulties*: about 70 per cent of these acts follow a distressing event, usually involving disharmony with another person. Long-term social problems, such as family or economic difficulties, are common.

• *Psychiatric disorder*: there is clearly a high prevalence of mental disorder among DSH patients, but it is difficult to generalize. All types of mental disorder are seen, including psychosis occasionally. Symptoms of low mood are common (over 50 per cent of cases), but most do not have a pervasive clinical depressive illness at follow-up. Personality disorder and substance misuse are also common (perhaps over 25 per cent).

Assessment

Before a valid psychosocial assessment can be carried out, the patient must have had time to recover from the immediate effects of the self-harm, such as drowsiness or confusion after an overdose. Three aspects require special attention:

• whether there was *serious suicidal intent*, as indicated by:
  – the subject claiming to have wanted to die and to regret survival
  – a premeditated act preceded by making arrangements for death, leaving a suicide note, and taking precautions against discovery
  – use of a method that the subject believed would be fatal
  – features associated with completed suicide, such as older age and social isolation

• whether *psychiatric illness* requiring treatment is present

• whether *social problems* are present.

It is not feasible, or necessary, for all cases to be assessed by a psychiatrist. Junior medical staff, nurses, and social workers in the general hospital can be trained to identify patients needing psychiatric referral. Standardized rating scales are available to aid the interview assessment.

Although many acts of DSH do not appear 'serious' on assessment, patients who have committed such acts nevertheless have a continuing elevated suicide risk. Accordingly, assessment will particularly focus on risk factors for suicide, which include male sex, living alone, previous deliberate self-harm, the presence of chronic mental or physical disease, and substance misuse.

Management

Over 50 per cent are judged to need psychiatric and/or social work follow-up as outpatients, but a high proportion fail to keep follow-up appointments. From

10 to 20 per cent of cases are judged to need psychiatric hospital admission because of psychiatric illness and/or continuing suicidal intentions.

Acute dilemmas may arise in the general hospital when self-harm patients are brought in but refuse medical treatments such as stomach washout or suture of lacerations. The Mental Health Act 1983 does not cover administration of medical treatment (as opposed to psychiatric treatment) against the patient's will; however, in a life-threatening emergency, it is permitted to give this under common law. The chosen course of action should be justified in the case notes, and full explanations to patients and/or relatives given.

Repeated DSH is a frequent feature of borderline personality disorder; every hospital or community mental health team will have a small number of regular attenders with the presentation. Often, the behaviour worsens if the patient is repeatedly admitted to hospital. Sometimes, management by behavioural means is appropriate; for example, patients sign a contract that if they self-harm they will be admitted to the hospital overnight and discharged the next day.

Prognosis

About 20 per cent repeat deliberate self-harm the next year, and around 1 per cent die by suicide the next year (nearly a 100-fold increase over the general population suicide rate). Up to 10 per cent die by suicide eventually.

Prevention

Primary preventive strategies are similar to those described above for completed suicide. Psychiatric treatment, social work, and counselling have been evaluated for secondary prevention in people who have already made an attempt. Although these interventions do help to reduce psychosocial problems, they have not been shown to reduce the repetition rate for deliberate self-harm.

References

Appleby, L., Shaw, J., Amos, T. *et al.* (2006). Suicide in mental health in-patients and within 3 months of discharge. *Br J Psychiatry* **188**, 129–134.

Bennewith, O., Gunnell, D., Peters, T. J. *et al.* (2004). Variations in the hospital management of self harm in adults in England: observational study. *BMJ* **328**, 1108–1109.

Hall, W., Mant, A., Mitchell, P. B. *et al.* (2003). Association between antidepressant prescribing and suicide in Australia, 1991–2000: trend analysis. *BMJ* **326**, 1008.

Harris, E. C. and Barraclough, B. (1997). Suicide as an outcome for mental disorders. A meta-analysis. *Br J Psychiatry* **170**, 205–228.

Hawton, K., Townsend, E., Deeks, J. J. *et al.* (2004). UK legislation on analgesic packs: before and after study of long term effect on poisonings. *BMJ* **329**, 1159.

Hunt, I. M., Kapur, N., Robinson, J. *et al.* (2006). Suicide within 12 months of mental health service contact in different age and diagnostic groups. *British Journal of Psychiatry* **188**, 135–142.

Mann, J., Apter, A., Bertolote, J. *et al.* (2005). Suicide prevention strategies. *JAMA* **294**, 2064–2074.

McClure, G. (2000). Changes in suicide in England and Wales, 1960–1997. *Br J Psychiatry* **176**, 64–67.

15 Eating disorders: anorexia nervosa and bulimia nervosa

Introduction

Anorexia nervosa (AN) and *bulimia nervosa* (BN) have been the principal eating disorders recognized in psychiatry. They are included in ICD–10. The existence of another eating disorder, *binge eating disorder*, has recently been suggested. *Obesity* far outweighs both AN and BN in its public health importance, but has not generally been regarded as a psychiatric disorder.

It is important to appreciate that AN and BN overlap to some extent, although a diagnosis of AN is held to take precedence over one of BN if they coexist. In addition, patients may, as it were, move from AN to BN, and back again, perhaps more than once, although the general trend is to move from AN to BN. Perhaps as many as half of those diagnosed with AN eventually become BN.

Anorexia nervosa (AN)

Definition

AN, named by Gull in 1874, is characterized by the following:

Hughes' Outline of Modern Psychiatry, Fifth Edition. David Gill.
© 2007 John Wiley & Sons, Ltd   ISBN 9780470033920

- *extreme weight loss* (at least 15 per cent) deliberately achieved by dieting and/or other means such as exercise or purgation

- *amenorrhoea* in females; *loss of libido* in males

- *abnormal attitudes* to food

- *distorted body image*, with morbid fear of fatness.

Prevalence

About 1 per cent of adolescent girls in the UK have the full syndrome, but milder partial versions are common, and prevalence has increased in recent years.

Epidemiology

- *Age*: most cases start in adolescence, but sometimes onset is before puberty or in adult life.

- *Sex*: 95 per cent are female.

- *Social class*: patients tend to come from families in social classes 1 and 2.

- *Occupation*: occupations which demand a slim figure, such as modelling, beauty therapy, and ballet dancing, are over-represented.

- *Nationality*: the condition mostly affects white subjects living in Western countries. Indeed, it has been suggested that eating disorders could be seen as a 'culture-bound' syndrome of Western societies.

Causes

- *Psychodynamic theories* view AN as a means of avoiding maturation, especially in sexual terms, or as a means of acquiring independence and/or a sense of achievement, through strict control of diet and weight. These attitudes may stem from disturbed family relationships, which are almost always evident in the established case, although they could then be the result of the condition rather than its cause.

- *Cultural theories* implicate the social and media pressures urging women to be slim and diet-conscious. For example, published fashion photographs are often stretched lengthwise to make the models look even thinner than they really are. Common to both these approaches is the idea that the anorexia develops, in response to family or peer influences, in a young person who lacks a secure sense of self.

• *Hormonal imbalance*: hypothalamic dysfunction is always present and is probably secondary to the weight loss.

Clinical features

A decision by a mildly overweight teenager to go on a slimming diet is a common starting point for this disorder.

• *Physical*: the patient loses weight by dietary restriction, and sometimes also by self-induced vomiting, taking laxatives or diuretics, and excessive exercising. Amenorrhoea may occur before there has been much loss of weight. Male patients show loss of sexual interest and impotence. Other common physical features are hypotension, bradycardia, constipation, mild hypothermia, and growth of downy (lanugo) hair. Vomiting or purging may result in disturbance of fluid and electrolyte balance. Bone fractures secondary to osteoporosis may occur in chronic cases.

• *Mental*: the patient is preoccupied with food and weight, takes pride in dieting, and feels guilty about eating more than small amounts. Most patients do not see themselves as unwell or underweight, but feel active, healthy, and fashionably slim. In chronic cases, greater insight may develop, often resulting in depression.

Differential diagnosis

• *chronic debilitating physical disease* such as cancer, pituitary failure, Addison's disease, TB, or AIDS

• *psychiatric illness*: depression, schizophrenia, and obsessive-compulsive disorder

• *hypothalamic* lesions.

Investigations will sometimes be necessary to rule out these other conditions; however, there is an important clinical pointer in that there will be no body image disturbance: only in anorexia will the patient, in actual fact seriously underweight, have an inappropriate belief of being overweight.

Physical complications

- *The following hormonal and biochemical changes may occur:*
  - reduction of sex and thyroid hormone secretion, secondary to hypothalamic and pituitary dysfunction
  - increase of growth hormone and cortisol secretion
  - increased insulin response to glucose loading
  - low basal temperature and impaired temperature regulation
  - low basal metabolic rate
  - high serum cholesterol
  - abnormal liver function tests
  - low serum zinc.

- *CT scan of the brain* may show ventricular and sulcal enlargement. These changes are not immediately reversible with weight gain.

- *Osteoporotic bones* may develop in chronic cases.

Treatment

This is often a chronic relapsing and remitting condition and repeated courses of treatment, including hospital admission, may be necessary.

- *Physical treatment*: the first priorities are restoration of weight and correction of physical complications. Severe cases require inpatient care, and compulsory treatment under the Mental Health Act 1983 is occasionally indicated. Weight gain is best achieved by winning the patient's agreement to eat more, and skilled nurses can usually manage this, although many patients will be unco-operative at first, secretly disposing of food or vomiting. Some units use a behavioural approach in which privileges such as watching TV or having visitors are conditional on regular weight gain, but many patients find this coercive and unhelpful. *Drug treatment* may include the use of major tranquillizers for agitation, and appropriate specific medication for coexisting psychiatric syndromes such as depression or obsessive-compulsive disorder. If antidepressants are indicated, tricyclics with their appetite-stimulating properties are more appropriate than SSRIs, which can cause weight loss.

- *Psychological treatment* includes cognitive or supportive therapy individually or in groups, and efforts to correct abnormal body image, perhaps with the aid of measurements or photographs. Psychodynamic approaches are usually unhelpful. Family factors must also be addressed, as in the case of a girl aged 16 who developed anorexia after her achievement of eight out of nine 'A' grades at GCSE was perceived by her family as a failure because of the single 'B'. She felt that the only thing she could succeed at was the control of her weight.

Prognosis

Recovery is judged by return to normal weight, return of menstruation, and improved psychological and psychosexual adjustment. After 5 years, about half these patients have recovered fully, and a quarter have improved to some degree. Some cease to be anorexic and go on to develop bulimic features. There is an increased risk of death from suicide, malnutrition, or physical complications. Poor prognostic features are a long history, older age of onset, abnormal pre-morbid personality, poor family relationships, and extreme weight loss.

Case example

A 16-year-old schoolgirl, intelligent but lacking in self-confidence, started to diet after a young man said that her tummy was too fat. The girl was working hard for exams at the time, and her parents were having some marital problems. While eating less and less, she became more and more interested in food and spent much time reading recipe books, and baking cakes for the rest of the family. She slept very little, and would get up early to run for an hour before school. Her weight dropped from 8 to 5 stone within about 3 months, and eventually her mother insisted on taking her to the doctor because her periods had stopped. The girl refused to talk about her condition or accept any medical treatment; however, she agreed to eat a little more within strictly controlled limits, taking an extra half-pint of milk and two slices of bread each day.

Her weight gradually increased again over the next few months but it was 6 years before menstruation resumed. She achieved a professional qualification, and held a responsible job throughout her 20s despite drinking half a bottle of vodka in private every night. The drinking decreased in her early 30s after she married an older man; they had no children. Now aged 50, she has continued to maintain her weight at 47 kg precisely and becomes very anxious if prevented, by circumstances such as going on holiday, from weighing herself twice a day.

Bulimia nervosa

Bulimia nervosa (BN), described by Russell in 1979, is characterized by the following:

- powerful and intractable *urges to overeat*
- efforts to *avoid the fattening effects of food* by inducing vomiting or abusing purgatives
- morbid *fear of fatness.*

BN and anorexia are closely related. Many anorexic patients exhibit bulimic symptoms, and 25–50 per cent of bulimic patients have a past history of anorexia.

Prevalence

Depending on diagnostic criteria, about 1–2 per cent of young women in the UK may be diagnosed as bulimic. Many cases can be successfully concealed because, unlike those with AN, bulimia sufferers look outwardly healthy.

Epidemiology

- *Sex*: most cases are female.
- *Age*: late teens or early 20s.
- *Marital status*: about 25 per cent are married.

Patients tend to be older, more sexually experienced, and more confident and outgoing than those with AN.

Clinical features

- *Physical*: bouts of eating vast quantities of food (bingeing) occur in response to an uncontrollable psychological urge. Self-induced vomiting often follows such episodes. Patients may have abrasions on the back of the hands where they have caught themselves on the teeth trying to induce vomiting. Between binges, most patients follow strict diets and may also abuse purgatives or take excessive exercise, so managing to keep their weight within the normal range.

- *Mental*: preoccupation with food and weight dominates patients' lives, but unlike many with AN, bulimic patients show good insight into their abnormal attitudes and behaviour. Depressive symptoms are common. Some patients abuse alcohol and a subgroup shows impulsive behaviour affecting many aspects of life.

Physical complications

Vomiting and laxative abuse may result in alkalosis; this dangerous complication may lead to cardiac arrhythmia (sometimes fatal), fits, and renal damage. Another serious but rare complication is acute dilatation or even rupture of the oesophagus or stomach. Swollen parotid glands, and dental damage due to frequent vomiting, may develop. Menstrual irregularity, or amenorrhoea, is common.

Treatment

- *cognitive-behavioural psychotherapy*, individual or group
- *antidepressants*, especially SSRIs in high dose.

Both these approaches are of proven effectiveness.

Prognosis

Few long-term studies are yet available, but the symptoms often persist for years, and mortality from suicide or physical complications may be up to 20 per cent.

Obesity

Obesity is not classed as a psychiatric disorder, but psychologically driven overeating may contribute to its development, and psychological problems may result from it. Increases in prevalence of obesity are of course a lifestyle issue (people are becoming less active) rather than a psychiatric one. Therefore, psychiatrists should perhaps concentrate on not making obesity worse by inappropriate prescribing of psychotropic medication for too long, or in too high doses. Patients on the newer antipsychotic drugs, especially olanzepine, need careful watching.

Further reading

NICE. Eating disorders. http://www.nice.org.uk/page.aspx?o=cg009niceguidance.

Palmer, B. (2006). Come the revolution – revisiting the management of anorexia nervosa. *Adv Psychiatr Treat* **12**, 5–12.

16 Disorders of female reproductive life

This chapter covers psychiatric disorder in relation to pregnancy, childbirth and motherhood, and the menstrual cycle.

It should be noted at some point that there are general effects of gender on health. Females consult more frequently for all health problems, including neurotic conditions, throughout life. Prevalence of neurotic conditions is higher in females than males. Males have an excess of conduct disorder as children, and of criminality and substance misuse as adults. Males with psychotic disorders such as schizophrenia do worse than females. Females live longer. It has been suggested that men may need special services (Kennedy, 2001).

Pregnancy

Broadly speaking, pregnancy appears to protect against psychiatric disorder, an effect having probable survival value in evolutionary terms. First onset of psychiatric disorder during pregnancy is rare, existing disorders tend to become less severe, and suicide rates during pregnancy and the puerperium are low. However, women with a history of chronic or recurrent psychiatric disorder require continuing assessment and care during pregnancy, and monitoring to detect and treat any worsening after childbirth, with the health and safety of both mother and baby in mind.

Hughes' Outline of Modern Psychiatry, Fifth Edition. David Gill.
© 2007 John Wiley & Sons, Ltd   ISBN 9780470033920

Psychotropic drug treatment during pregnancy, although best avoided for the baby's sake, is sometimes essential for the mother's mental health. There is no evidence that antipsychotics, tricyclic antidepressants, or benzodiazepines cause serious harm to the foetus, although a newborn whose mother had been taking benzodiazepine might exhibit a transient withdrawal syndrome. The key point is that organogenesis is largely complete by 3 months; hence, it is most unlikely that medication taken from then on could cause malformation, the adverse effect most feared by parents and prescribers.

Hence, the undoubted desirability of the mother's being drug free throughout pregnancy sometimes has to be set aside. It then becomes a matter of balancing a potential risk to the baby from intrauterine exposure to psychotropic medication against the mental health needs of the mother. Frequently, the baby's need to have a well mother after birth tips the balance toward cautious use of medication during pregnancy if other treatment measures have proved insufficient.

However, lithium should be avoided, because it may cause foetal thyroid enlargement and, if taken in the first trimester, foetal cardiac malformation. It is important that the mother receives full information about proposed drug therapy, and gives informed consent (see *British National Formulary* guidelines on prescribing in pregnancy).

ECT can safely be given in pregnancy.

Unplanned pregnancies sometimes occur in women whose judgement is affected by psychiatric illness or learning disability, and may remain undiagnosed until a late stage.

Hyperemesis gravidarum refers to unusually prolonged and severe forms of the normal experience of vomiting ('morning sickness') during the early stages of pregnancy. While there may be physical causes, such as multiple pregnancy, psychosocial aspects – especially anxiety – are often prominent.

Pseudocyesis is 'phantom pregnancy'; that is, the woman develops symptoms and even signs of pregnancy, including abdominal distension, in the absence of a pregnancy. It is, however, now rare in UK practice. *Couvade* refers to an analagous syndrome in the man, who develops these features, as it were, in sympathy with the mother. Again, it is rare.

Puerperal psychosis

Definition

This is customarily defined as psychosis beginning within 12 weeks of delivery. Most cases are now 'functional', that is, a form of mental illness without organic factors. In previous generations, and possibly still in developing countries, the psychosis was frequently organic in origin (due to confusion consequent on infection or other medical causes).

Frequency

The frequency is about 1–2 per 1000 births.

Predisposing factors

- past history of psychosis
- past history of puerperal psychosis: 20 per cent risk of recurrence in subsequent pregnancies
- family history of psychosis
- primiparity.

Causes

- *Medical disorders*: pelvic infections, thromboembolism, and other physical complications of childbirth, although not common nowadays, need to be excluded in every case. The clinical picture would in this case be one of delirium – in other words, it would be an organic psychosis. In early cases, the defining feature of confusion, reduced conscious level, may be apparent only on detailed cognitive testing.

- *Hormone changes*: it is speculated that the abrupt fall in oestrogen and progesterone concentrations that occurs after delivery might precipitate psychosis in predisposed women.

- *Psychosocial stress*: childbirth as a major 'life event' could precipitate psychosis in predisposed women.

Clinical features

Premonitory symptoms may occur in late pregnancy, but onset of frank psychosis is usually sudden, 2–14 days after delivery. Even in the majority of cases that do not have an identified physical cause, symptoms such as bewilderment, emotional lability, and perplexity are often prominent. Depressive and manic syndromes are commoner than schizophrenic ones, although mixed pictures often occur. The thought content, and any delusions or hallucinations present (for example, 'I am too wicked to be a mother'; 'this baby's body is rotting inside') occasionally lead the patient to harm or even kill herself and/or her child.

Treatment

These illnesses can be severe and unpredictable. The safety of the mother and particularly of the baby must always be paramount. Hospital admission is usually necessary, preferably to a specialized mother and baby unit.

Treatment is in principle the same as would be used for the equivalent psychosis occurring apart from the puerperium. However, ECT should more readily be considered, for manic and schizophrenic syndromes as well as depressive ones. ECT often relieves symptoms more quickly than drugs, and most psychotropic drugs enter breast milk, a potential (though sometimes overemphasized) concern if the mother is breast-feeding. High-dose progesterone is reported to be helpful but has not been tested in a clinical trial. The issue of contraception may need addressing if the illness is prolonged.

Prognosis

Short-term prognosis is good, but there is a 20 per cent chance of recurrence after any subsequent pregnancy, and a 50 per cent chance of later recurrence not related to pregnancy.

Post-natal depression and other neurotic syndromes

Any neurotic disorder can occur in the post-natal period. In addition to post-natal depression and 'maternity blues', the two syndromes (see below) most frequently described, anxiety disorders and obsessive-compulsive disorders sometimes occur. Symptomatology usually centres on the baby. Affected mothers often try to hide their symptoms because they know they are expected to be happy at this time, feel ashamed of their negative attitudes toward their baby, or are afraid the baby will be taken into care.

Maternity blues

About 50 per cent of mothers experience irritability, lability of mood, and tear-fulness following delivery, maximal at about 4 days, and tending gradually to resolve by about day 10. Such symptoms may be considered normal in the sense of being extremely common; however, they can cause considerable distress to the patient and family, and there is evidence of a weak linkage with psychiatric disorder. This is an appropriate subject for prenatal education, and supportive care from family, midwife, and GP. If the syndrome fails to resolve, mental health services may be required.

Post-natal depression

Depression more persistent than 'maternity blues' occurs after 10–20 per cent of births. It tends to present later than puerperal psychosis. Many cases represent the continuation, exacerbation, or recurrence of depression that was present before the birth or even before the pregnancy: psychosocial factors are of particular importance.

A subgroup of women suffer depressive illness specifically related to childbirth, and their rates of depression at other times are not raised. Psychological difficulties in adjusting to motherhood, coping with the added responsibilities and changed social role, especially when there are social problems such as lack of support from the child's father or poor housing, may contribute to these depressive states. Minor hormone imbalance might also be involved.

Clinical features are not distinct from other depressive illnesses, and may include depression of mood, anxiety, panic attacks, fatigue, loss of libido, anorexia, and insomnia. Some of these symptoms are difficult to distinguish from the inevitable changes in sleep, eating pattern, and sexual function brought about by giving birth and caring for a child. Thoughts of hating or wishing to harm the baby are common, and should always sensitively be asked about; the mother will feel very guilty about any thoughts of this kind, and may be much helped by talking about them, and understanding that she is not alone in experiencing them. Actual harming of the baby is rare unless the mother is psychotic. The illness may last for months or years, especially if, as is often the case, it goes undetected and untreated. This chronic ill health in the mother is believed to hinder cognitive and emotional development in the child.

Case example

A 29-year-old professional woman lived comfortably with her husband and two small children. Her third pregnancy was unplanned, but the couple seemed to accept it well. Midway through the pregnancy, the husband was made redundant, and they began to experience some marital difficulties. During the third trimester, the patient became increasingly tearful and tired. She had a prolonged and painful labour, but the baby was well, and breast-feeding was established satisfactorily.

At home over the next 2 weeks, the health visitor noticed the patient became very distressed when her baby cried and seemed not to know what to do. She appeared mildly perplexed and was not taking much care of herself or her surroundings. On questioning, she confirmed that she could hardly sleep, she had little appetite, her weight was dropping fast, and she could not enjoy her baby as she had enjoyed the other two. She admitted feeling 'ugly' and 'dirty' (because of dribbling milk) and had considered leaving home because she was such a bad mother and wife. She scored 18 (high) on the Edinburgh Postnatal Depression Scale.

The health visitor called the GP, who visited the family and confirmed the diagnosis of depression, prescribed a tricyclic antidepressant (compatible with breast-feeding), and encouraged the health visitor to offer supportive counselling in addition to monitoring the baby's well-being.

Within 6 weeks the patient's mood had lifted, and she was restored to her former competent self, returning to work part-time while her husband stayed at home to look after the children. She continued on medication for another 6 months, during which time the couple came to accept their new circumstances and re-established a good emotional and sexual relationship.

Treatment includes a combination of the following:

- *social support*: training in childcare, contact with named midwives and health visitors, and introduction to other mothers of young children. Such measures in pregnancy have been shown to have preventive value, and health visitors given special training can provide valuable supportive counselling after the birth.

* *antidepressant drugs*

* *psychotherapy*: individual, marital, family, or group.

Abortion

The Abortion Act 1967, with its subsequent amendments, permits abortion before 24 weeks' gestation in the case of risk to the mother's life, the mother's physical health or mental health, or the health of her existing children; later abortion is permitted in the case of foetal abnormality. Most abortions are carried out on the grounds of risk to the mother's mental health, but usually without a psychiatric opinion.

Postpartum psychosis after a previous delivery is usually regarded as a justification for abortion if the woman wants one, but since the risk of recurrence of postpartum psychosis after a single previous episode is only 20 per cent, abortion should not necessarily be advised in such cases.

Abortion seldom has serious psychiatric sequelae, but about 25 per cent of women experience significant guilt or depression afterward, especially if they were ambivalent about the abortion or pressured to accept it.

Stillbirth and perinatal death

Mothers of babies who were stillborn, or died soon after birth, almost always develop grief reactions as found after other forms of bereavement. They are at high risk of prolonged depression and have an increased suicide rate. Fathers are also affected but have not been so thoroughly studied. Management after neonatal bereavement should include opportunities for the parents to see and touch the dead child, encouragement to give the baby a name, take a photograph, hold a funeral, receive an explanation for the death and obstetric/genetic advice about future pregnancies, and bereavement counselling from an experienced professional. Such measures have been shown to reduce the duration of psychiatric morbidity.

Premenstrual syndrome

Many women report depressed mood, irritability, or anxiety, often combined with physical symptoms such as breast tenderness, headaches, bloated feelings, and weight gain, for up to 2 weeks before the onset of menstruation. Premenstrual tension has been used successfully as a defence in criminal trials, although this is exceptional. Regarding treatment, a wide variety of interventions has been systematically reviewed (http://www.clinicalevidence.com/ceweb/conditions/woh/0806/0806.jsp): diuretics and pyridoxine are considered to have good evidence of effectiveness. 'Likely to be beneficial' treatments include non-steroidal anti-inflammatory drugs; SSRIs have 'a trade-off between benefits and harms'. Some popular treatments, including evening primrose, are of 'unknown effectiveness'.

The menopause

Epidemiological studies do not demonstrate any increase in major psychiatric morbidity in women of menopausal age. However, mild to moderate depression or anxiety may develop at this time of life; perhaps secondary to hormone changes, perhaps reactive to physical symptoms, or perhaps reflecting life changes such as children leaving home, death of parents, and awareness of ageing.

Again, a variety of treatments has been used (http://www.clinicalevidence.com/ceweb/conditions/woh/0804/0804.jsp), especially hormone replacement therapy (HRT): progesterone alone is 'beneficial', but oestrogen alone or in combination with progesterone causes 'improved menopausal symptoms but increased risk of breast cancer, endometrial cancer, stroke, and venous thromboembolism after long term use', and there is a 'trade-off between benefits and harms'. Antidepressants are of 'unknown effectiveness'.

Hysterectomy

Depressive reactions may occur after hysterectomy; some women having this operation are distressed by the loss of their childbearing capacity and/or their sense of femininity. However, follow-up of women having hysterectomies for menorrhagia of benign origin shows the majority to be pleased with the results, and overall psychiatric morbidity significantly lower after the operation than before, although still higher than in the general population.

Reference

Kennedy, H. (2001). Do men need special services? *Adv Psychiatr Treat* 7, 93–99.

17 Sexual problems

Sexual problems may present in various medical settings: primary care, general or specialist psychiatric practice, gynaecology, urology, and genitourinary medicine (GUM), as well as in non-health settings such as Relate (formerly the Marriage Guidance Council). Whether or not certain variants of sexual behaviour or function are perceived as 'problems' will depend on the expectations, and moral values, of the individual and of his or her social group. Topics in this chapter are arranged as follows:

- *sexual dysfunctions*, in which sexual performance fails to satisfy the subject or partner
- *sexual deviations*, in which sexual practice departs from convention in a way that distresses the subject or offends others
- *gender-identity disorders*
- *homosexuality*, which is not a disorder, but is conveniently considered here.

Sexual dysfunctions

These conditions, in which some aspect of sexual performance fails to satisfy the subject or partner, may be categorized in several ways but perhaps most clearly by relating them to the five stages in the model of normal sexual response described by Masters and Johnson.

Hughes' Outline of Modern Psychiatry, Fifth Edition. David Gill.
© 2007 John Wiley & Sons, Ltd   ISBN 9780470033920

	Male	Female
Desire	Reduced libido	Reduced libido
Excitement	Erectile dysfunction	Unresponsiveness
Intercourse	Loss of erection	Vaginismus
Orgasm	Premature/delayed ejaculation	Anorgasmia
Resolution	Priapism	
All stages	Dyspareunia	Dyspareunia

Reduced libido in women, and erectile and ejaculatory problems in men, are among the most common reasons that couples present for advice. The terms 'frigidity' and 'impotence' are imprecise and judgemental, and should be avoided.

Causes

- *Background factors*: anxiety or ignorance about sex, past experience of sexual abuse, general disharmony between the couple concerned, a constitutional discrepancy in sex drive between the two partners, or a lack of physical attraction between them.

- *Ageing*: sexual drive and performance in both sexes decrease with age, although the decline is more marked in males. For example, the prevalence of erectile dysfunction in men is about 2 per cent at age 40, and 25–30 per cent at age 65.

- *Psychiatric illness*: most psychiatric illnesses, especially depressive illness and anxiety states, reduce sexual drive, performance, and pleasure. The exception is mania, in which sexual interest and activity increase.

- *Organic brain disease*: the dementias, and lesions of the frontal lobe may produce sexual disinhibition.

- *Genital and pelvic pathology*: for example, congenital abnormality, infection, and injury to the genitalia or spinal cord.

- *Endocrine and metabolic disorders*: for example, diabetes, sex hormone deficiency, hyperprolactinaemia, hypertension, arteriosclerosis, and renal failure.

- *Drugs*: psychotropic drugs, especially antidepressants and neuroleptics, may affect sexual function and so may many of the drugs used in general medicine, such as antihypertensives and diuretics. The most common culprits are SSRIs, which frequently reduce libido and/or produce anorgasmia in both sexes.

- *Alcohol*: impaired sexual function may result from intoxication, peripheral neuropathy, disturbed sex hormone metabolism due to cirrhosis of the liver, marital conflict, or treatment with disulfiram.

Assessment

If both partners attend, they should, if they agree, be interviewed separately and then together. The two parties frequently differ in their view of what the problem is, and in their desire for treatment, and it is important to be clear about such differences. The duration of the problem, and whether it is present with other partners and in masturbation, should be established. A medical history, psychiatric history, and physical examination should always be obtained, followed by laboratory investigations if indicated. It is especially important to use a sensitive, non-judgemental style when interviewing people with sexual problems.

Treatment

- *Underlying causes*, such as psychiatric or medical illness, should be managed appropriately.

- *Psychological approaches*: simple explanation and counselling may be all that is required, and sometimes can be best provided from the many useful books and videos available to the public. More complex cases may need formal psychotherapy, individually or as a couple.

- *Sex therapy*: this derives from the methods of Masters and Johnson. The couple are usually treated together. Treatment begins with a 'sensate focus' phase during which intercourse is not attempted, so that the couple stop repeating an experience of failure, but spend a set time alone together each day to concentrate on talking about relationship issues and exchanging non-genital physical affection. In stages, the couple then work toward genital stimulation, followed by intercourse. They may be taught specific techniques according to the type of dysfunction present; for example, the 'squeeze technique' for premature ejaculation, or extended foreplay in orgasmic delay.

Case example

A man aged 52, happily married for 23 years, was referred to psychiatric outpatients by his GP, who said his patient was distressed by 'progressive impotence', and had recently watched a television programme about Viagra, which he was keen to try. The man himself seemed rather embarrassed by the referral. He attended without his wife, and had not told her about it; she had 'not seemed especially keen on sex' after the menopause, and they had been having intercourse about every 2 weeks in recent years, largely at his request. He had recently taken an antihypertensive drug, and had been finding it more difficult to sustain an erection; although his blood pressure had since settled and he was able to stop this medication, his erectile difficulty had not entirely resolved. Direct enquiry established that there was less of a problem during masturbation.

The psychiatrist could detect no physical or mental disorder, and blood tests including prolactin were normal. He advised that the problem would probably continue to resolve, and that specific treatment was not required at present, although sildenafil (Viagra) would be effective, if it was necessary to use it in the future.

At follow-up, the patient was invited to ask his wife to attend. There had been some further improvement in his erections, but it emerged that his underlying fear was that he was 'failing in his marital duties'. The psychiatrist advised that their sexual relationship, in particular their frequency of intercourse, was not abnormal for their age. Although it was possible that the wife was suffering from some oestrogen deficiency symptoms, including vaginal dryness, that might well have responded to hormone replacement therapy, the couple declined further appointments, saying they were 'reasonably happy with things as they are'.

- *Systemic drugs*: these are appropriate when a specific medical indication is present. Examples include:
  - oestrogen/progesterone hormone replacement therapy in postmenopausal women
  - the phosphodiesterase type-5 inhibitors sildenafil (Viagra), tadalafil, and vardenafil increase cyclic guanosine monophosphate (cGMP), leading to penile smooth muscle relaxation. Taken 1 hour before sexual activity, they

have revolutionized the treatment of erectile dysfunction. Although generally well tolerated, they occasionally cause priapism, however, which is a medical emergency for which the patient must be advised to go immediately to hospital. For erectile dysfunction, these drugs have largely replaced agents such as yohimbine tablets and penile injection treatments (although these treatments were never widely used). They are being tried for premature ejaculation and also for female sexual dysfunction, although there is as yet no clear evidence of effectiveness.
   - androgen treatment for reduced sexual drive in men who have low testosterone levels
   - bromocriptine for male sexual dysfunction secondary to hyperprolactinaemia.

* *Local treatments for female partner*:
   - topical lubricants/oestrogens for vaginal dryness
   - vaginal dilators, of progressively larger size, for vaginismus.

* *Local treatments for males with erectile failure*:
   - intracavernosal injection of vasoactive drugs such as papaverine and prostaglandin E_1 (aprostadil)
   - vacuum devices using suction to establish erection, which is then maintained by a ring
   - surgical implants.

Prognosis

It is difficult to generalize, but most patients seen for advice about sexual problems improve to some extent. The advent of sildenafil will certainly have improved outcomes overall.

Sexual deviations

Most variants of sexual orientation and behaviour, sometimes called 'paraphilias' or 'alternative sexual practices', are no longer classed as psychiatric disorders, and more liberal attitudes in society during recent years have reduced the frequency of psychiatric involvement with them. However, sometimes these variants are associated with psychiatric disorder, social maladjustment, or transgressions of the law.

   Psychiatric treatment is only indicated in carefully selected cases. When a sexual deviation leads to the patient's developing secondary psychiatric problems, such as depression or substance misuse, psychiatric assessment may be appropriate. However, the boundaries have to be clear. The patient must be clearly told that he retains responsibility for his behaviour. In deviations which lead to conflict with the law, such as paedophilia, mental health services have to be extremely cautious about involvement, in case they are blamed – probably wrongly, but mud sticks – if the subject reoffends.

Causes

The cause of sexual deviations is generally unknown. These preferences, which are much commoner in males than females, are usually present by early adulthood or before. They may therefore be regarded as a permanent feature of the personality that may become more marked with the passage of years or at times of stress. Some of these behaviours are associated with difficulty in forming normal relationships; for example, indecent exposure may occur in men with poor social skills and/or learning disability. Availability is also a factor, as in bestiality among men with ready access to animals. There may be a genetic component. In rare cases, a first onset in later life may be due to functional psychiatric illness or organic brain disease.

Psychodynamic theorists have suggested that these behaviours are due to abnormal parental attitudes, such as excessive dominance of one parent, or parental desire for a child of the opposite sex. In the behavioural model, deviant sexual behaviour is conceived as being learned by conditioning or modelling, and maintained by reward in the form of orgasm and anxiety reduction. Behavioural factors probably underpin cases where the person spends longer and longer viewing pornography, such as that available on the Internet; however, these cases may also have features of obsessive-compulsive disorder and/or addictive behaviours.

Individual deviations will now be briefly described.

Sadism and masochism

Sadism is sexual gratification from inflicting cruelty on the partner. Masochism, which often coexists in the same individual, is sexual gratification from being subjected to cruelty. Minor forms of both tendencies are common. Extreme forms of sadism can lead to sexual crimes.

Fetishism

A group of conditions in which sexual desire is focused on a body part other than the genitals (for example, the feet) or an inanimate object (for example, a particular type of garment). If treatment is indicated at all, behaviour therapy is the treatment of choice.

Bestiality

Bestiality is intercourse with animals, and is most common among male farm workers. It is illegal.

Indecent exposure

Indecent exposure (exhibitionism) is illegal exposure of the genitals to another person, usually carried out by a man in the presence of a girl or woman unknown to him. Most exhibitionists are young men who expose a flaccid penis; these are anxious, inhibited personalities whose sexual adjustment is poor, and who feel guilty about exposing. They often cease the behaviour after detection. A minority are sociopathic men who expose an erect penis while masturbating, and derive pleasure and excitement from the act. This group is more likely to repeat the behaviour, and to progress to more serious offences.

Paedophilia

Paedophilia is sexual preference for children. Sexual contact with a child under 16 is an imprisonable offence. This usually involves men, and less often women, who have difficulty forming sexual relationships with adults. Many have themselves been abused as children. Homosexual and heterosexual types exist. Behaviour ranges from a superficially affectionate relationship with a known child to the homicidal rape of a strange one. Dangerous paedophiles require secure care and antilibidinal drugs.

Incest

Incest is sexual intercourse with a parent, sibling, child, or grandchild, and is an imprisonable offence. The most common forms are between father and daughter, and between brother and sister. It is often associated with learning disability, social deprivation, overcrowding, and/or a poor sexual relationship between the parents in the family. Some girls involved in incestuous relationships have sexual difficulties in later life, but the frequency of long-term ill effects is unknown. However, there is certainly a raised incidence of mental disorder, especially personality disorder. There is a greatly increased risk of genetic defects in children conceived through incest.

Treatment

- *Behavioural and cognitive therapy*: older techniques, such as aversion therapy, were designed to discourage unwanted desires and behaviours, but are now little used because of ethical objections. (A mild type of aversion therapy that might be acceptable would be a mild aversive stimulus administered by the patient, such as snapping an elastic band round the wrist when the unwanted thoughts occur.) Modern approaches place greater emphasis on positive conditioning by encouraging preferable alternatives. For example, paraphilias may be treated with 'orgasmic reconditioning', in which, during masturbation, the subject is encouraged to concentrate on acceptable fantasies. For deviations which appear to be a substitute for adult heterosexual relationships, social skills training may help.

- *Group therapy* is often used for offenders, who are thereby encouraged to confront the effects of their behaviour on victims. This may be within correctional facilities and run partly by warders and partly by a prison psychologist.

- *Drugs*: antilibidinal drugs for male sexual offenders include the anti-androgen *cyproterone acetate*, the major tranquillizer *benperidol, oestrogens*, and the gonadorelin analogue *goserilin*. These drugs may cause impotence, infertility, and breast enlargement. Thus, they should be used only for dangerous sex offenders. Occasionally, they may be used under the Mental Health Act. If so, this requires the support of two approved consultant psychiatrists as well as the subject's own informed consent.

- *Psychodynamic psychotherapy* explores possible origins of the sexual deviation in disturbed relationships or repressed events in childhood. This option is less used nowadays, because of the move toward evidence-based treatments.

Few of the above treatments have been rigorously demonstrated to be effective, and it is particularly important to remember this in forensic cases. Therapeutic optimism has led to some recidivist sexual offenders being removed from the criminal justice system into the health-care system, and subsequent reoffending wrongly attributed by the media to failures of psychiatric care rather than the elective behaviour of the offender. Some sex offenders express a wish for psychiatric help because they hope to avoid a prison sentence.

Gender-identity disorders

Transvestism

Transvestism is a wish or compulsion to wear clothing of the opposite sex. Most transvestites are male, and most are heterosexual, but sometimes the condition is associated with homosexuality, transsexualism, or sexual deviations. Transvestism is common and not illegal.

Transsexualism

Transsexualism is a rare disorder of sexual identity in which there is a strong wish to change to the opposite sex, with a belief of having been born into the wrong sex, present since early childhood. Most subjects are biologically male. Many are married men with children. Some are homosexual.

Transsexuals usually present for treatment because they want surgical sex reassignment. Such surgery is (in the UK) done only in one or two centres. The subject should have received thorough information and counselling, and successfully lived in the role of the opposite sex for an extended period (perhaps using non-surgical measures the while, such as hormone treatment), and be free of psychiatric disorder. Most subjects who fulfil these criteria are said to be pleased with the results of surgery. The male-to-female operation, involving removal of the penis and scrotum and creation of an artificial vagina, is more satisfactory than the female-to-male version and should enable the subject to experience sexual intercourse as a woman (but not, of course, to bear children as a few naive subjects expect). The operation is combined with breast surgery, hormone treatment to change the secondary sex characteristics, and tuition in behaviour appropriate to the new sex.

In law, the sex has remained the original one as stated on the birth certificate, although there are pressures to amend this.

Homosexuality

Homosexuality, an exclusive or predominant sexual preference for the same sex, is no longer classed as a psychiatric disorder. It is mentioned here because it may be associated with increased rates of depression, alcoholism, and neurosis, probably because of the associated social stigma. Social attitudes to male homosexuality have become well publicized since the advent of HIV and AIDS.

Female homosexuality was not illegal in the UK, as, when such a law was mooted to Queen Victoria, she declined to believe that it existed. Male homosexual acts were illegal until 1967, when they were legalized between consenting males over the age of 21 (in private). Recently, the age of consent has been changed to 16 in the UK (17 in Northern Ireland). Male homosexuality remains illegal in many jurisdictions, however.

Homosexual interests or experiences are common in adolescence. According to community surveys, up to 4 per cent of adult males are exclusively homosexual (gay) and an additional minority of men are bisexual to some degree. The percentages for females are similar. Some homosexuals resemble the opposite sex in their physical habits, mannerisms, or dress.

Causation of homosexuality, like heterosexuality, remains unclear. Reported biological factors include a genetic component, as demonstrated by twin studies. Hormone differences in the prenatal period have been suggested. Psychodynamic factors have also been postulated. The review by Bancroft (1994) concluded that 'it remains difficult, on scientific grounds, to avoid the conclusion that the uniquely human phenomenon of sexual orientation is a consequence of a multifactorial developmental process in which biological factors play a part, but in which psychosocial factors remain crucially important.'

In the past, various interventions, including psychotherapy, behaviour therapy, and hormone treatments, were tried in order to modify homosexual orientation, all to little effect. This is no longer considered appropriate, and modern approaches are designed to aid adaptation to the homosexual state, any coexisting psychiatric disorder being treated in standard fashion. For homosexuals facing other difficulties, services organized by gays themselves, such as telephone advice and self-help groups, may be appropriate sources of support.

Further reading

Bancroft, J. (1994). Homosexual orientation. *Br J Psychiatry* **164**, 437–440.
Tomlinson, J. (2002). *ABC of Sexual Health*. Oxford: Blackwell.

18 Child and adolescent psychiatry

Child and adolescent psychiatrists deal with patients up to school-leaving age. Most psychiatric disorders of childhood involve a quantitative rather than qualitative abnormality of emotion, conduct, or rate of development. Emotions or conduct considered abnormal at one age may be normal at another.

Community surveys have indicated that 7–20 per cent of children can be diagnosed as having psychiatric disorder. Prevalence is higher in inner-city areas than rural ones. There is a strong association with socio-economic deprivation. Only about 10 per cent of affected children receive psychiatric treatment.

Before puberty, boys have more psychiatric disorder than girls, and conduct disorders are more common than emotional disorders. During adolescence, the rates increase, with more girls affected and a higher proportion of emotional disorders.

Predisposing factors

Most cases probably have a multifactorial causation, including genetic predisposition to psychiatric disorder, biological factors such as poor nutrition before and/or after birth, and a psychologically stressful and/or deprived environment. Individual factors associated with childhood psychiatric disorder include the following:

Hughes' Outline of Modern Psychiatry, Fifth Edition. David Gill.
© 2007 John Wiley & Sons, Ltd   ISBN 9780470033920

- organic brain disease

- chronic physical disease

- low intelligence

- child abuse (see below)

- discord within the family, and undesirable parental attitudes, which include overprotection as well as hostility or neglect

- physical or mental illness in another family member, especially the mother; in the case of psychiatric disorder, the child's mental health may be at risk because of genetic factors as well as disruption of the home environment

- separation from the mother, especially if there is no adequate substitute; Bowlby's work on maternal deprivation formed the basis of 'attachment theory', emphasizing the importance of a consistent caregiver, who is usually but not necessarily the biological mother, during early life

- adoption

- single parent family

- lower social class

- poverty

- antisocial behaviour in family

- large family

- ethnic minority.

Classification

In clinical practice, disorders are usually grouped as follows:

- emotional/neurotic disorders

- conduct disorders

- psychoses

- specific delays in development

- symptomatic.

It is useful to consider a *multiaxial* approach, including the following:

- clinical psychiatric syndrome

- developmental level

- intellectual level

- medical conditions

- psychosocial situation.

History taking and examination

The child and both parents (or other main carers) need to be interviewed, either together or separately depending on the age of the child and the preferences of those concerned. Most of the history has to be obtained from the parents if the child is young. A separate interview with the parents may reveal problems of their own that are affecting the child, or have arisen through living with a disturbed child.

History

- *complaint*

- *history of present difficulties*

- *family*: age, occupation, and mental and physical health of parents and siblings; personal history of the parents including their own childhood; emotional atmosphere of the household

- *developmental history*:
  - pregnancy; whether planned, obstetric complications
  - milestones
  - illnesses
  - separations from parents, and reactions to these

- *school*: academic achievements, relations with other children and with teachers

- *life events* and *social difficulties*.

Interview with child

The older the child, the more he or she will be able to give a direct account of the problems. Although information from younger children may have to be obtained indirectly through play, drawing, or asking the child to tell a story or give 'three wishes', direct enquiry about the problems as perceived by the child should never be omitted.

Mental state

Observation of mental state is carried out under the same headings used in adult psychiatry. Particular attention should be given to signs suggesting minor neurological impairment: over- or underactivity, poor coordination, short attention span.

Physical examination

Neurological examination should be included.

Psychological testing

This may be done by the educational psychology service provided by local authorities to schools, or by the health service; it includes the following:

- intelligence
- educational achievements
- personality assessment
- motor and perceptual development.

Independent informant

- schoolteacher
- social worker
- general practitioner/health visitor.

A telephone call to a professional with knowledge of the family will frequently clarify a problem impossible to sort out in the consulting room.

Treatment

Psychological therapies, whether using a psychodynamic approach or a cognitive-behavioural one, have traditionally predominated over drug treatments in child psychiatry. The whole family should preferably be involved in therapy, since family functioning appears to have a marked influence on most psychiatric disorders of childhood. Sometimes, although the child is presented as the patient, the primary problem turns out to lie with another family member, such as a mother suffering from depression. In other cases, parents or siblings are being secondarily affected by the child's emotional disturbance.

Child psychiatry is usually practised in the community, with a team approach, often called Child and Adolescent Mental Health Services (CAMHS). Inpatient admission is rare. In child and family therapy centres, a team of professionals including child psychiatrists, educational psychologists, social workers, child psychotherapists, and community nurses carry out multidisciplinary treatment. Child psychiatrists and their colleagues also practise in general hospitals, special schools, social services assessment units, and remand homes.

Both assessment and management require collaboration between health, education, social, and legal services. Liaison child psychiatry is concerned with physically ill children, both in hospital and community settings.

Relationship with adult disorder

Prospective follow-up studies indicate that children with conduct disorders often continue to behave antisocially in adult life. Neurotic disorders have a better prognosis, but are weakly associated with adult neurosis of the same type. Childhood psychosis has a poor long-term outcome. Retrospective studies of adults with major mental illness, schizophrenia, and bipolar affective disorder show an excess of both conduct and neurotic disorders in childhood. However, only a minority of emotionally disturbed children develop major mental illness when they grow up.

The main clinical syndromes will now be described.

Neurotic (Emotional) disorders

Classical forms of neurotic illness, such as anxiety states or obsessive-compulsive disorder, sometimes occur in childhood, but mixed syndromes are more usual. Isolated phobias and rituals are common in otherwise well-adjusted children.

School attendance problems

School refusal is reluctance to attend school, due either to fear of teachers or other children (*school phobia*), or fear of leaving the mother (*separation anxiety*). The mother often covertly encourages it because she herself is depressed or immature, and reluctant to be separated from the child. The child may complain of headache or abdominal pain on school mornings. Treatment includes psychotherapy for the child and mother, dealing with any contributory factors at school, and encouragement to attend.

School refusal should be distinguished from *truanting*, which is staying away from school to do something more enjoyable, and is classed as a conduct disorder.

Affective disorders

Depression

Depressive symptoms, often reactive to a loss or other life stress, are common in young children but the full-blown picture of depressive illness is rare before puberty. Somatic symptoms like anorexia, abdominal pain, or headaches are a frequent presentation.

The treatment of depression in this age group has become controversial; cases have been widely reported in which links were claimed between suicide and the prescription of antidepressant medication. The question has recently been reviewed by NICE (2005), and a 'stepped care' approach was recommended. Professionals in primary care are advised against the prescription of antidepressant medication; it is considered that they should concentrate on support and risk assessment. Only in moderate to severe depression is antidepressant medication (fluoxetine) recommended, and then only in specialist hands.

Bipolar affective disorder occasionally starts in childhood, with either depressive or manic episodes. *Mania* may be misdiagnosed as conduct disorder or hyperkinetic syndrome (see below).

Suicide in early childhood is rare but suicide in adolescents, especially males, is increasing.

Conduct disorders

Conduct disorders involve persistent antisocial behaviour: stealing, lying, vandalism, truancy, aggression, and sexual disturbances. They are associated with adverse social circumstances, and with brain damage, and are about four times more common in boys than in girls. Treatment involves social casework and/or psychotherapy, family therapy being increasingly used. Behaviour therapy may modify a circumscribed problem.

Delinquency

'Juvenile delinquency' is law-breaking behaviour in children over the age of 10. Delinquency is strongly associated with social factors: disturbed families, large families, criminality in other family members, poverty, and residence in certain city neighbourhoods. In some areas, about 20 per cent of boys show delinquent behaviour. Delinquency is also associated with individual factors: low intelligence, brain damage, and minor physical deformities. Management of serious cases may involve supervision by a probation officer, local authority care, or a period of community service, but it is uncertain whether such measures influence the outcome. About 40 per cent of persistently delinquent teenagers become criminals in adult life.

Attention deficit disorder

Attention deficit disorder (hyperkinetic syndrome) is characterized by restlessness, impulsiveness, inability to concentrate, and short attention span. It is more common in boys. There is often a history of birth trauma or other cerebral insult in early life. Aggressive behaviour, low intelligence, epilepsy, minor motor abnormalities, and minor EEG changes are sometimes present. Food additives, as in coloured sweets or drinks, may exacerbate the symptoms.

This is a real syndrome but it has tended to be over-diagnosed, especially in the USA, the term 'minimal brain dysfunction' being applied to cases with no demonstrable abnormalities on examination or investigation.

Differential diagnosis includes mania.

A behavioural-modification programme combined with special teaching methods at school is the treatment of choice. Avoiding food additives may be helpful. The most effective short-term drug treatment is, paradoxically, with a cerebral stimulant such as dextroamphetamine, methylphenidate, or pemoline. These drugs have many adverse effects, including stunting growth, and they may be addictive, so are best reserved for occasional or short-term use. They are only lisensed for use as part of a multidisciplinary care package. Spontaneous improvement by adolescence is usual. Problems arise when children leave CAMHS for adult services and request continued prescription of stimulants, as they are not licensed in adults.

Psychoses

Childhood psychosis is rare, affecting 40 per 100 000 children. Types of such psychoses include *disintegrative (developmental) psychosis*, in which a child aged 2–8 years, previously normal, becomes emotionally withdrawn, loses speech, deteriorates intellectually, and shows emotional and behavioural disturbance. *Schilder's disease, lipoidosis*, and *SSPE* (subacute sclerosing panencephalitis, due to the measles virus) are among the causes of this rare condition.

Schizophrenia occasionally starts in childhood.

Autism is believed to be associated with abnormalities of cerebellar and brainstem function. Twin studies suggest a genetic predisposition. Prevalence is 20 per 100 000 children, and it is more common in boys. Learning disability, often due to a specific cause such as rubella, is present in 70 per cent of cases, whereas parental intelligence is in the normal range. Neurological impairments are found in 25 per cent, and 30 per cent develop epilepsy during adolescence.

Symptoms start within the first 30 months of life and include abnormal response to sound, failure to understand speech, either mutism or abnormal forms of speech (echolalia, nominal aphasia, or pronoun reversal), aloofness from people, and insistence on rituals and routines.

Autism seldom recovers and affected children often have substantial care needs, although their life expectancy is normal. The lower the IQ, the worse is the prognosis. Special education, behavioural methods, and psychotropic drug treatment may produce some improvement. *Kanner's syndrome* is autism with a normal IQ. *Asperger's syndrome*, or schizoid personality of childhood, may be a mild form of autism and comprises eccentric isolated behaviour with circumscribed interests and stilted speech: 'autistic traits'. The phrase *autistic spectrum disorder* may better describe the range of cases.

Delays in development

Educational underachievement

Causes include:

- *low IQ*

- *specific delays in development*. *Specific reading retardation*, or *dyslexia*, is an isolated difficulty in learning to read and write, more common in boys and sometimes associated with clumsiness and conduct disorder. *Specific arithmetical disorder* and *specific motor retardation* are also described as isolated syndromes. These disabilities may be improved by special teaching methods

- *physical handicaps*: problems with vision or hearing, epilepsy

- *poor relationships* with parents or teachers, or low parental expectations

- *boredom* in bright children

- *drug or solvent use*.

Nocturnal enuresis (bedwetting)

Bedwetting is a common problem, present in 15 per cent of 5-year-olds and 10 per cent of 10-year-olds and a small proportion of teenagers. Its causes include the following:

- *slow maturation,* which may have a genetic component, and is most common in boys from large and socially disadvantaged families

- *emotional disturbance*

- *medical disorders* such as urinary infection and diabetes

- *physical malformation* of the urinary tract.

Treatment is best directed toward the cause. Symptomatic measures include the following:

- *practical: limiting fluids* before bed, *toileting* before bed, and *lifting* the child at night

- *token economy regimes* such as a 'star chart' to reward dry nights

- *buzzer and pad* device

- *tricyclic antidepressants*, effective because of their anticholinergic properties; imipramine syrup is often used

- *desmopressin* nasal spray.

Encopresis (faecal incontinence)

Bowel control is normally achieved by the age of 4 years. Faecal incontinence affects 1 per cent of school-age children. Its causes include the following:

- *constipation with overflow* due to physical disorders such as anal fissure and Hirchsprung's disease

- *diarrhoea*, due to infection or other physical causes, or anxiety

- *psychological problems* such as neurotic disorders or disturbed family relationships

- *learning disability*.

Symptomatic disorders

Tics and Gilles de la Tourette syndrome

A tic is a repetitive, purposeless movement such as blinking or grunting, partly under voluntary control. Tics may develop in normal children, and are exacerbated by emotional disturbance. They are best ignored, and usually disappear spontaneously, but, if not, then behaviour therapy may help.

Gilles de la Tourette syndrome comprises multiple tics and compulsive utterances. Tics first affect the facial muscles, and then spread to other parts of the body. Involuntary utterances then occur, such as barking noises, and later obscene words or short phrases (coprolalia). Echolalia and echopraxia may be present. Onset is usually in childhood, and boys are affected three times more often than girls. The syndrome has a genetic component, and may be associated with organic brain disease or the presence of minor neurological signs. Medication with haloperidol, pimozide, or clonidine, and/or behaviour therapy, may be effective.

Eating disorders

Anorexia (loss of appetite) is usually the result of physical ill health. Excessive parental concern about food can result in anorexia, or lead the child to use food refusal or vomiting to manipulate the parents. Depression is another cause. *Anorexia nervosa* (see Chapter 15) occasionally affects prepubertal children but more often starts in adolescence.

Overeating is often a compensation for emotional deprivation. Overeating in adolescence usually causes obesity (and hence further emotional difficulties); obesity in youth is a growing public health problem, but not, of course, primarily a psychiatric one.

'Pica' is eating the inedible. Exploration of objects with the mouth is normal up to 2 years of age, but may continue for years in children who are blind, have learning disability, or lack environmental stimulation. Sucking lead-painted objects may cause mental and physical damage.

Child abuse

Abuse of children may be physical, sexual, and/or emotional. In recent years, there has been increased awareness of child abuse, and its actual frequency may also have increased. Up to 5 per cent of children are reported to professional agencies because of suspected abuse.

Most child abuse is carried out by the parents. Such parents are typically young, immature, and poor, and were abused during their own childhood. The 'cycle of abuse' is a phrase which expresses this tendency for abuse to run in families. A small minority is mentally ill. There is a raised incidence of factors likely to impair bonding between parents and child: unwanted pregnancy, complications during pregnancy or birth, separations between parents and child, and ill health in the child.

Physical abuse (non-accidental injury, baby battering)

Fractured bones, periosteal haemorrhage, bruises, retinal haemorrhage, and cigarette burns are common manifestations. The child is often retarded in both mental and physical development. The parents themselves may bring the child for treatment, claiming the injury was accidental. Some cases lead to the death of the child.

A variant is *Munchausen syndrome by proxy*, in which a carer, usually the mother, fabricates illness in a child by giving a false medical history and/or inflicting deliberate physical harm. It is criminal behaviour, not an illness, although perpetrators will need a psychiatric assessment.

Sexual abuse

This is a topical and controversial subject. Sexual abuse of children appears to be a common problem, but poses diagnostic difficulties because it is so often concealed. Both over- and under-diagnosis may have serious consequences for both (alleged) victim and (alleged) perpetrator. Possibly about 10 per cent of children undergo sexual abuse, ranging from touching to penetrative intercourse.

Most victims are girls, abused by their fathers, brothers, or other male relatives. Sexual abuse of boys is more often carried out by men outside the family, either an authority figure such as teacher, clergyman, or scoutmaster, or a stranger who offers bribes. Occasionally the perpetrator is female.

Some cases come to light because the child, or mother, seeks help directly from a treatment agency. More often the presentation is indirect, such as genital bruising or infection, early teenage pregnancy, a crisis such as an overdose or running away from home, vague neurotic symptoms, or inhibited development. Many cases remain concealed.

Victims of child sex abuse appear to be at increased risk of certain psychiatric disorders in adult life. These include psychosexual difficulties, neuroses, personality disorders, eating disorders, somatization, and deliberate self-harm. The proportion of victims who suffer serious long-term effects of this kind is not known; however, most authorities agree that sexual experience with adults is almost always harmful to the child. Even if it takes place in the context of a superficially affectionate relationship, the surrounding secrecy and coercion are likely to induce fear or guilt in the child.

Emotional abuse and neglect

Children whose parents are habitually critical and rejecting, and neglect physical and/or emotional care, may present with delays in development, recurrent minor physical ailments, or disordered behaviour.

Management of abuse

If there is considered to be a risk to a child, all health-care staff are under a legal obligation to notify the local authority child protection team, so that the risk can be assessed and any appropriate action taken. Sometimes, this duty to inform the local authority may involve a potential breach of confidentiality, as in respect of an adult psychiatric patient who is a parent. (This can lead to difficulties, so it is wise to discuss such matters within one's team or with a colleague or professional adviser.)

If there is immediate risk, the child can be received into foster care, or taken to a place of safety; sometimes this is with the agreement of the parents ('voluntary accommodation'); on other occasions, the local authority will apply to a magistrate under the Children Act.

Medical assessment of suspected cases of physical or sexual abuse should only be carried out by a senior paediatrician or child psychiatrist with relevant experience, because of the sensitive nature of this work and the diagnostic difficulties that may arise.

Social services departments are responsible for prevention and management, and keep a register of children at risk. This would be followed typically by a multidisciplinary case conference, attended by social workers and other professionals such as police, health visitor, GP, paediatrician, and child psychiatrist. Under the Children Act 1989, the child's interests receive priority over other considerations.

Close surveillance combined with family and individual psychotherapy may enable the family to remain intact, but in some cases it is necessary to remove the perpetrator to prison and/or take the abused child into care.

The tragic death of Victoria Climbie was followed by an inquiry (http://www.victoria-climbie-inquiry.org.uk/); among its recommendations was the establishment of a Children's Commissioner to oversee services and make sure that children's needs are included.

Psychiatry of adolescence

Psychiatric disorder is present in 15–20 per cent of adolescents. 'Adolescent turmoil' (identity crisis), when the process of maturation involves mood swings, rebellious behaviour, or experimentation with contrasting lifestyles, is a common phenomenon that may be confused with psychiatric illness.

Schizophrenia, affective disorders, neuroses, eating disorders, substance misuse, and deliberate self-harm may all begin during adolescence, and personality disorders may become clearly evident at this time. Drug misuse and completed suicide in adolescents are becoming increasingly common.

Distinguishing adolescents with formal psychiatric illness from those whose problems stem from disturbance of adjustment and relationships, or substance misuse, can require prolonged observation.

Treatment of seriously disturbed adolescents may be carried out in a residential unit. Length of stay is usually several months and treatment methods are predominantly psychotherapeutic, whether or not involving the patient's family.

Reference

NICE (National Institute for Health and Clinical Excellence) (2005). Depression in children and young people. www.nice.org.uk/CG028.

Further reading

Barker, P. (2004). *Basic Child Psychiatry* (7th edn). Oxford: Blackwell Scientific.
Viner, R. (2005). *ABC of Adolescence.* Oxford: Blackwell/BMJ Books.

19 Learning disability

The terms *learning disability* (LD) and *learning difficulties* are now used in preference to older ones such as *mental handicap*, *mental retardation*, or *mental subnormality*. Sometimes, patients with LD need to be admitted to hospital compulsorily under the Mental Health Act 1983; if so, the grounds are 'abnormally aggressive or seriously irresponsible conduct', and *mental impairment* is the term used.

For practical purposes, LD is defined in terms not only of low IQ (intelligence quotient) test results, but also difficulty in coping independently and/or behavioural problems. Below 70 is the most frequently used marker for LD. Corresponding IQ levels are about 50–69 for mild cases, and below 49 for severe ones, but many people with IQs below 70 lead independent lives and do not need special medical or social care.

Frequency

An IQ below 70 is found in 2.5 per cent of the general population, and 0.4 per cent have an IQ below 50. Severe LD is 25 per cent more common in males than females, mostly due to X-linked conditions.

Causes

About 70 per cent of mild cases belong to the 'non-specific' or 'subcultural' group, in which handicap results from a poor genetic intellectual endowment

Hughes' Outline of Modern Psychiatry, Fifth Edition. David Gill.
© 2007 John Wiley & Sons, Ltd   ISBN 9780470033920

combined with a physically, educationally, and/or emotionally deprived up-bringing. Mild LD is associated with poverty, overcrowding, large family size, and family disruption. Child abuse is an important but often unrecognized factor.

About 30 per cent of mild cases, and nearly all severe cases, result from a specific organic pathology. About 35 per cent of severe cases have a gene or chromosome abnormality, Down's syndrome being most frequent, and about 65 per cent have acquired brain damage. Specific causes can be classified as follows:

- *chromosome or gene abnormalities*, as in Down's syndrome and phenylketonuria

- *primary maldevelopments of the brain of obscure aetiology*, such as spina bifida with hydrocephalus, and microgyria

- *prenatal factors affecting the mother*, such as rubella, cytomegalovirus, toxoplas-mosis, syphilis, radiation, malnutrition, alcoholism, and teratogenic drugs

- *perinatal damage*, as caused by birth trauma, anoxia, rhesus incompatibility, or extreme prematurity

- *post-natal damage*, as caused by encephalitis, meningitis, lead poisoning, or head injury.

Diagnosis of learning disability

Severe cases are usually obvious from infancy, because developmental delay and physical abnormalities are present. Mild cases may remain undetected until learn-ing difficulties become apparent at school. Differential diagnosis includes deaf-ness and emotional disturbance.

Investigation should aim to find the cause and effects of the LD, and of any associated psychiatric disorder. It includes medical history, family history, physical examination, mental state examination, chromosome studies, and testing of blood and urine for abnormal metabolites. Discovery of a specific cause enables genetic counselling for the family, and occasionally permits specific treatment for the child, such as special diets for certain enzyme defects. Even if no specific cause is found, a detailed psychological, medical, and social assessment will permit informed decisions on aims and methods of management.

Associated phenomena

- *Physical health problems,* including motor disorders, malformations, and impairments of sight and hearing, are present in about 30 per cent of severe cases.

- *Epilepsy* is seen in about 25 per cent, being more frequent the lower the IQ.

- *Psychiatric illness* is seen in up to 40 per cent. Patients may not have the linguistic ability to describe psychiatric symptoms, so they present with behaviour disturbance. There is a raised incidence of all common mental health problems, including both affective and psychotic illnesses (Smiley, 2005).

- *Behaviour disturbance.* Causes include:
  - a manifestation of the underlying brain damage
  - a manifestation of the underlying genotype (behavioural phenotype)
  - psychiatric illness
  - physical illness
  - excessive, insufficient or inappropriate medication (psychotropics, anticonvulsants)
  - frustration with a boring or repressive environment
  - communication difficulties
  - adjustment reactions following stressful events, such as change of residence or bereavement. People with LD may be just as much affected by such psychological stresses as anyone else, and also may need a longer time to adjust to them.

Behaviour disturbance in the form of aggression, overactivity, or self-mutilation is present in about half of severe cases, and is often the reason for families requesting institutional care for a child with LD. Behaviour disturbance is also found in adults with milder impairments who are living in the community, and often leads to conflict with the law.

Failure to learn desirable behaviour of which the patient is potentially capable, such as speech and self-care, may also be considered as a type of behaviour disturbance.

Management

A multidisciplinary approach is appropriate, with a view to helping people with learning disabilities to integrate into the general community ('normalization') and meet such personal needs as close relationships and appropriate occupation.

Medical management includes diagnosis and treatment of physical and psychiatric problems. In clinical practice, the presence of LD in a given patient will be well known in most cases, but what requires to be dealt with may be a change in behaviour or the development of overt psychiatric symptoms.

Methods of *assessment* and treatment may need to be modified from those used for people without intellectual impairment (Bradley and Lofchy, 2005). However, it is important to talk to the patient as much as possible directly, not just to the caregivers, and to involve him in the assessment.

If psychotropic drugs are used, the optimum regimen has to be found by titrating the dose against the target problems, perhaps over a period of several months. LD patients tend to be very sensitive to the effect of medication; doses must therefore start low and be increased only cautiously and gradually, if necessary. Unwanted effects are also more frequent; it is a question of balancing the benefits and drawbacks of medication in an individual patient.

Psychologists are involved in assessing patients' overall intelligence, and any specific defects or abilities. They help to plan individual behavioural treatments, which can be useful even in severe cases for teaching self-care, practical skills, and social behaviour. Desirable behaviour or the acquisition of skills is given positive reinforcement by a tangible reward or approving attention. Undesirable behaviour may be a means of seeking attention, in which case it is best ignored, or it can be managed by occupying the patients with interesting alternative activities.

Social and educational aspects are important. Improving the environment of children from deprived backgrounds has been shown to lead to increases in IQ, although it is uncertain whether this improvement is maintained into adult life. Many parents of affected children prefer to keep them at home, and this is frequently possible with help from community services. Alternatives include sheltered accommodation such as locally based hospital units (LBHUs), community homes, and hostels provided by the local authority. Long-term hospital care is now discouraged, except for very severe cases or those with extremely 'challenging behaviour', but people with LD and superadded psychiatric or behavioural disorders may well require acute admission to specialist units from time to time.

Children with mild LD are placed in ordinary schools if possible. They will be 'statemented' by the local education authority, ensuring extra help in the classroom from learning-support assistants. Special schools exist for severe cases. Further training after school-leaving age is provided in adult training centres. Some patients can hold ordinary jobs, and others are employed in sheltered workshops.

Prognosis

Mild cases have a good prognosis and are usually capable of living independently in adulthood. Some are 'late developers' who eventually achieve an IQ within the normal range.

Life expectancy for severely affected patients used to be short, but many now survive into middle or old age.

Prevention

Many cases of LD could be prevented by the following measures:

- *improved antenatal and obstetric care*, such as rubella immunization for girls, treatment of rhesus incompatibility, and special care of low-birthweight babies

- *screening of neonates*, to detect such metabolic conditions as phenylketonuria and hypothyroidism

- *improved infant welfare*, including immunization programmes, and early detection of mild LD and impaired sight and hearing

- *genetic counselling*, which has become more important with recent advances in molecular genetics. For parents who have already produced a child with a gene or chromosome abnormality, it may be possible to calculate a precise risk of any future children being affected. In the case of recessive conditions, the carrier state in relatives can be determined. Genetic counselling should preferably be carried out as a planned procedure, rather than delayed until a new pregnancy is already in progress

- *prenatal diagnosis*: whereby many congenital abnormalities can now be detected at an early stage of pregnancy, allowing the option of aborting an affected foetus should the mother choose this course.

Techniques include the following:

- *ultrasound*: to confirm gestational age and detect major structural abnormalities.
- *serum alpha-fetoprotein (AFP)*: offered to pregnant women: raised levels suggest a neural tube defect such as anencephaly or myelomeningocele. Low levels can suggest Down's syndrome.
- *amniocentesis*: offered if AFP is abnormal. Amniotic fluid is sampled by the transabdominal route. Foetal chromosomes are examined, and specific genetic defects excluded by enzyme estimations or gene probes. Amniocentesis carries a small risk of causing miscarriage, infection, or damage to the child.
- *chorionic villus biopsy* (CVB): offered at 6–8 weeks for high-risk pregnancies only. Chromosome and gene abnormalities can be detected. Chorion sampling is carried out by the transvaginal or transabdominal route, and carries a small risk of causing miscarriage.

Before such tests are carried out, the mother (and father) should be informed about their purpose, their accuracy, the implications of both positive and negative results, and any risks attached to them.

Some important specific causes of LD will be described in the text. The box gives a fuller list, but is not complete; new genetic syndromes are continually being identified.

Box 19.1 Some Specific Causes of LD

Autosomal chromosome abnormalities:
    Down's syndrome*
    Trisomy D (trisomy 13; Patau's syndrome)
    Trisomy E (trisomy 18; Edwards' syndrome)
    'Cri du chat' syndrome
Sex chromosome abnormalities:
    Males:
        Fragile X syndrome (Martin–Bell syndrome)*
        XYY syndrome*
        XXY syndrome (Klinefelter's syndrome)*
    Females:
        XO syndrome (Turner's syndrome)*
        XXX syndrome*

Autosomal dominant gene abnormalities:
  Tuberous sclerosis*
Autosomal recessive gene abnormalities
  Phenylketonuria*
  Homocystinuria – aminoaciduria
  Hartnup disease – aminoaciduria
  Maple syrup urine disease – aminoaciduria
  Galactosaemia*
  Tay–Sachs disease*
  Gaucher's syndrome – lipid storage disorder
  Niemann–Pick disease – lipid storage disorder
  Hand–Schueller–Christian disease – lipid storage disorder
  Hurler's syndrome (gargoylism) – mucopolysaccharide storage
    disorder
  Laurence–Moon–Biedl syndrome*
  Congenital hypothyroidism*
Sex-linked recessive gene abnormalities
  Lesch–Nyhan syndrome*
  Hunter's syndrome – mucopolysaccharide storage disorder
Prenatal infection
  Cytomegalovirus*
  Toxoplasmosis*
  Rubella*
  Syphilis*
Birth complications
  Birth injury*
  Rhesus incompatibility*
Post-natal damage
  Encephalitis, meningitis
  HIV infection
  Severe head injury
  Lead poisoning*
Miscellaneous
  Hydrocephalus*
  Microcephaly*

*See following text.

Chromosomal abnormalities

Abnormalities of the autosomal chromosomes usually cause severe LD combined with widespread anatomical deformities, but the effect of sex chromosome abnormalities is more variable.

Autosomal chromosomes

Down's syndrome is caused by one of two conditions, trisomy 21 or translocation of chromosome 21. It is the most common specific cause of LD, occurring in 1 per 650 pregnancies.

Trisomy 21 does not generally run in families, but becomes more frequent with increasing maternal age, as shown in the following table:

Maternal age	Frequency of trisomy 21 (per 1000 births)
under 35	1
35–39	4
40–44	13
over 45	35

Translocation of chromosome 21, which is not related to maternal age, may result from mosaicism in either parent, in which case there is a likelihood of future pregnancies also being affected. This disorder also occurs sporadically.

LD, often severe, is always present. Physical features include a typical facial appearance with slanting palpebral fissures, short little finger with only one palmar crease ('trident hand' and 'simian crease'), hypotonic muscles, cardiac defects (10 per cent of patients), and high susceptibility to chest infections, lymphatic leukaemia, and premature ageing. Patients used to die young, but many now live to middle or old age, often developing Alzheimer's disease in their 40s (an observation which helped to locate an Alzheimer's gene to chromosome 21).

There are differing opinions as to whether all pregnant women should be offered antenatal screening for detection of Down's syndrome; certainly, older mothers, and those with a previously affected baby, should have the option to be screened.

Sex chromosomes

Sex chromosome abnormalities are described here although they are not always associated with LD.

Male phenotype

Fragile X (Martin–Bell syndrome) is the next most common genetic cause of LD after Down's syndrome. The long arm of the X chromosome appears to have a fragile tip when grown in special media, due to a gene with multiple abnormal DNA triplicate repeat sequences (of CGG). Fragile X syndrome is a common cause of severe LD in males, and causes lesser degrees of disability in some carrier females. Affected males have large testes (macroorchidism), 'bat ears', and long faces. Psychotic symptoms, aggressive or socially impaired behaviour associated with social anxiety, and language impairments are common. Screening in pregnancy for women from affected families offers the possibility of aborting foetuses with Fragile X.

XYY syndrome is associated with low IQ, infertility, neurological disorders, tallness, skeletal disorders, and myopia, but some cases are phenotypically normal.

XXY syndrome (Klinefelter's syndrome) comprises hypogonadism, infertility, tallness, effeminate body shape, and usually low IQ. Testosterone therapy may render the appearance more masculine.

Female phenotype

XO syndrome (Turner's syndrome) comprises ovarian dysgenesis, short stature, webbed neck, and sometimes coarctation of the aorta. IQ may be normal or low, and visuo-spatial disorders are often present. Patients are infertile, but oestrogen therapy may render their appearance more feminine.

XXX syndrome (triple X, 'superfemale') is sometimes associated with low IQ and physical abnormalities, but other cases are phenotypically normal. Patients are not infertile, but their children may have various chromosome abnormalities. Women with more than three X chromosomes have LD and numerous physical defects.

Gene abnormalities

Autosomal dominant

Tuberous sclerosis is characterized by LD (in about 40 per cent of cases), epilepsy (in about 60 per cent of cases), and facial angiofibromas. Nodules of neuroglia, sometimes calcified, occur in the brain and show on a brain scan. Muscular and vascular tumours may occur in various organs, and 'café au lait spots' and 'shagreen patches' on the skin. Disease-determining gene loci have been found on chromosomes 9 and 16.

Autosomal recessive

Phenylketonuria occurs in 4 per 100 000 live births. It results from a defect in phenylalanine hydroxylase, the enzyme that converts phenylalanine to tyrosine, or from enzyme defects in the subsequent metabolic pathway. Phenylpyruvic acid and other abnormal metabolites of phenylalanine are present in the urine after 3 weeks of age, enabling a screening test to be carried out. Carriers of the gene can be detected by a phenylalanine loading test for genetic counselling purposes. Patients have fair colouring, because melanin production is impaired. Untreated cases have severe LD, but if a low-phenylalanine diet is started in infancy and continued until age 10, intellectual development may approach normal.

Galactosaemia results from a defect of galactose 1-phosphate uridyltransferase, the enzyme that converts galactose to glucose. Vomiting, jaundice, and hepatosplenomegaly are present from infancy, and cataracts develop later. It can be detected by finding galactose in the urine. A diet free from milk and other galactose-containing foods ameliorates the symptoms.

Tay–Sachs disease is a degenerative condition of the central nervous system due to an abnormality of lipid metabolism. It occurs mostly in Jewish families. A cherry-red spot appears on the macula after a few months of age and is followed by optic atrophy and blindness. Epileptic fits develop, and patients usually die about the age of 2 years.

Hurler's syndrome (*gargoylism*) is a disorder of the metabolism of mucopolysaccharides, which accumulate in the brain and other organs, causing hepatosplenomegaly. Aggressive temperament may be associated.

Laurence–Moon–Biedl syndrome comprises LD, retinitis pigmentosa, polydactyly, obesity, and hypogonadism.

Congenital hypothyroidism, due to deficiency of one of the enzymes involved in thyroxine synthesis, causes general retardation of development with lethargy and a puffy appearance. Symptoms can be alleviated by lifelong thyroxine replacement therapy.

Sex-linked recessive

Lesch–Nyhan syndrome results from a defect of purine metabolism, with accumulation of uric acid. There is severe LD, self-mutilation, spasticity, and choreo-athetosis. 5-Hydroxytryptophan treatment may ameliorate the behaviour disorder.

Acquired handicap

Prenatal infections

Cytomegalovirus is the commonest form of intrauterine infection to cause LD. The mother is usually symptom-free. The child has microcephaly, necrotizing haemorrhaging encephalitis, and intracerebral calcification, and may die in early life.

Toxoplasmosis is a protozoal infection that causes LD, choroidoretinitis, and miliary intracranial calcification. Maternal infection can be detected by serological testing in pregnancy.

Rubella, if contracted by a woman during the first trimester of pregnancy, can cause LD, deafness, cataract and cardiac lesions in the child. Such cases are preventable by vaccination of girls who have not developed natural immunity to rubella in childhood.

Congenital syphilis, now rare, causes LD, deafness, keratitis, and malformed teeth, and general paralysis of the insane (GPI) develops in adolescence. Serological tests may be negative. It can be prevented by screening pregnant women and giving antisyphilitic treatment if required.

Birth complications

Birth injury or rhesus incompatibility may cause LD associated with either spasticity or athetoid movements of one or more limbs (cerebral palsy).

Post-natal damage

Lead poisoning may result from exposure to high concentrations of petrol fumes, or from sucking lead-painted objects, as children already handicapped by low IQ or sensory impairments are particularly likely to do. It causes mild intellectual impairment, anaemia with basophil stippling of red cells, and a 'lead line' on the gums and epiphyses.

Miscellaneous

Hydrocephalus has various causes: congenital malformation of the fourth ventricle associated with spina bifida, meningitis, or brainstem tumour in childhood, or rarely a sex-linked inherited condition. Insertion of a shunt ameliorates brain damage.

Microcephaly may result from a recessive autosomal gene and comprises severe LD, overactivity, and a low cephalic index, which gives a bird-like appearance. Microcephaly may also result from other causes such as radiation or cytomegalovirus infection *in utero*.

References

Bradley, E. and Lofchy, J. (2005). Learning disability in the accident and emergency department. *Adv Psychiatr Treat* **11**, 45–57.

Smiley, E. (2005). Epidemiology of mental health problems in adults with learning disability: an update. *Adv Psychiatr Treat* **11**, 214–222.

20 Psychiatry of old age

The psychiatry of old age is of growing importance, because the proportion of elderly people in the UK population is increasing. 'Old age' services, as opposed to 'general adult' services, may take patients over the age of 65 or 70, depending on local arrangements. In some districts, patients with long-term mental health problems from adult life are kept on by general psychiatry, with elderly psychiatry taking cases which present after 65 or other agreed cutoff.

Psychiatric illness becomes more common with advancing age, because elderly people have a high prevalence of cerebral and systemic diseases that can cause organic brain syndromes, and because they are often subject to emotional stresses and loss. These include the deaths of spouse, siblings, and friends; loss of occupation, company, and income after retirement; deterioration in bodily functions; the prospect of further ageing and death; and, sometimes, both within private households and institutions, mistreatment by those with the responsibility for care ('elder abuse').

Frequency

Community surveys show the following approximate prevalence figures for psychiatric illness in people over the age of 65:

Hughes' Outline of Modern Psychiatry, *Fifth Edition*. David Gill.
© 2007 John Wiley & Sons, Ltd   ISBN 9780470033920

Depression   15%
Anxiety and phobias   15%
Dementia   10%

Prevalence rises sharply after about the age of 75.

Clinical syndromes
Depression

Depression (see Chapter 5) is the most common psychiatric disorder in old people, and first admission rates for depression are highest in the 50–70 age group. Mixed anxiety-depressive states frequently present in primary care with psychiatric symptoms, insomnia, physical problems, or social difficulties ('failure to cope'). Most depressive episodes recover in the short term, but long-term prognosis is worse than for younger patients. At least 70 per cent develop further episodes.

Suicide rates rise with age, and suicide in elderly people is often associated with clinical depression as well as with social isolation.

Depression in old people may be associated with cognitive impairment and therefore be difficult to distinguish from early dementia. A careful history, mental state examination, and brain scan often help to make the distinction, but the two disorders may coexist.

Antidepressant drugs are effective, but low doses should initially be used because unwanted effects, such as postural hypotension with tricyclics, are more severe than in younger adults. If successful, antidepressants should be continued for 1–2 years in old people, perhaps even for life, because of the high likelihood of relapse. ECT is readily considered in the elderly, as it acts more quickly than medication and, apart from transient mental confusion, often has fewer unwanted effects. ECT may be lifesaving in a severely depressed patient who is dehydrated due to refusal to eat and drink.

Mania (see Chapter 5)

Although first admission rates for mania show a slight increase with age, it remains an unusual presentation. It is important to exclude physical causes such as a brain tumour, cerebrovascular disease, or medication such as steroids, especially if a careful search (old case notes, interviewing relatives) fails to reveal any previous history. Patients with long-standing bipolar illness tend to suffer less mania and more depression if they survive into old age. Transient depressive symptoms occur during most manic illnesses in the elderly. Physical illness or injuries often result from self-neglect and overactivity, so inpatient treatment is desirable.

Schizophrenia (see Chapter 4) *and paranoid disorders* (see Chapter 8)

A small proportion of psychotic illnesses (probably less than 10 per cent) start after the age of 65. This is usually the paranoid form with good preservation of general personality. (The term *paraphrenia* may be used.) It is important to check for sensory impairment, which may be contributing to the problem by increasing the patient's isolation and reinforcing any paranoid tendency. Social activity, as through a day centre or residential home, may be helpful if the patient will accept it. Antipsychotic drugs are used, but results are sometimes disappointing.

Case example

A widower aged 73 had lived an increasingly isolated life since retirement. His GP was called to see him as an emergency by the police, to whom he had made frequent 999 calls alleging that his neighbours were trying to murder him with gas. Apart from his obvious delusions, he was otherwise in good health. He did not believe that he was in any way unwell. He was compulsorily admitted, after a domiciliary visit from the duty psychiatrist, to a psychiatric ward under the Mental Health Act 1983. He was unwilling to take oral medication, but his symptoms partially resolved with a small dose of a depot antipsychotic injection. Although he could be discharged, he remained isolated and generally suspicious, and his community psychiatric nurse frequently had difficulty in persuading him to have his injection.

Neurotic disorders (see Chapter 6)

Reactions to bereavement or other stressors may produce brief adjustment disorders in the elderly, just as in younger people; however, it is unusual for a prolonged neurotic condition to become established in an elderly person who has previously been free of such symptoms. Such a first presentation in an elderly person should raise suspicion of organic disorder or depressive illness.

Dementia, delirium, and other organic brain syndromes

(see Chapter 10)

Case example

A woman of 83 had been diagnosed as suffering from moderate to severe dementia of Alzheimer's type, but was able to remain at home because of the devoted care of her 62-year-old daughter. Her behaviour became much more agitated and confused over a period of 2 days, alternating with periods of drowsiness; her urine had become foul-smelling over this time. The GP and community psychiatric nurse diagnosed acute-on-chronic confusion due to urinary tract infection, and continued to look after the patient at home, for her daughter wished to avoid hospital admission. With antibiotics, a change of catheter, and some sedation with small doses of chlorpromazine, the patient's condition returned to normal over a few days. Her daughter nevertheless appeared exhausted, and regular respite care admissions were arranged to ease her burden.

Alcohol and drugs

Alcohol misuse (see Chapter 13) may become a problem in old age, but is often concealed. Depression, loneliness, and boredom, perhaps following the death of a spouse, are common precipitants. Drug misuse (see Chapter 12) usually involves prescribed drugs, such as benzodiazepines, which often cause ataxia and cognitive impairment in this age group. If an elderly person with unrecognized alcohol or drug dependence develops an intercurrent illness and/or is admitted to hospital, withdrawal symptoms may ensue.

Assessment

Although it is important to reach a psychiatric and/or medical diagnosis, identification of the practical problems facing the patient may be the most urgent requirement. Often the point at issue is whether he or she is able to cope at home. This may hinge on something as mundane as, for example, whether a neighbour who does the shopping is prepared to continue doing so.

An assessment in the patient's home surroundings is more meaningful than one carried out in hospital, and an interview with an informant is highly desirable, especially if there is any question of cognitive impairment. The timespan of the illness can be crucial in making a diagnosis; an acute confusional state will usually come on over hours or days, a mental illness such as depression over weeks, and dementia over months or years.

Psychiatric history and mental state are recorded in the usual way (see Chapter 3). Particular emphasis should be placed on medical factors and social circumstances, and it is essential to test cognitive function. Physical examination may well reveal undiagnosed pathology that needs attention.

Standardized instruments for interviewing elderly patients include the CAMDEX (Cambridge Examination for Mental Disorders of the Elderly) and the GMSS (Geriatric Mental State Schedule). Short questionnaires for assessing cognitive function include the Mini Mental State Examination.

Specific treatments

Psychotropic drugs (see Chapter 23) should be used in small starting doses because of the following facts:

- Metabolism and excretion are slow.

- Both therapeutic effects and unwanted effects may be found with low doses.

- Medical conditions necessitating caution in drug use may be present.

- Interactions with other medication may occur.

Forgetfulness and other factors may lead to poor compliance, so single-drug therapy in once-daily dosage is desirable. The prescriber should become familiar with a small number of preparations and their unwanted effects, make a special effort to gain the trust of the patient, and pay great attention to explanation and detail. For example, someone with severe arthritis of the hands may not be able to take tablets dispensed in a 'blister pack'; and a change in colour of tablet, or from tablet to capsule, may be especially worrying for an elderly person.

Antidepressants: either *tricyclics* or *SSRIs* may be used. Tricyclics are cheaper, have predictable unwanted effects, and can be started at very low doses. Some authorities recommend drugs of secondary tricyclic structure, such as *nortripty-line*, because anticholinergic and hypotensive effects are less than with tertiary tricyclics such as amitriptyline.

The major advantage of the SSRIs is their lack of toxicity in overdosage. However, they frequently cause worsening in anxiety and gastrointestinal upset, although it is not possible to predict which patients will be affected.

Lithium is used in prophylaxis of depression and mania.

Sedatives for use in psychosis or agitation include the following:

• *Promazine* is an effective sedative but weak antipsychotic.

• *Haloperidol* is often effective in doses as low as 1 mg, but it has marked Parkinsonian side-effects.

• *'Atypical' antipsychotics*, such as olanzepine and risperidone, have, since the last edition of this book, come and gone for use in the elderly. They rapidly became popular on introduction, because of a perceived reduction in extrapyramidal side-effects. However, it has now become clear that olanzepine and risperidone are associated with an increased risk of stroke in elderly patients with dementia, and the CSM has advised that risperidone and olanzepine should not be used for treating behavioural symptoms of dementia.

• *Hypnotics and 'minor' tranquillizers* were overprescribed in the past, creating a large population of elderly long-term users. However, it is possible that the pendulum has swung too far against these drugs; provided they are used judiciously in line with *British National Formulary* recommendations, they remain a safe and effective treatment for transient neurotic states such as insomnia after bereavement.

ECT (see Chapter 24) may be used if the patient is fit for anaesthetic, and is often better tolerated than antidepressant drugs, but many patients need long-term drug prophylaxis also.

Psychological treatments (see Chapter 22)

Psychotherapy in its briefer forms may be helpful, but not in dementia (Burns *et al.*, 2005). Intensive exploratory work is inappropriate because major changes in personality or attitudes are not likely to be achieved. Individual or group treatment may be focused on adaptation to bereavement or the other losses of old age. *Marital therapy* may be indicated, because conflicts in a marriage often become more obvious when the partners are brought into constant contact by retirement or restricted mobility. Special techniques for this age group include *reality orientation* (RO) and *reminiscence therapy*.

Practical memory aids (e.g. PDAs) may be of benefit for dementia patients.

Organization of services

The vast bulk of psychiatric disorder is coped with by patients themselves, their relatives, and their carers; some cases are recognized and treated in primary care, but only the minority reach secondary care. GPs have sometimes been criticized for not knowing about such problems in patients on their list, but there are indications that GPs avoid making these diagnoses if they feel, as is often, unfortunately, the case, that local psychiatric services for the elderly are overstretched.

Multidisciplinary teams in old-age psychiatry, as in general adult psychiatry (see Chapter 26), include doctors, nurses, psychologists, social workers, and occupational therapists. They work in liaison with primary health-care teams, social services, and gerontology departments.

Many of the problems identified in a comprehensive assessment are *social* rather than psychiatric, and require practical interventions accordingly. For example, a depressed patient living alone in poor accommodation will be unlikely to make a good recovery with antidepressant medication alone. Attending a day centre might combat loneliness and improve nutrition, and a social worker would advise about housing and social security benefits.

Physical problems also need to be addressed. Undiagnosed medical illness, inappropriate medication, and dietary deficiencies are common in this age group.

Hospital admission is frequently valuable to treat illness or, commonly, to relieve a social crisis. However, hospitalization should not be undertaken too lightly. Many old people survive in their own homes through a complex network of informal care and company from relatives, friends, church, the voluntary sector, and domestic pets, and this network may prove impossible to reassemble following an admission. If the patient does go into hospital, a gradual discharge with increasing periods of home leave is the rule.

Occupational therapy assessment is often important, to see whether the patient can manage day-to-day tasks such as cooking, cleaning, and shopping.

Inpatient facilities include assessment wards for functional psychiatric illness and for dementia patients. These are separate from the wards for younger adults, but some facilities may be shared with physicians for the elderly.

Respite admissions at regular planned intervals are particularly valued by relatives, and provide patients themselves with care and company, and an opportunity for thorough medical and nursing review.

Day hospital care is often preferable to inpatient admission, and also less costly.

Home care, a 'package' of 'community care', not only supports people with continuing difficulties, but can also be used as a treatment, with increased support at times of crisis.

Most care is now provided in the community. However, old-age psychiatry remains a 'Cinderella' specialty with many unmet needs; it is clear that the health and social services would be entirely unable to cope were it not for unpaid carers and the voluntary sector.

A major change has been the new responsibility of local authority social services to 'purchase' appropriate care for individuals. This care may range from provision of home helps, laundry, and meals-on-wheels, to residential accommodation. Such measures can no longer be directly prescribed by health services, so good local, day-to-day working relationships with social workers are vital. Integrated teams of health and social services staff are now the norm.

Supported accommodation, such as warden-controlled housing, can be very helpful in maintaining independent living. Alternatives include nursing or residential homes, almost all privately run now. Long-stay hospital provision for dementia patients is now almost extinct.

Reference

Burns, A., Guthrie, F., Marino-Francis, E. *et al.* (2005). Brief psychotherapy in Alzheimer's disease: randomized controlled trial. *British Journal of Psychiatry* **187**, 143–147.

Further reading

Jacoby, R. and Oppenheimer, C. (2002). *Psychiatry in the Elderly* (3rd edn). Oxford: Oxford University Press.

21 Forensic psychiatry

Strictly speaking, 'forensic' psychiatry could refer to any aspect of psychiatry with a legal dimension. In practice, however, the term 'forensic psychiatry' applies mainly to the interface between psychiatry and offending (criminal) behaviour.

For convenience, risk assessment and report writing, both of which are relevant to all of psychiatry, are discussed in this chapter.

Forensic psychiatrists are psychiatrists (mostly general adult but some child and adolescent as well) with special knowledge of offending behaviour among the mentally disordered, and the law relating to this. Their role includes:

- assessment and care of patients in prisons, Medium Secure Units, and Special Hospitals

- psychiatric reports on criminal matters for courts and lawyers

- court diversion schemes for mentally disordered offenders (MDOs)

- supervision of patients in the community, such as those on restriction orders (s37)

- consultation service to general psychiatrists.

Considerable political and media interest in forensic psychiatry has followed a succession of well-publicized individual 'scandals'; for example, crimes by MDOs

Hughes' Outline of Modern Psychiatry, Fifth Edition. David Gill.
© 2007 John Wiley & Sons, Ltd   ISBN 9780470033920

have led to calls for them to be detained permanently in psychiatric hospitals. Measures such as the Supervision Register and Care Programme Approach have been introduced, in part in response to such pressures, although the Supervision Register was soon abolished again.

Offending behaviour

Community surveys show that offending behaviour is extremely common, and that the vast majority of the population has broken the law in some way at some time. Generally speaking, offending behaviour is commoner in males than females, and peaks during the teenage years, gradually becoming less frequent thereafter. Most cases involve minor property offences such as theft and vandalism. Only a proportion is reported, and only a fraction of this results in any conviction. Of people convicted, the proportion going on to become persistent serious offenders is small.

Causes of offending behaviour are predominantly social and environmental, rather than psychiatric. Conduct disorder in children ('juvenile delinquency') often persists into adulthood as criminality and/or antisocial personality. Criminality tends to run in families. Twin and adoption studies indicate some specific genetic component of this inheritance, and up to half of antisocial behaviour may have a genetic basis. However, other factors such as coming from a large impoverished family, poor parenting, a culture of criminal behaviour in the neighbourhood and school, and low intelligence are thought to be of greater influence.

Male offenders outnumber female ones about 10-fold, and male prisoners outnumber female ones about 30-fold. Both cultural and biological factors contribute to this discrepancy. Female prisoners have more mental and physical disease than male ones.

Mental disorder in offenders

Because of the difficulty of obtaining representative samples of offenders in the community, surveys on mental disorder among offenders have mainly been done on those in prison. The prevalence of mental disorder among prisoners, whether remanded or sentenced, is much higher than in the community. Figures have obviously varied between different populations studied, but a fifth of women prisoners and a third or more of male prisoners have antisocial personality disorder; prisoners were 10 times likelier than the general population to have psychosis or personality disorder (Fazel and Danesh, 2002). Fifty per cent or more may have abused substances at some time.

Criminality and violence in psychiatric patients

There is an excess of offending, including violence, among those with mental disorder. However, antisocial personality disorder and substance misuse are stronger risk factors than mental illnesses such as schizophrenia. The bulk of offending in general, and violence in particular, has nothing to do with mental illness. A recent study, for example (Fazel and Grann, 2006), found that about 5 per cent of violent crimes were committed by those with psychosis (which has a prevalence of about 1 per cent); the association was stronger in females.

Predicting violence and dangerousness

Dangerousness varies according to the situation, and is impossible to predict with complete accuracy in individual cases. Nevertheless, general guidance can be given. Risk factors for repeated violence include the following:

- *past history of violence*: by far the most important guide to present and future risk

- personal/family history of criminality/substance misuse/suicidal behaviour

- preoccupation with, or threats of, violence

- psychiatric disorder, especially with paranoid delusions or command halluci-nations regarding violence

- cold/callous explosive/antisocial personality traits

- impulsivity/irritability/emotional arousal

- ready availability of a weapon and a victim.

In a potentially violent situation in psychiatric practice, consider the above factors with due regard for intuition and common sense. If the interviewer feels anxiety or fear, it is prudent to adjourn the interview to seek assistance and advice.

Managing risk

'Risk assessment' is an important part of the work of mental health professionals. In forensic psychiatry, risk to others is a concern as well as risk to self. It is the responsibility of all practitioners and of the system they work in to assess risk continuously, and to try to manage it so as to reduce it as far as possible. Risk assessment should be integrated into all aspects of modern psychiatry. The use of printed or computerized forms can help to ensure that assessments are done, recorded, and, most importantly, communicated to others. Following adverse events, it has been frequently found in inquiries that important decisions, such as discharge of a patient from hospital, had been taken by staff who were not in possession of all the key risk information about that patient.

Risk assessment is especially important when something is changing in the patient's care, such as reduction of frequency of observation on a ward or discharge from hospital.

When things do go wrong, there should be non-judgemental efforts to find out why, so that improvements can be made.

Psychiatric aspects of specific offences

Homicide

'Unlawful homicide' includes *murder*, *manslaughter*, and *infanticide*. The legal definition of murder requires that the crime was premeditated and the accused was fully responsible for the act. If these conditions are not fulfilled, the offence becomes manslaughter.

There are 800–900 homicides per year in England and Wales. In about 75 per cent of cases, killer and victim are well known to each other. Alcohol and other substances are often a factor, both in the background and at the time of the offence. Up to 15 per cent of killers commit suicide soon after their crime. A recent review (Oyebode, 2006) indicates that there are about 40 homicides per year by people in contact with mental health services in the 12 months prior to the event. (To put this in context, this is roughly the same number as those done by (non-psychiatric) offenders on probation.) However, surveys indicate that up to 50 per cent of killers could be diagnosed with a mental disorder of some kind – mainly personality disorder and substance misuse, although depressive disorder and psychosis also occur.

The legal finding of *diminished responsibility* (see below) applies in less than 5 per cent of homicides. The law classifies diminished responsibility, infanticide, homicide in a failed pact of suicide, and *not guilty by reason of insanity* (see below), as 'abnormal homicides'. Fewer than one in six homicides is classified as 'abnormal'. The presence of a mental disorder may permit a murder charge to be reduced to manslaughter on the grounds of diminished responsibility. A verdict of murder always carries a sentence of life imprisonment, but manslaughter may receive any sentence, including a hospital order under the Mental Health Act 1983, or even a non-custodial sentence.

A rare plea, in practice reserved for murder cases, is '*not guilty by reason of insanity*' when the offender fulfils the MacNaughten Rules; that is, he either did not know the nature and quality of his act, or did not know that it was wrong. A deluded patient is assumed to be under the same degree of responsibility as if the delusions were true. If this plea is successful, the accused is sent to a psychiatric hospital under the equivalent of section 37 of the Mental Health Act.

About half of those accused of murder claim amnesia for the event, but this is not an adequate defence, nor is voluntary intoxication with alcohol or drugs. Automatism, in epileptics or sleepwalkers, can constitute an acceptable defence.

Infanticide is a defence when a child less than a year old is killed by its mother who is 'suffering from a mental imbalance attributable to the effects of giving birth or to the consequent lactation'.

Mental disorders which can contribute to homicide are as follows:

- *personality disorder*

- *alcohol and drug misuse*

- *psychoses, usually with delusions,* as depressed people may kill their children or other close relatives because of a delusion that they were going to suffer an even worse fate. Psychosis may lead to homicide through paranoid delusions; even here, the victim is often known; stranger killing (e.g. http://www.zitotrust. co.uk/), the type so feared by the general public – or at any rate so prominent in the media – is rare. Puerperal psychosis accounts for some, but not all, cases of infanticide.

- *morbid jealousy*

- *learning disability,* in which frustration may be expressed by violence

- *epileptic automatism*: a rare phenomenon

- *automatism during sleep*, in which individuals prone to sleepwalking or night terrors occasionally kill during sleep – a rare defence hard to prove

- *organic brain disease.*

Fitness to plead

It has always been recognized that the accused person has to have a basic understanding of the legal process in order to have a fair trial. Standard tests have grown up in order to determine 'fitness to plead'. The grounds for a patient being considered unfit to plead are inability to:

- understand the charge, or

- give instructions to a lawyer about his defence, or

- understand the difference between pleading guilty and not guilty, or

- challenge a juror, or

- follow the proceedings of the case in court.

Psychiatric reports are important in helping the court to determine the question of fitness to plead.

If the person is found unfit, a 'trial of facts' follows. If it is found that the person did commit the offence, the court can dispose of the case by making an order, such as for admission to hospital, as in section 37 of the Mental Health Act, with or without a restriction order. If the patient goes to hospital, receives treatment, improves, and becomes fit to plead, there is provision for him to be brought back to be tried by the court in the normal way.

The question of fitness to plead used to come up only rarely, and in the most serious cases, because persons found unfit to plead were sent to a Special Hospital without limit of time. However, in recent years, the court has had flexibility in how it 'disposes' of such cases, including community disposals and absolute discharge with no order. It seems, perhaps unsurprisingly, that the question of fitness to plead is now raised more frequently by the defence in a range of much less severe cases.

Rape

Rape is sexual intercourse with a person who does not consent. Many cases are probably not reported to the police. Most rape victims are women, but male rape is an increasingly recognized problem. Victims of rape may develop psychiatric disorders, such as post-traumatic stress disorder or sexual dysfunction. Sympathetic treatment in special sexual assault centres can help to reduce the distress associated with reporting this crime, which may require intimate examination to obtain evidence.

Various psychiatric classifications of rapists have been proposed in the past ('violent', 'sadistic', etc.) but these are not now regarded as helpful: rape is an offence not an illness. If assessment is requested, the offender should be assessed in a standard way. Personality disorder, substance misuse, and low intelligence are often found in rapists; mental illness is infrequent.

Antilibidinal drugs may be used in the management of rapists. However, this is a very difficult area medico-legally, as the prescriber may be blamed for any reoffending. If such drugs were to be considered, it would only be as part of an overall package of offender management.

Arson

Arson is taken very seriously by the criminal justice system, for obvious reasons. Occasionally, one may see a patient who has committed a string of minor offences, and the system appears to have bent over backward to keep them out of prison. But if they commit arson, even without serious consequences, the attitude of the justice system can immediately become very different.

Arson may be committed by

- *criminals* – for example, to obtain insurance money or conceal evidence of another crime

- *psychotic* patients motivated by delusions

- those with *sociopathic personality* and/or *low intelligence* who start fires for excitement, sexual stimulation, or revenge. They often repeat the offence and may require secure detention.

- children and adolescents with *conduct disorder*.

Theft from shops ('shoplifting')

The law does not distinguish shoplifting (theft from shops) from other kinds of theft, but it has been studied separately by psychiatrists. In the cases described, it is predominantly a crime of women. Types include the following:

- straightforward *theft*

- search for *excitement* by those of sociopathic personality

- *psychiatric disorders*, including depressive illness (especially in middle-aged women), mania, schizophrenia, dementia, and learning disability

- *absent-mindedness* due to medical conditions such as epilepsy or hypoglycae-mia, or prescribed drugs such as benzodiazepines

- shoplifting by *addicts*, who may steal from shops in order to fund their habit.

Other topics with forensic implications include antisocial personality (see Chapter 7), sexual deviations (see Chapter 17), juvenile delinquency (see Chapter 18), child abuse (see Chapter 18), and the Mental Health Act (see Chapter 26).

Treatment: general considerations

If a clearly identified mental illness appears directly related to the offending behaviour, the prognosis could be good for both the illness and the offending behaviour. For example, a man with schizophrenia who smashes up a television shop because he believes it is transmitting harmful rays will be unlikely to repeat this behaviour if his delusions resolve with treatment. However, mental disorder may coexist with offending behaviour without being a significant causative factor, so that treatment of the disorder has little impact on the behaviour.

Substance misuse is very common among offenders. If, for example, a chronic alcoholic can be rehabilitated, he will be less likely to commit drunkenness and public order offences. Many prisons run AA groups for this reason. However, it is not always appropriate to remove a person from the criminal justice system on the grounds of substance misuse alone. Motivation to stop substance misuse may appear higher before an impending court appearance than later proves to be the case.

Psychological or behavioural treatments have been tried, irrespective of the presence or absence of mental disorder, for a variety of habitual offenders, such as those convicted of car theft, 'road rage', and assault. Few if any of these treatments have been shown to be effective in randomized, controlled trials, and they tend to be regarded cautiously by psychiatrists. If they are to be provided, prison psychology services, probation, or social services are the best source.

Facilities for mentally disordered offenders

Forensic psychiatry services

There has been a move away from thinking about forensic psychiatry mainly in terms of special inpatient units. Well-developed forensic psychiatry services are now characterized by a multidisciplinary, team-based, community approach, including:

- consultant forensic psychiatrist, and junior doctor(s)
- community psychiatric nurse and social worker
- psychologists
- administrative support.

They provide a range of services to courts and prisons, see referrals from general psychiatry colleagues, and work closely with probation. They carry a caseload of outpatients, and may be based partly at a Regional Secure Unit (see below).

Regional Secure Units

Regional Secure Units (RSUs) have been set up around the country, in line with current policy to expand the number of 'medium secure' beds in each health district. This is so that the majority of psychiatric patients with violent behaviour, and of psychiatrically disturbed offenders, can receive treatment locally and only the most dangerous ones be sent to Special Hospitals.

A typical RSU might have 20 beds, under the supervision of a consultant forensic psychiatrist and associated multidisciplinary team. Inpatient beds are frequently full, with pressure to accept referrals of 'difficult-to-manage' (not necessarily forensic) patients from general psychiatric services. Such patients can be difficult to contain in modern psychiatric wards, which frequently lack intensive care beds (see Chapter 25).

Prison Medical Service

Just as most mental disorder in the community as a whole is managed in primary care, so most mental disorder among prisoners has been managed by the Prison Medical Service. There are moves to make health care in prisons part of the general NHS, and, increasingly, NHS purchasers (currently known as Primary

Care Trusts, although changes in nomenclature and organization are frequent) are being given responsibility for health care in prisons.

From the point of view of mental health care, this is highly desirable. If a patient with mental health problems enters prison, it is desirable that knowledge about his diagnosis and treatment should follow him in; conversely, a patient with mental health problems being managed in prison should be able to have this management continued when he is released. Integrating prison medical services within the general NHS will be likely to help to reduce the discontinuities in mental health care on reception into or discharge from prison, which have been frequent under the arrangement of having a separate prison medical service.

Because of the high rates of mental disorder in prisons, most prisons also have regular input from general adult and/or forensic psychiatric services. They will advise on diagnosis and management, either in the general wings or the prison hospital. In some units, there are dedicated facilities, set up by mental health services, and staffed and managed by them.

Compulsory treatment under the Mental Health Act 1983 (see Chapter 27) is not, however, permitted in prisons. Sometimes it is necessary to transfer an inmate to psychiatric hospital, not necessarily under conditions of security, and the psychiatrist is able to assist in placement. There are appropriate sections of the Mental Health Act, regarding both sentenced (s47) and remanded (s48) prisoners.

As previously indicated, surveys of prisoners indicate that up to 50 per cent or more can be diagnosed as having some sort of mental abnormality. Sociopathy and substance misuse are the main diagnoses, but learning disability, functional psychosis, organic brain disease, and epilepsy are also found in excess. In some cases this disorder has not been recognized. Others are in prison because no psychiatric hospital place can be found for them. However, the presence of certain psychiatric disorders, such as personality disorder, substance misuse, or treated chronic mental illness, does not necessarily mean that prison is inappropriate.

Diversion schemes

In some magistrates' courts, regular attendance by psychiatrists or other trained staff allows psychiatrically disturbed persons coming before the court to be diverted as appropriate from the criminal justice system into the health-care system. Diversion also happens at an even earlier stage; for example, the custody sergeant at a police station may ask the police surgeon to examine an arrested person, and, if a mental disorder is present, the help of local psychiatric services is sought. Section 136 of the Mental Health Act also assists: it provides for someone who is disturbed in a public place to be taken to a place of safety for an assessment of their mental health.

Social and probation services

Social and probation services have a close relationship with forensic psychiatry, including:

- social and probation reports on offenders before the court
- resettlement of offenders
- probation and bail hostels.

For example, a mentally disordered person convicted of a crime may be put on probation, with psychiatric treatment as a condition of this. Failure to cooperate with treatment would be a breach of the probation order and result in the offender's being brought back before the court. This has sometimes been criticized as making psychiatry part of the criminal justice system. There would then, for example, be concern that what was said in medical confidence to a doctor might be made known to the criminal justice system.

For minor offences, probation with a condition of psychiatric treatment has fallen out of favour for this and other more practical reasons: it would place mental health services in an impossible situation if they had to inform probation every time a patient did not, for example, collect a prescription. For more serious matters, the advantages can outweigh the disadvantages, and it is still used.

Primary care

Many offenders, especially released prisoners, may not be registered with a GP. This situation often adds to the difficulties of providing adequate medical care for this population, with its high rate of both physical and psychiatric illness.

Special Hospitals

Special Hospitals exist for treatment of patients with mental disorder, mainly psychosis, sociopathy, or learning disability, who have committed violent crimes.

They comprise Broadmoor, Rampton, and Ashworth in England, and Carstairs in Scotland. All patients are compulsorily admitted and detained under the Mental Health Act 1983, the majority from the courts, and some from prisons or psychiatric hospitals. Violence to others, sex offences, and arson are the most frequent reasons for admission. Prospective admissions are assessed by Special Hospital staff, the main criteria being the presence of mental disorder and a 'grave and immediate' risk to others. Most patients stay several years, but about 50 per cent eventually become fit for transfer to a local psychiatric unit in preparation for discharge to the community.

These hospitals have been staffed jointly by prison and health staff. There has been some confusion over how much of their purpose was care, and how much confinement. Recently, there have been moves to bring the Special Hospitals within the mainstream of health services, so that, for example, at the time of writing, Broadmoor Hospital is now part of a London Mental Health Trust.

Psychiatric reports: criminal

Court reports should be written in non-technical language, as they will be used by lawyers and other lay persons. All technical words, even those commonplace to psychiatrists, such as 'schizophrenia', should be explained.

Before beginning work, the wise psychiatrist obtains the written agreement of the person requesting the report to pay his fee, as this work is not part of NHS practice. A proper letter of instruction is essential. This must set out the points on which the psychiatrist is to report. A general request for 'a report' is not adequate.

The commonest type of report relates to a patient for whom the psychiatrist provides NHS care. In this case, the report has clearly arisen out of NHS practice, and only a modest fee would be appropriate. For example, the patient concerned may be one with an existing mental disorder who has been arrested for a minor public order offence. Here the need is for an expeditious and brief report. Two A4 sheets are ample for most such cases.

Reports are frequently requested by courts, and by defence lawyers. It is crucial to establish clearly the question behind the request; for example, is the court asking about fitness to plead or advice about sentencing? The following scheme is appropriate:

- name, age, address, occupation, and marital status

- sources of information: when and where the psychiatrist interviewed the defendant, other informants interviewed, and documents consulted

- index offence

- forensic history

- medical and psychiatric history, including history of present illness (if any)

- personal background, including family history

- present social circumstances

- substance use

- circumstances of index offence, including opinion on mental state at the time of offending

- present mental state

- opinion, including advice on specific points raised by the person requesting the report

- advice as to disposal. This is traditionally phrased in appropriate language, recognizing that the authority rests with the court; for example, 'I respectfully offer the Court the following suggestions as to disposal, for its consideration.'

Case example

An unemployed man aged 38 presented himself to casualty with the complaint of 'hearing voices'. He admitted to recent drug use, and the likely diagnosis seemed drug-induced psychosis. He was admitted to a psychiatric ward informally, and rapidly improved with oral antipsychotic medication, but discharged himself before a full assessment had been made. He did not attend follow-up, but presented again with similar symptoms shortly afterward. On this occasion, no beds were available, and he was sent home with medication. Two weeks later, his consultant was surprised to receive a request from the local magistrates' court for a psychiatric report 'to assist in sentencing for a number of motoring offences'.

After old notes had been consulted, it emerged that this man had been brought up in a large and chaotic family, of long-standing criminal tendencies, and had been subject to a mixture of neglect and abuse. He had spent his life taking, selling, repairing, and even living in cars, and had multiple convictions for vehicle offences; none of a variety of sentences had influenced this behaviour. His only psychiatric history was the complaint of hearing voices during his last term of imprisonment; he had been transferred to hospital, only to abscond shortly afterward. His probation officer indicated to the psychiatrist that the court was very keen for him to be taken on for medical treatment, as it felt that other disposals would be ineffective.

At interview, residual psychotic symptoms were still apparent, but resolving. The man was frank about his drug use, and also about his intentions to continue with his offending behaviour.

The psychiatrist's report indicated that his personality appeared to have been damaged by his unsatisfactory upbringing, and that he continued to have a psychotic illness, partly due to illicit drug use and partly due to the stress of impending imprisonment.

The court accepted the psychiatrist's recommendation of a community disposal, with the condition of psychiatric treatment. It also imposed a suspended prison sentence. The patient accepted depot antipsychotic medication, which seemed to help the psychosis, but he continued to offend. He therefore breached the terms of his suspended sentence, and was imprisoned.

In respect of more serious offences and civil litigation (personal injury, employment tribunal, family courts, etc.) or insurance claims, reports will be more extensive. They will need to summarize other documents (for example, GP notes) and proceed by reasoned argument to a conclusion. Here, the psychiatrist may be practising as an expert witness, and his primary duty is not to those instructing him, but to the court (http://www.dca.gov.uk/civil/procrules_fin/contents/parts/part35.htm).

References

Fazel, S. and Danesh, J. (2002). Serious mental disorders in 23 000 prisoners: a systematic review of 62 surveys. *Lancet* **359**, 545–550.

Fazel, S. and Grann, M. (2006). The population impact of severe mental illness on violent crime. *Am J Psychiatry* **163**, 1397–1403.

Oyebode, F. (2006). Clinical errors and medical negligence. *Adv Psychiatr Treat* **12**, 221–227.

Part III Treatment

22 Psychological treatment

The term *psychological treatment* is largely synonymous with *psychotherapy*, defined by Storr as 'the art of alleviating personal difficulties through the agency of words and a personal professional relationship'. Some psychotherapeutic techniques make use of actions, exercise, music, or art as well as words. Psychotherapy may be carried out with individuals, groups, couples, or families.

Historical background

Medicine has always recognized the importance of the patient's confiding relationship with the physician, as enshrined in the Hippocratic oath of ancient Greece. This non-specific psychological aspect of treatment is especially important in psychiatry. Through the years, more specific psychological approaches have been conceptualized, ranging from medieval notions of the 'casting out of demons' in mad people to the 'animal magnetism' of Mesmer in the nineteenth century.

It was only a little over 100 years ago, however, that a systematic theoretical base for psychological treatment was developed in Sigmund Freud's 'psychoanalysis'. Although now little used in practice, psychoanalysis has been paramount in establishing the importance of psychological matters with the general public, and in providing one of the most enduringly interesting models of the mind. The work of Freud and the post-Freudians is briefly described below.

Hughes' Outline of Modern Psychiatry, Fifth Edition. David Gill.
© 2007 John Wiley & Sons, Ltd   ISBN 9780470033920

Many of these ideas now look dated, seeming more like cultural movements than medical or scientific theories. Indeed, if one accepts the position that the definition of a scientific theory is that it is capable of being disproved by experiment, little of what is in the next section would be defined as science. However, many people continue to find these theories of great interest, and they have certainly been an important part of the development of psychiatry. The time has not yet arrived when it will be possible to have a proper training in psychiatry without at least an acquaintance with the terms.

Sigmund Freud (1856–1939)

Freud's system of psychoanalysis formed the basis of psychodynamic psychotherapy. During psychoanalysis, in which 50-minute treatment sessions take place 3–5 times a week for several years, the patient talks about past and present events, emotions, dreams, and fantasies, and uses 'free association' to recall repressed or forgotten material to conscious awareness. The therapist's interpretations relate to Freud's concepts, which include the following:

- *The model of the mind:* the structure of the mind is seen as having three parts: *id* (inherited, instinctive, largely unconscious, motivated by the 'pleasure principle'), *ego* (largely conscious, acting according to the 'reality principle' and using the ego defence mechanisms), and *superego* (derived from introjection of authority figures, and equivalent to conscience).

- Stages of psychosexual development: in each of the *oral, anal, oedipal,* and *genital* stages, the *libido* or sexual energy (asserted by Freud to be of prime importance in all areas of mental activity) is attached in a particular direction.

- *Transference:* attitudes derived from early relationships are projected onto the therapist.

- *Resistance:* the patient avoids exploration of a topic which is the subject of unconscious conflicts.

- *Ego defence mechanisms:* these are unconscious processes to reduce anxiety. They include *denial, repression, rationalization, projection, reaction formation, displacement, sublimation, intellectualization, conversion, fixation, regression,* and *introjection* (see Glossary; they are particularly associated with the name of Anna Freud).

- *Dreams*: in these, the real or 'latent' content is converted into the 'manifest' content by the mental 'censor' through the mechanisms of *condensation, displacement*, and *symbolism*.

- *Parapraxes*: these are mistakes and memory lapses in everyday life that have unconscious significance ('Freudian slips').

Carl Jung (1875–1961)

Jung's system of psychotherapy, called *analytical psychology*, emphasizes the exploration of dreams and the unconscious, and aims at 'individuation' of the patient; this involves achieving harmony between the conscious and unconscious, and full experience of the self. Jungian concepts include the following:

- *Libido*, or general psychic energy, flows between pairs of opposites such as progression–regression, conscious–unconscious, and extroversion–introversion. If it is blocked in one direction, pathology results; for example, excess energy in the unconscious manifests as psychiatric illness.

- *The unconscious mind* is revealed in dreams, with both personal and collective aspects, the latter including instincts, archetypes, and universal symbols.

- *Personality* depends on the degree of extroversion and introversion and which of the 'four functions' – thinking, feeling, sensation, and intuition – is most highly developed. There is an outward personality, or 'persona', and an unconscious 'shadow' which has opposite characteristics.

Jung's book *Man and His Symbols* gives a readable, illustrated account of his life and work.

Melanie Klein (1882–1960)

Klein worked with children under 2 years old, and believed that failure of psychological development at this time was the origin of neurosis in later life. She described developmental stages: the *paranoid-schizoid position* related to the child's perception of its mother's breast first as a 'good object', which is introjected, and then as a 'bad object' onto which aggressive feelings are projected. This is followed by the *depressive position* when the child becomes aware that the good and bad mother are the same and must cope with the depressive anxiety of having attacked the needed good object.

Other 'neo-Freudians' include Adler, Fromm, Reich, Erikson, Sullivan, Horney, Anna Freud, Winnicot, and Fairbairn.

Principles of psychotherapy today

Types of psychotherapy

Supportive psychotherapy involves discussion of problems at a simple, practical level, which may include offering advice. Any good doctor–patient relationship includes an element of supportive psychotherapy. Psychotherapy can be usefully combined with antidepressants or other psychotropic drugs for patients with formal psychiatric illness. Many psychotherapists prefer to speak of 'clients' rather than 'patients'; however, the term 'patient' is retained here for the sake of consistency with the rest of the book.

A wide variety of talking treatments is in use in the UK. Outside health services, many patients consult counsellors and other types of therapists. Many patients pay alternative or complementary practitioners, but, clearly, this is beyond the scope of the present book. I will concentrate below on the three main types of talking treatment provided in UK health services: *counselling, cognitive-behavioural therapy (CBT)*, and *dynamic psychotherapy*.

Many other named techniques exist, such as *cognitive-analytical therapy* (Ryle), *interpersonal therapy* (Klerman), *client-centred therapy* (Rogers), *Gestalt therapy* (Perl), *psychodrama* (Moreno), and *transactional analysis* (Berne), although some are largely practised in the private sector rather than through the NHS. Current opinion emphasizes the similarities between different schools of psychotherapy, rather than their differences.

Indications for psychotherapy

The patients who respond best are those suffering from neurotic symptoms or mild personality disorders who are well motivated to change, firmly committed to treatment, able to understand psychological concepts, prepared to take responsibility for decisions, reasonably intelligent, and verbally fluent. (Sceptics might say that patients with all these laudable qualities are not in pressing need of therapy!) Contrary to previous belief, older patients can benefit as well as younger ones.

Contraindications for psychotherapy

Patients who have psychotic illnesses, are misusing substances, or have severe personality disorders are usually considered unsuitable.

Unwanted effects of psychotherapy

- *Excessive dependence* on therapy or the therapist may develop.

- *Intensive techniques may cause distress* and, occasionally, precipitate acute psychiatric breakdown.

- *Disorders for which physical treatments are required*, such as severe depression, or medical illness presenting with psychological symptoms, may be missed, especially by non-medical therapists.

- *Ineffective psychotherapy wastes time and money* and lowers morale.

Unwanted effects should be infrequent with skilled assessment, and well-trained therapists in proper supervision.

Training of psychotherapists

Therapists usually train after initial qualification and experience in another profession such as psychiatry, psychology, nursing, other health-care disciplines, and social work. Training requirements vary widely according to the school of therapy, and a period of personal therapy is required by some. Desirable qualities in a therapist are the ability to be sympathetic but detached, non-judgemental, and honest. Therapy is more likely to be successful if patient and therapist like one another, so that a strong 'therapeutic alliance' can develop.

NHS provision of psychotherapy

Most mental health-care services are organized around particular clinical problems and/or patient groups; only departments of psychotherapy are based on a particular form of treatment. This somewhat 'special' status has extended to the type of psychotherapy offered, which, until recently, was mainly psychodynamic, carrying considerable prestige and exerting a strong influence on psychiatric education and training.

Recent years have seen a reaction against psychodynamic psychotherapy, however. Prospective, randomized, controlled trials have not generally shown superiority of this treatment over comparison conditions, such as waiting-list controls. In contrast, brief, structured psychotherapies of the cognitive and cognitive-behavioural types do appear more effective than control conditions. Trends are therefore toward increased use of, and funding for, the latter types. It seems reasonable that health-care resources should be focused on treatments that have been shown to be effective ('evidence-based medicine'), especially considering the greater cost of long courses of dynamic therapy. However, part of this movement may represent another swing in the history of psychiatry of the biological/psychological pendulum; too marked a shift away from the fascinating, if 'unscientific', notions of psychodynamic psychotherapy may in the future be seen as counterproductive.

Planning and practical organization of therapy

NHS psychotherapy sessions usually take place weekly and last 50 minutes. All sessions should preferably be at the same time on the same day of the week in the same place. Punctuality by both patient and therapist is important. Interruptions, including phone calls, should be prevented. These practical rules provide patients with a secure framework in which to explore difficult issues.

Some therapists draw up a contract at the beginning to specify the patient's problems, goals of treatment, and proposed number of sessions.

Notes are written immediately afterward, but not during the session itself. Details of the content of sessions should not be revealed to other people except in the context of supervision seminars.

Some individual types of psychotherapy will now be described.

Counselling

A great deal of *counselling* is done in general practice and in other settings. It has expanded greatly over the past 20 years or so. It is very popular with patients and GPs, and clearly fulfils a need for patients to talk things over with a trusted adviser.

Probably, this popularity is only partly to be seen in mental health terms. Social factors such as family instability and reduction in involvement in organized religion may have meant that many individuals in distress do not have such ready access to their own means of support as did previous generations. Expectations and values have changed as well, the virtues of reticence (the traditional British 'stiff upper lip') being replaced by a notion that it is intrinsically 'good to talk'.

Counselling forms part of the valuable work done with patients by organizations such as the Citizens Advice Bureau (practical problems such as debt, housing, benefits, etc.), Cruse (bereavement), and Relate (relationship problems).

Primary care counsellors need to be appropriately accredited and qualified, and to have regular supervision. They usually offer a limited number of sessions, typically six to eight, and practice in a non-directive, supportive, 'reflective' way. Most patients probably do well.

From the perspective of secondary care, where patients who have not improved with counselling may be referred, there can be a perception that counsellors do sometimes inappropriately stir up old problems from the past. This can lead to patients becoming more distressed and perhaps requiring referral, when they would not otherwise have done so. Certainly, there is no evidence that provision of counselling and primary care leads to a reduction in workload in secondary care.

As regards effectiveness, in a large, randomized trial in the UK, both counselling and CBT were more effective for depression than usual GP care, with no difference between the two types of talking therapy (Ward *et al.*, 2000).

Cognitive-behavioural therapy (CBT)

CBT has become established as the psychotherapy of choice, being perceived as effective and cost-effective. It remains important to understand the twin strands of CBT. *Behaviour therapy* per se is now less prominent. However, cognitive therapists are happy to admit that their treatment involves components of behaviour therapy, such as activity scheduling, and that the term 'cognitive therapy' is effectively shorthand for CBT.

The principles of *cognitive therapy* and *behavioural therapy* will now be described, followed by an account of how they are brought together in CBT.

Cognitive therapy is based on the work of Aaron Beck. Like most American psychiatrists of his era, his training was psychodynamic. However, he became frustrated with the lack of progress of patients under his care, in relation to the amount of input. He thus sought to address practically and directly, rather than through the convolutions of psychoanalysis, the maladaptive beliefs and attitudes presumed to contribute to current symptoms.

Cognitive (Latin *cogito*: 'I think') therapy is based on the principle that thought influences mood, so that depression, anxiety, and other symptoms arise from, or are perpetuated by, faulty thought patterns and beliefs. The aim in therapy is to identify *automatic negative thoughts* that appear to be contributing to the symptoms, and to encourage the patient to reconsider them in the light of the evidence, and to try alternative viewpoints and behaviour patterns. This process should lead to better understanding of the symptoms, and more control over them. For some patients, exploration of visual images is an appropriate variant of this technique.

Beck originally described several types of maladaptive thinking patterns to be addressed in therapy, including the following:

- *selective abstraction*: dwelling on only the negative aspects of a situation

- *overgeneralization*: a single matter wrongly assumed to have wide-ranging implications

- *magnification*: a trivial matter exaggerated out of proportion

- *all-or-none reasoning*: issues seen as 'black or white' with no middle ground

- *arbitrary inference*: things assumed, without good evidence, to be negative.

Behaviour therapy is based on learning theory, a model of human and animal behaviour originating in the field of pure (non-clinical) psychology. In the 1950s, workers such as Eysenck, Lazarus, Wolpe, Bandura, Marks, and Rachman began to introduce these ideas into clinical practice as behaviour therapy. This involves the acquisition of desirable new behaviours as well as the loss of unwanted ones.

Behavioural therapy is a structured method, employing practical strategies to overcome current symptoms. The principle is changing behaviour, rather than addressing presumed underlying causes or accompanying thoughts and feelings. It is related to Pavlovian principles, in which external changes have significant effects on the responses of the individual.

Common parlance such as 'get back on the horse' or 'use makes master' encapsulate the principle that doing a feared activity or entering a feared situation of itself causes subsequent fears to be less. This illustrates the principle of behaviour therapy.

Behaviour therapy was originally applied to neurotic symptoms that could be regarded as 'maladaptive learned responses', as in monophobia (phobia restricted to one specific object or situation) developing after a frightening experience. Behavioural techniques have since been applied to a much wider range of disorders, including generalized anxiety states, obsessive-compulsive disorder, eating disorders, sexual problems, and the management of chronic disability caused by brain damage or schizophrenia.

Problems are defined and objectives of therapy agreed at the beginning. Progress during therapy is regularly assessed by measurable criteria: for example, frequency of occurrence of a particular behaviour pattern, or questionnaires to monitor mood change.

Critics have claimed on theoretical grounds that, because the past events or unconscious conflicts which produced the symptoms are ignored, behaviour therapy cannot produce a lasting cure, and that 'symptom substitution' will occur. In practice, this seldom happens.

Behaviour therapy appears comparable in efficacy to other forms of psychotherapy, it is often less time-consuming than other methods, and the patient need not be intelligent or verbally fluent to benefit. Specific techniques include the following:

- *Systematic desensitization (graded exposure)*: progressive introduction to a feared object or situation, using an agreed hierarchy. For example, a person with a fear of spiders agrees with the therapist to encounter them first in imagination, then in pictures, and then as a plastic one, before finally seeing a real one.

- *Flooding*: immediate exposure to the feared stimulus in its full form. This is claimed to be as effective as graded exposure, but many patients find the prospect unacceptable.

- *Modelling*: the patient imitates the therapist's behaviour, for example, in social skills or assertiveness training.

- *Biofeedback techniques*: to modify physiological variables such as heart rate, blood pressure, and muscle tension. Some people find this helpful in controlling anxiety or pain.

- *Response prevention*: for compulsive behaviour. For example, the therapist prevents the obsessional patient from repeated hand washing; the patient's anxiety initially rises, but then decays naturally when the feared consequence (such as infection) does not occur.

- *Thought stopping*: for obsessional thoughts. The patient learns to stop an obsessional train of thought, usually by 'switching' to another. This is very similar to the cognitive technique of 'distraction'.

- *Massed practice (satiation)*: the unwanted behaviour is repeated so often that the patient no longer wants to continue it.

- *Aversion therapy*: traditional forms are now seldom used for ethical reasons. They involved coupling an unwanted behaviour, such as substance misuse or deviant sexuality, with an unpleasant stimulus such as drug-induced vomiting or electric shock. Milder self-administered forms may be helpful; for example, snapping an elastic band worn around the wrist can provide distraction from obsessional thoughts or from an unwanted behaviour such as overeating.

- *Covert sensitization*: aversion therapy carried out in imagination only.

- *Shaping (chaining)*: the separate learning of each stage in a complex process; for example, a brain-damaged or learning-disabled patient learning to dress.

- *Token economy regimes*: rewards are given for desirable behaviour, and privileges withdrawn for undesirable behaviour. The approach has been used in the rehabilitation of chronic schizophrenics, but ethical considerations apply.

- *Relaxation training*: used in a variety of problems, mainly to manage anxiety. The patient tenses up and then progressively relaxes all muscle groups, while breathing regularly and deeply. This is a gradually acquired skill, which can be taught individually or in groups, or with the aid of commercially available audio- and videotapes.

A course of behaviour therapy would typically involve several of the above components; for example, a spider phobic might take part in a programme of graded exposure, and be given relaxation training to cope with attendant anxiety. It seems likely that most behavioural treatments include some cognitive component, although some purists might not accept this.

CBT in practice

CBT is brief (6–12 sessions) and problem-oriented, and it demands active participation both from the therapist, who provides a structured approach and sometimes a substantial educational input, and from the patient. Structure is provided by several factors, including the following:

- prior agreement on the *number of sessions*
- setting of *agreed, tangible goals* (such as a patient with social phobia going shopping alone)
- *planned structure* for each session
- *homework*.

A typical session includes:

- greeting
- setting agenda for session
- review of homework
- review of events since previous session
- feedback on last session
- problems to be addressed in session
- setting homework
- feedback.

Components of the therapy include the following:

- *cognitive techniques*, such as the following:
  - questioning negative automatic thoughts
  - distraction techniques to take the patient's attention away from negative thoughts

- *behavioural techniques*:
  - keeping a diary: simple notes on thoughts/feelings/activity to establish the influence of thoughts on mood
  - activity scheduling: planning pleasurable experiences/activities.

Many of these are first tried out within the session, and then practised as agreed specific homework tasks.

The skill of the therapist lies not only in using these techniques and structures, but doing so in a sensitive and supportive way, for the building of good rapport between patient and therapist is as essential here as in all kinds of therapy. Trust in the therapist will encourage the patient to engage in prescribed tasks that are often anxiety-provoking or even unpleasant in themselves, such as going out for the socially phobic person, or challenging a negative self-concept for the depressed.

Indications

Randomized, controlled trials have shown that CBT is effective in mild to moderate depression (Butler *et al.*, 2006). Other trials have shown it to be effective for anxiety disorders (Bisson, 2006; Gale and Browne, 2006; Kumar and Browne, 2006), bulimia nervosa (Hay and Bacaltchuk, 2006), and possibly somatoform disorders, and even psychotic disorders. As well as treating an index episode, this therapy may have prophylactic value in preventing future episodes (secondary prevention).

Case example

A man who had been made redundant from his job as bank manager developed depressive illness; retaining his private medical insurance for a limited time, he saw a psychiatrist privately. Declining medication, he was referred for cognitive therapy; the insurer agreed to pay for 10 one-hour sessions. The patient considered himself an utter failure at work, and extended this belief to all other aspects of his life (overgeneralization), perceiving rejections where none were intended, and becoming even more depressed in consequence. Objective consideration revealed that his redundancy was one of many in the bank, occasioned by transfer of jobs to foreign parts, rather than a personal rejection, as he had assumed (arbitrary inference). Keeping a mood diary quickly convinced him of the connection between his thoughts and his depressed mood. He made rapid progress in the first three sessions, but then 'got stuck'. Further cognitive work increased his insight but did not improve his mood. The therapist noticed his reluctance to set practical goals, and placed more emphasis on activity scheduling, especially pleasurable activities outside the home. By the end of therapy, he had made further progress, and was happy with the outcome: patient and therapist agreed that residual symptoms (mainly social anxiety, lack of energy, and poor concentration) would continue to improve if he continued to practise the new thinking skills he had learnt, and to build up his social activities, which had previously been mainly related to his work.

Psychodynamic psychotherapy

Assessment

Psychodynamic (interpretative)

Exploration of early life and re-experiencing habitual patterns in the current relationship with the therapist are used to explain and relieve symptoms. Modern psychodynamic methods, although based on those of Freud and the post-Freudians, use shorter and more eclectic treatment, such as cognitive analytic therapy (Ryle).

Before a patient is taken on for psychodynamic therapy, a detailed initial assessment should be carried out by an experienced therapist. Presenting symptoms should be considered in the light of early experience, use of psychological defence mechanisms, and personality traits. Subsequent treatment may, in training units, be carried out by a more junior therapist under supervision. Duration of treatment in the NHS, previously a year or more, now tends to be measured in months.

Technique and mechanisms of change

The therapist should take the role of a professional but sympathetic listener, avoid asking too many questions, and avoid imposing his or her own feelings and opinions through making moral judgements or giving direct advice. In contrast to cognitive and behavioural therapies, there is no explicit planned agenda in the sessions. While improvement of current symptoms may result simply from the opportunity to talk and express feelings, more fundamental change usually requires the use of interpretations designed to help the patient be more aware of emotions and express them more clearly, as in the following:

- *Identifying and challenging defences* against unacknowledged feelings: use of mental defence mechanisms (see Glossary).

- *Pointing out discrepancies* between stated wishes and actual behaviour; for example, a patient may repeatedly say that he wishes to end an unsatisfactory relationship, but take no practical steps to do so.

- *Pointing out links* between earlier life experiences and current problems; for example, a patient's silence in the face of marital problems might parallel his response as a child to difficulties between his parents.

- *Comments on the transference* between patient and therapist as revealed by the patient's behaviour within the session itself. Transference means that the patient feels and behaves toward the therapist as toward important figures in the past. Transference can develop more easily if the therapist's real personal attitudes and circumstances are not revealed.

- *Counter-transference*: the therapist's feelings and behaviour toward the patient, may also be utilized constructively if properly recognized. If not recognized, they can hinder the therapy.

Evaluation of results

As discussed above, randomized, controlled trials suggest that psychodynamic therapy has little or no therapeutic effect additional to that of comparison conditions, in contrast to the more structured cognitive and behaviour therapies, which have consistently demonstrated positive treatment outcomes. Psychodynamic therapists have responded by pointing out that there are difficulties in evaluating the outcome, because:

- Neurotic disorders often remit spontaneously.

- Specific effects of psychotherapeutic technique are difficult to distinguish from non-specific benefits of regular individual attention.

- The content of treatment sessions is difficult to standardize because it varies with the individual characteristics of patient and therapist.

- Benefits of a subtle kind may not be detectable by standard questionnaires.

However, these considerations have not prevented CBT from being demonstrated to be effective. Perhaps the only valid response is that the outcome criteria are not agreed between the two broad schools of psychotherapy; many psychodynamic patients do not fit into a formal diagnostic category, and may wish for therapy for personal development rather than symptom relief. In either case, it is becoming increasingly hard to justify expenditure of limited NHS psychiatric resources on individual psychodynamic therapy, although it is still available in the private sector.

Group therapy

Group therapy is more powerful than individual therapy for some patients, and more economical of resources. Groups may use any of the analytical, cognitive, and behavioural techniques described above.

Selection criteria are similar to those for psychotherapy in general. Group therapy is especially suitable for patients whose main problems concern relationships with others, and patients with a shared problem: alcohol or drug misuse, anxiety, and childhood sexual abuse, for example. Shy patients who find it difficult to participate in group discussion may not benefit, whereas talkative patients may monopolize a group and arouse hostility from the other members, but a skilled therapist can encourage both types to play a more balanced part.

The therapist should facilitate trust and open disclosure, and encourage regular attendance. Factors likely to impede the group's success, such as dropping out, lateness, absences, socialization outside the group, breaches of confidentiality, and subgrouping, should be discouraged.

Some therapists act as detached leaders; others participate more actively. Some groups have two co-therapists, preferably of equal status.

Mechanisms of change

The same mechanisms operate as in individual therapy, but those treated in groups have the advantage of being able to share their problems and ways of coping with others similarly affected.

As the introduction of newcomers may retard progress and arouse hostility, 'closed' groups with a fixed lifespan and the same members throughout are ideal, if not always practicable. A good size is 5–10 members. Outpatient groups usually meet once a week for 1–2 hours. Groups run on psychoanalytic lines may continue for 2 years or more. Groups using behavioural or cognitive techniques, such as anxiety management groups, last only 6–12 weeks. Inpatient units run on 'therapeutic community' lines use daily group therapy as the main method of treatment.

Family and marital therapy

Psychiatric symptoms are often exacerbated by a dysfunctional relationship between marriage partners, or within a larger family group. Common problems include the following:

- *scapegoating*, in which one family member is automatically blamed for problems

- extremes of *authority and dependency*

- *ambiguous communication styles*

- *family secrets*

- *gratification* of one person through the illness of another

- *a shared stress*, such as bereavement, affecting the whole family.

'Systems theory' has been influential; it views the family as a self-contained system, in which changes in one element are compensated for by complementary changes in others. Thus, problems in one family member can be addressed not only directly, but also by changing the response of the others.

There are various types of family therapy; *systemic therapy* has been influential: the family is seen as a self-contained system, whereby a change in one member, by a process of feedback, is bound to affect other members. *Strategic therapy* emphasizes the role of the therapist in designing and evaluating the effects of therapy.

Recent trends within society, such as the replacement of traditional marriage by 'serial monogamy', more mothers working outside the home, more men unemployed, and fewer older people in close contact with their children and grandchildren, have influenced the type of presenting problems and expectations of outcome.

Therapy involves regular meetings between family members and therapist(s). As with group therapy, a particular technique can be adopted, but general principles include:

- encouraging *clear communication* between family members

- setting *practical goals* agreed by all parties

- emphasizing *positive aspects* of relationships and encouraging rewarding behaviour

- discouraging *criticisms*, especially repetitive ones about the past.

Role-play may be used to enable better appreciation of others' points of view.

Good motivation by all participants, and a reasonable degree of goodwill and honesty between them, are prerequisites for success and the therapists should avoid taking sides.

Recent advances

Psychotherapy continues to develop, fuelled partly by notions – not totally realistic – that it represents a more fundamental solution to problems than other therapies, such as medication, which may be seen as 'merely drugging the problem'. Indeed, the provision of mass CBT has even been suggested as a solution for social problems (http://www.strategy.gov.uk/downloads/files/mh_layard.pdf).

Dialectical behaviour therapy for borderline personality disorder (Palmer, 2002) represents a novel way of seeking to help some of the most damaged and inaccessible psychiatric patients.

Certain software packages are already officially recommended for milder states of depression and anxiety (NICE, http://www.nice.org.uk/page.aspx?o=TA97). The Internet offers a potentially confusing mixture of harmful and helpful information for patients (Tantam, 2006); already, online CBT is in development (e.g. http://www.moodgym.anu.edu.au).

References

Bisson, J. (2006). Post-traumatic stress disorder. *Clinical Evidence* (15th edn), pp. 1453–1469. London: BMJ Books. http://www.clinicalevidence.com/ceweb/conditions/meh/1005/1005.jsp.

Butler, R. *et al.* (2006). Depressive disorders. *Clinical Evidence* (15th edn), pp. 1366–1406. London: BMJ Books. http://www.clinicalevidence.com/ceweb/conditions/meh/1003/1003.jsp.

Gale, C. and Browne, M. (2006). Generalised anxiety disorder. *Clinical Evidence* (15th edn), pp. 1407–1418. London: BMJ Books. http://www.clinicalevidence.com/ceweb/conditions/meh/1002/1002.jsp.

Hay, P. and Bacaltchuk, J. (2006). Bulimia nervosa. *Clinical Evidence* (15th edn), pp. 1315–1331. London: BMJ Books. http://www.clinicalevidence.com/ceweb/conditions/meh/1009/1009.jsp.

Jung, C. (1971). *Man and His Symbols.* New York: Laurel.

Kumar, S. and Browne, M. (2006). Panic disorder. *Clinical Evidence* (15th edn), pp. 138–139. London: BMJ Books. http://www.clinicalevidence.com/ceweb/conditions/meh/1010/1010.jsp.

(NICE) National Institute for Health and Clinical Excellence. (2006). Depression and anxiety – computerised cognitive behavioural therapy (CCBT). http://www.nice.org.uk/page.aspx?o=TA97.

Palmer, R. (2002). Dialectical behaviour therapy for borderline personality disorder. *Adv Psychiatr Treat* **8**, 10–16.

Tantam, D. (2006). Opportunities and risks in e-therapy. *Adv Psychiatr Treat* **12**, 368–374.

Ward, E., King, M., Lloyd, M. *et al.* (2000). Randomized controlled trial of non-directive counselling, cognitive-behaviour therapy, and usual general practitioner care for patients with depression. I. Clinical effectiveness. *BMJ* **321**, 1383–1388.

Further reading

Bateman, A., Brown, D. and Pedder, J. (2000). *An Introduction to Psychotherapy* (3rd edn). London: Routledge.
Hawton, K., Salkovskis, P. M., Kirk, J. and Clark, D. M. (eds) (1989). *Cognitive Behaviour Therapy for Psychiatric Problems: A Practical Guide.* Oxford: Oxford University Press.
Storr, A. (1990). *The Art of Psychotherapy* (2nd edn). Oxford: Butterworth Heinemann.

23 Psychopharmacology

General principles of using psychotropic drugs

Psychotropic drugs are immensely valuable in the treatment of mental illness. They are not, however, a substitute for psychological treatments and social care; best results are often achieved by some combination of all these approaches. Relevant questions about psychotropic drug use include the following.

When is drug treatment indicated?

Clear-cut psychiatric illness often responds well to drugs, but medication may be less effective for milder illness, personality disorders, behaviour problems, and reactions to stress. In primary care, much psychiatric symptomatology is brief and self-limiting, and medication may not be necessary, although it is often prescribed.

Do the therapeutic effects outweigh any negative aspects?

All effective drugs have side-effects, usually unwanted ones. Many psychotropics react adversely with *other drugs* or *alcohol*, and impair *driving skills*. *Elderly patients*, women who are *pregnant or breast-feeding*, and *patients with medical disorders* are at greatest risk of unwanted effects. *Tolerance and/or dependence* seldom cause problems except with benzodiazepines, but patients are often

Hughes' Outline of Modern Psychiatry, Fifth Edition. David Gill.
© 2007 John Wiley & Sons, Ltd   ISBN 9780470033920

needlessly worried about 'getting addicted' to other psychotropics, especially antidepressants. Patients with suicidal tendencies may use psychotropic drugs for *overdose* if issued with large quantities. The *financial cost* of drug treatment is another significant factor, although likely to be considerably less than the cost of inadequately treated mental illness.

What if drug treatment seems appropriate, but has not worked?

Many patients take their drugs irregularly, or not at all. Compliance can be improved by using single-drug regimens, taken once daily. Most psychotropic drugs persist at therapeutic levels for at least 24 hours, giving little rationale for divided doses.

If drug treatment seems appropriate but has not worked, has the drug been given in adequate dosage for long enough?

Depressive illness treated with antidepressants and schizophrenia treated with antipsychotics may take 4–6 weeks to respond. With antidepressants, use of subtherapeutic doses for too short a time is a common error.

How long should treatment be continued?

Benzodiazepines for anxiety and insomnia should be given for only a few weeks at a time, because of the risk of tolerance and dependence; but antidepressants, if effective, should be continued for several months to prevent relapse. Lithium for prophylaxis of affective disorder, and antipsychotics for maintenance treatment of schizophrenia, are usually continued for several years and sometimes are needed for life.

With difficult or atypical cases, it may be necessary to experiment with different pharmacological groups in order to find the best drug or combination of drugs. Changes should be made one at a time, and not before each one has been given a chance to work.

Which route of administration?

Oral medication is of course the rule. Liquid rather than solid formulations are easier for some patients to swallow – and harder for uncooperative ones to hide in their mouths. Intramuscular injections include ordinary short-acting ones, such as haloperidol 10 mg for severe agitation in a psychotic patient, and long-acting 'depot' preparations where the active medication is esterified and suspended in an oily form from which it is released slowly, such as haloperidol decanoate 100 mg every 4 weeks to keep chronic schizophrenia in remission. Intravenous injections are rarely used, and are unsafe with some psychotropic drugs.

Proprietary or generic formulation?

Lithium is one of the few psychotropic drugs where this matters pharmacologically, as the same dose of different preparations may produce very different levels in the patient, so the prescriber must specify and stick to a particular one. This consideration does not apply to most other drugs, so generic prescribing to reduce costs is officially encouraged. However, generic prescribing has the disadvantage that different formats (size, shape, colour, and taste) of tablets containing the same dose of the same drug are available, causing patients potentially to be alarmed if the appearance of their medication changes when a fresh supply is dispensed.

The need for explanation

Prescription of drugs should always be accompanied by clear explanation and discussion about the need for medication, why a particular compound has been chosen, the likely benefits and risks, and the effects both wanted and unwanted. Such talks take only a short time, are highly valued by patients, and have been shown to improve compliance. Written information leaflets are also helpful.

What about the new drugs?

There has been a wave of new drugs, both antipsychotics (atypicals) and antidepressants (SSRIs, etc.), as well as others. The manufacturers have claimed that these new drugs are as effective as older drugs, but have fewer side-effects. They do seem to have a more favourable side-effect profile in some cases, although their adverse effects are now beginning to emerge: for example, weight gain and diabetes with olanzepine. In medicine, as in life, one does not get anything for nothing, however, and clinical experience is that the newer drugs are less powerful. Although they may be satisfactory for milder cases, they may not be as effective in more severe cases in more disadvantaged areas.

This chapter describes the main groups of psychotropic drugs, with reference to some commonly used examples. The *British National Formulary* (*BNF*) is the standard daily reference, but it must be remembered that it is primarily written for GPs; the *Maudsley Prescribing Guidelines* offers more detailed guidance, specifically for mental health.

Antipsychotics

Antipsychotics (*neuroleptics, major tranquillizers*) specifically ameliorate psychotic symptoms (delusions and hallucinations), as well as having a general sedative action. *Chlorpromazine* was first introduced in the 1950s, as an antihistamine; a French surgeon noted its marked sedative action on surgical patients, and it was then tried out on psychiatric patients, often with dramatic results. Many other compounds are now available (Box 23.1).

Box 23.1 Antipsychotic Drugs in Common Use

Generic name	Proprietary name	Chemical group
Chlorpromazine	Largactil	Phenothiazine
Clozapine	Clozaril	Dibenzapine
Fluphenazine decanoate*	Modecate	Phenothiazine
Flupenthixol decanoate*	Depixol	Thioxanthene
Haloperidol	Serenace	Butyrophenone
Haloperidol decanoate*	Haldol	Butyrophenone
Olanzepine	Zyprexa	Atypical
Pimozide	Orap	
Diphenylbutylpiperidine		
Promazine	Sparine	Phenothiazine
Risperidone	Risperdal	Atypical
Sulpiride	Dolmatil	Benzamide
Trifluoperazine	Stelazine	Phenothiazine
Zuclopenthixol decanoate*	Clopixol	Thioxanthene
Zuclopenthixol acetate†	Acuphase	Thioxanthene

*Long-acting intramuscular injection.
†Medium-acting intramuscular injection.

Indications

* *schizophrenia*

* *mania*

* *severely agitated or violent behaviour* associated with any psychiatric disorder or organic brain syndrome

* *anxiety* that has failed to respond to other treatments

* in general medicine as *antiemetics* and to *potentiate analgesics and anaesthetics.*

Pharmacology

Most antipsychotics are thought to work at least partly through blocking dopamine receptors in the brain. Serum prolactin level is a measure of this dopaminergic blockade. However, different antipsychotic drugs have different effects at the various subtypes of dopamine receptors. Most antipsychotics also have antiadrenergic, anticholinergic, and antihistaminic actions.

Chlorpromazine is regarded pharmacologically as a 'dirty' drug; that is, it has actions on several neurotransmitter systems. As indicated above, its antihistamine action produces sedation, which is often useful in acute psychiatric presentations. By contrast, haloperidol is a 'cleaner' drug, with actions predominantly on the dopamine system. Because it does not have actions on the histamine and acetylcholine systems, it may not be strongly sedative in some patients; it may therefore need to be supplemented in clinical use by prescription of minor tranquillizers such as the benzodiazepines.

Recently, 'atypical' antipsychotics have been introduced and have rapidly become popular. They were initially promoted as being free from side-effects, but, inevitably, after a few years, their side-effects have become apparent. Risperidone can cause extrapyramidal side-effects. Olanzepine, especially, but also other atypicals are associated with weight gain and diabetes. They also carry a specific risk of stroke, causing them to be discouraged in the elderly.

Prescribers must remain alert to sudden changes in medication availability and indications. Lack of a sufficient market caused the company concerned suddenly to stop supplying droperidol. Action by the Committee on the Safety of

Medicines caused the very useful and gentle drug thioridazine (Melleril) to be abruptly withdrawn as a first-line treatment of schizophrenia, on the basis of reported cardiovascular problems. And more recently, as indicated above, the supposedly safe atypicals have been warned against in the elderly, in whom they may cause stroke.

Administration

Acute psychosis may be treated with oral medication given three or four times daily. There is a calming effect from the start, but control of delusions and hallucinations may take 3–4 weeks, and sometimes the full benefit is not seen for 6–12 months. In schizophrenia, the positive symptoms respond better than the negative ones. A recently introduced, medium-acting intramuscular preparation, *Clopixol Acuphase*, which exerts its effects over 2–3 days, is useful in very disturbed patients.

Chronic schizophrenia is often treated by slow-release, intramuscular injections (depots) every 1–4 weeks. Such injections may have a pharmacological advantage for some patients in whom oral medication is incompletely absorbed or undergoes rapid first-pass metabolism in the liver, but their main advantage is ensuring regular medication and follow-up for a group of patients whose compliance with oral treatment tends to be poor.

For some cases of schizophrenia that do not respond to conventional doses of drugs, clozapine should be considered at an early stage, as responses to this drug are seen that do not seem to occur with other agents. High-dose regimens are much less commonly used nowadays, especially since the advent of clozapine. In patients with treatment-resistant psychosis, it is better to add a drug from another class, usually a benzodiazepine, or consider ECT.

Unwanted effects

Antipsychotic drugs have a great many potential unwanted effects. Most common and troublesome are those involving the *extrapyramidal nervous system*, as follows:

- *Parkinsonism*, with tremor, rigidity, bradykinesia, and sialorrhoea

- *akathisia*, with mental agitation and motor restlessness

- *acute dystonia,* including torticollis, other abnormal postures, and oculogyric crisis.

All these extrapyramidal effects respond to *anti-Parkinsonian* drugs such as *benzhexol* or *procyclidine*, but these extra drugs should not be given unless required because they may cause sedation and confusion, and exacerbate psychotic symptoms and anticholinergic effects; moreover, they (especially procyclidine, because of a temporary mood-altering effect) may be abused.

Tardive dyskinesia is another syndrome of abnormal movements that develops in up to 20 per cent of patients on long-term antipsychotic drug treatment. Elderly, female, and brain-damaged patients are most likely to be affected. Involuntary movements of choreiform or athetoid type affect the orofacial muscles and sometimes the limbs or trunk. The cause may be proliferation or hypersensitivity of dopamine receptors after prolonged blockade by antipsychotic drugs, or imbalance between dopamine and its antagonists acetylcholine and GABA. There is no effective treatment; anti-Parkinsonian drugs help some patients. Reducing or, paradoxically, increasing the dose of the responsible antipsychotic may help. Prevention is better, and may be achieved by using the lowest antipsychotic dose that is effective.

Other unwanted effects of antipsychotic drugs include *hypotension, cardiac arrhythmia,* either *dry mouth* or *excessive salivation (sialorrhoea), constipation, weight gain, reduced fertility, bone marrow depression, blurred vision, retention of urine, impotence, jaundice, rash, photosensitivity,* and *hypothermia* especially in the elderly.

Neuroleptic malignant syndrome is a rare, but potentially fatal, acute complication of antipsychotic drug use. Symptoms include catatonia or extrapyramidal movements, and hyperpyrexia. Affected patients require intensive medical care.

Antipsychotics are mainly metabolized in the liver. Their main drug interaction is to potentiate the sedative effects of other psychoactive substances, most importantly alcohol, antidepressants, and benzodiazepines. Liver damage is the main contraindication. Regarding use in pregnancy, no serious adverse effects on the foetus are known. Antipsychotic drugs enter breast milk in tiny amounts, but usually, if there is clear indication for their use, the benefit of having a healthy mother outweighs any potential risk to the infant. Antipsychotic drugs lower the convulsive threshold slightly, so caution is required in patients with epilepsy. They sensitize the skin to sunburn, so advice and sunblock preparation are needed in sunny periods.

Tolerance and dependence do not occur.

Choice of drug

The newer drugs appear to offer an advance in the treatment of schizophrenia, at least in expanding the range of choice of available drugs. They are recommended by NICE (http://www.nice.org.uk/page.aspx?o=289559) to be 'considered in the choice of first-line treatments for individuals with newly diagnosed schizophrenia'. In other words, the evidence reviewed did not allow NICE to recommend that the newer drugs should generally be used as first-line treatment, or that they should be reserved for use when a typical drug has failed.

Some psychiatrists still regard *chlorpromazine* as their first-line antipsychotic; however, they are now in a minority. Clinical experience is that the majority of UK psychiatrists do now regard atypical antipsychotics as first-line drugs, and most will reserve the older drugs for when atypical drugs have not worked.

Overall, the advantage lies with the prescriber becoming familiar with two or three key drugs, which he can prescribe with confidence and which work in his hands.

In my own practice, I find *olanzepine* be a satisfactory initial treatment for acute psychotic episodes. Often a suitable starting dose is 5 mg at night. There are liquid and quick-dissolving tablets, formulations that are helpful if there is doubt about whether the patient can be trusted to swallow conventional pills. It is a sedative drug, and this is helpful to patients (and nurses) in the acute stages. It does not, however, seem to be the most powerful drug against the core symptoms of psychosis, delusions, and hallucinations. I find that a combination of olanzepine with a small dose of haloperidol (1.5–5 mg, for example) can be helpful if there are residual psychotic symptoms. Such doses of haloperidol are well tolerated, and the combination may be better in the long run than the alternative of persisting with maximum doses of olanzepine, with the attendant risk of weight gain.

The main disadvantage of olanzepine is its association with weight gain and even with diabetes; if it is used as a maintenance treatment, therefore, the dose should be reduced to a minimum, and monitoring of weight is important.

Risperidone can produce extrapyramidal effects, more so than olanzepine, but less so than the typical antipsychotics. It is less associated with weight gain and olanzepine. There is an injectable preparation, which offers an alternative to the traditional depot antipsychotics; some patients do well on it. However, it seems not to be as strong a drug as the 'typical' antipsychotics for the most severely affected.

Aripiprazole and *quetiapine* are other atypicals available; they are felt to have benign profiles of unwanted effects, but to be of limited effectiveness in severely ill patients.

If the first drug chosen does not work, it is logical to change to one of a different chemical group. If two drugs have failed, clozapine should be considered.

Clozapine is a highly effective antipsychotic but is licensed only for use in resistant cases that have failed to respond to first-line drugs. Because of its risk of agranulocytosis, it is only available on a named-patient basis on condition that regular blood counts are satisfactory. The full benefit of clozapine may not be seen for at least a year.

Thioridazine causes few Parkinsonian effects, and is sedative, but is more likely to cause confusion – all these because of its strong anticholinergic properties. It has been described as 'the first atypical'. Unfortunately, because of cardiovascular side-effects, it is no longer regarded as suitable for routine use.

Haloperidol is pharmacologically 'cleaner', with fewer actions outside the dopaminergic system; it has a reputation of being prone to cause extrapyramidal effects. This may be due to its previous use in very high doses, perhaps in an effort to produce the sedation that its mainly dopamine-focused actions mean is inherently unlikely.

However, even small doses of haloperidol (1.5–5 mg) are profoundly antipsychotic, and at this dose, haloperidol is well tolerated. It can be supplemented with benzodiazepines (or olanzepine) if additional sedation is required. Such regimens offer an alternative, probably underused, to automatic prescription of the very much more expensive atypicals.

Amisulpiride was thought to have specific effectiveness against negative symptoms, but unfortunately, this has not generally been borne out in use. It appears to be a fairly gentle, although not especially strong, antipsychotic.

Antidepressants

Three classes of antidepressants are generally distinguished, on the basis of chemical structure or presumed pharmacological mechanism of action: the tricyclics (structure of three rings), the selective serotonin reuptake inhibitors (SSRIs), and the monoamine oxidase inhibitors (MAOIs). However, certain antidepressants cannot be fitted neatly into this somewhat arbitrary classification. Some features of these three classes are given in the table:

Class	Example	Characteristics
Tricyclics	Trimipramine (Surmontil)	The most effective antidepressants in severe depressive states Anxiolytic, analgesic, and hypnotic properties, which are predictable, dose-related, and helpful Wide dose range
MAOIs	Phenelzine (Parnate)	Grossly underused due to fears of 'cheese reaction' and consequent dietary restriction; effective in atypical and refractory depression
SSRIs	Fluoxetine (Prozac)	Widely prescribed by GPs for emotional problems, often effectively as a placebo Frequently but unpredictably cause agitation, gastrointestinal upset, and sexual dysfunction Less effective for severe cases Limited dose range Reports of suicidality and withdrawal symptoms

Antidepressants: tricyclic group

Tricyclics were for many years the standard first-line drug treatment for depressive illness, but they have been supplanted by the SSRIs in this regard in general practice. *Imipramine* and *amitriptyline* are the longest established drugs of the tricyclic group but many others exist (Box 23.2), some having a tetracyclic or other chemical structure.

Indications

- *depressive illness*

- *depression* associated with other psychiatric conditions

- *anxiety states* and *panic disorder*

- *nocturnal enuresis*

- *chronic pain*, especially of 'neuropathic' type.

Box 23.2 Tricyclic and Related Antidepressants in Common Use

Generic name	Proprietary name	Structure
Amitriptyline	Tryptizol	Tricyclic
Amoxapine	Asendis	Tricyclic
Clomipramine	Anafranil	Tricyclic
Dothiepin (now called dosulepin)	Prothiaden	Tricyclic
Doxepin	Sinequan	Tricyclic
Imipramine	Tofranil	Tricyclic
Lofepramine	Gamanil	Tricyclic
Maprotiline	Ludiomil	Tetracyclic
Mianserin	Bolvidon, Norval	Tetracyclic
Nortriptyline	Allegron	Tricyclic
Trazadone	Molipaxin	Novel
Trimipramine	Surmontil	Tricyclic

Pharmacology

One mechanism of antidepressant action is believed to be prevention of reuptake of amine neurotransmitters into neurons. Changes in the number or sensitivity of postsynaptic receptors may also be involved. Most antidepressants affect both the noradrenaline and 5-HT systems, but others act selectively on one or the other. They have peripheral anticholinergic effects.

Administration

These drugs should be started in a small dose, increased every few days if well tolerated. The oral route is almost always used; some parenteral preparations exist but do not have any clear advantage and are now rarely used. It is often possible to give the total dose at night; this helps with sleep and improves compliance.

Many patients in fact begin to improve within days rather than weeks, possibly owing to the anxiolytic and hypnotic effects of these drugs, which are immediate. However, there may be a delay of 2 or more weeks before the antidepressant effect is manifested, and it is essential to counsel patients about this, especially as side effects are most prominent in the first week.

Even if a depressive episode seems to have recovered completely with drug treatment, the drug should be continued in full therapeutic dose for at least 6 months before dose reduction is considered.

Unwanted effects

A long list of possible unwanted effects, many of them due to the tricyclics' anticholinergic properties, are listed here, but in practice only a few commonly occur.

Sedation may be beneficial if the patient is anxious or sleeping badly, but can be a nuisance during the day. Fortunately, it wears off over a few days in most patients with true depressive illness. While affected, patients must be advised not to drive or use machinery. Sedation is made worse by alcohol.

Dry mouth, *blurred vision*, and *constipation* are common, and *urinary retention* may occur. *Postural hypotension* may be dose-limiting, especially in the elderly. Tricyclics can also cause *confusion* in elderly patients, or those with organic brain disease. Tricyclics lower the *convulsive threshold*, but this effect should not stop their use in a depressed epileptic, where the benefits of effective treatment far outweigh the risk of precipitating a fit.

Less commonly, tricyclics, especially amitriptyline, can cause *cardiac arrhythmia* or *heart block*, precipitating sudden death in some patients with cardiac disease. Other rare but potentially serious effects are precipitation of *glaucoma*, and *hepatic* and *haematological* reactions.

Weight gain is common, and deters some patients from taking these drugs.

Tricyclics are metabolized in the liver. They have additive interactions with MAOIs, barbiturates, phenothiazines, anticholinergics, and anticoagulants, as well as with alcohol. The main contraindications are cardiac disease, glaucoma, and prostatic enlargement. Use in pregnancy is relatively safe, as no serious adverse effects on the foetus are known, and tricyclics enter breast milk in small amounts only. Tolerance and dependence are not a significant problem, and it is important to reassure patients of this; however, sudden withdrawal of a tricyclic may cause nausea, headache, sweating, and insomnia.

Tricyclics – except lofepramine – are toxic in overdose, and this has been one of the reasons for SSRIs, which are generally not toxic, becoming more popular. It has not been shown that tricyclics cause an excess of suicides; on the other hand, concerns have been expressed that SSRIs can cause suicidality, linked probably to their propensity to cause agitation in some patients. The key to seeking to minimize suicide is good overall care with risk assessment and risk management; choice of drug should be dictated by clinical effectiveness.

Choice of drug

Patients in whom depression is accompanied by agitation or insomnia are most likely to benefit from one of the more sedative tricyclics such as *amitriptyline*, *dothiepin*, or *trimipramine*, whereas patients with psychomotor retardation may be better on a non-sedating drug such as *imipramine*, *lofepramine*, or *nortriptyline*.

The side-effect profile may determine the choice of drug, especially in patients with co-existing medical disorders. Compounds such as *amitriptyline* tend to produce more unwanted effects than the newer ones, yet, for some patients, they appear to be more effective as antidepressants.

If depression proves resistant to tricyclics, another drug may be added. *Lithium* augmentation is sometimes helpful. Combined therapy of a tricyclic with an *SSRI* or *MAOI* (see below) is another option but may be hazardous, so it should be used only by experienced specialists.

Antidepressants: SSRI group

SSRIs (selective serotonin reuptake inhibitors) (Box 23.3) have been available on the UK market since 1989, and have been widely prescribed.

Their prescription to child patients; however, has become very controversial, because of lack of evidence of effectiveness in this patient group, and also concern over increased suicide risk. Recent NICE guidance is that 'antidepressant medication should not be used for the initial treatment of children and young people with mild depression'; even in moderate to severe depression; the place of medication is given as 'brief psychological therapy +/− fluoxetine' (http://www.nice.org.uk/page.aspx?o=cg028niceguidelineword).

On the face of it, there seems to be some discrepancy between this and the NICE guidance for adults: 'When an antidepressant is to be prescribed in routine care, it should be a selective serotonin reuptake inhibitor (SSRI)' (http://www.nice.org.uk/page.aspx?o=cg023niceguidelineword). However, NICE is really preaching to the choir on this. SSRIs have been vigorously promoted, and have been commercially successful. Many GPs use them as first-line treatment for depressive illness, on the basis of claimed therapeutic advantages that have not always stood up to critical examination.

In specialist care, there is seldom much point in initiating SSRI prescription, as most patients referred with depression will already have been tried on them in primary care. If they have had a good trial of an SSRI, there would be no point in trying a different SSRI, as the similarities far outweigh the differences.

If there has been no response, a different drug class (TCA or MAOI) should be tried. If there has been a partial response, a second drug (for example, trimipramine at night, especially if sleep remains a problem) can be added; this is a safe manoeuvre in specialist hands.

Occasionally, an SSRI may be added to the treatment regimen of a patient who has made a partial response to tricyclic antidepressant (TCA) medication; for example, adding fluoxetine 20 mg mane to the treatment of a patient taking trimipramine 150 mg nocte may have a modest effect in improving mood, and the alerting effects may also be useful.

Box 23.3   SSRI Antidepressants

Generic name	Proprietary name
Citalopram	Cipramil
Escitalopram	Cipralex
Fluoxetine	Prozac
Fluvoxamine	Faverin
Paroxetine	Seroxat
Sertraline	Lustral

Points of comparison between TCAs and SSRIs include:

Efficacy

Clinical trials suggest that SSRIs and tricyclics are about equal in their antidepressant properties, although some patients respond better to one or other type of drug. However, patients included in commercial drug trials tend to be toward the milder end of the spectrum. Some trials have excluded, for example, those with suicidal risk or comorbid conditions. Clinical experience is that severely depressed patients, especially those whose sleep is disturbed, respond better to a sedative tricyclic or other drug than to an SSRI.

Unwanted effects

SSRIs are claimed to have fewer unwanted effects than tricyclics, but the picture is mixed: 'one systematic review . . . found that about twice as many people taking TCAs compared with SSRIs had dry mouth, constipation, and dizziness but that slightly more people taking SSRIs had nausea, diarrhoea, anxiety, agitation, insomnia, nervousness, and headache' (Butler *et al.*, 2006).

Although not physically addictive in the sense that they do not give rise to tolerance, with a constant need to increase the dose to achieve the same effect, some patients do find it difficult to get off them. They report anxiety, tremor, and a variety of other symptoms. There is of course a good deal in common between these alleged discontinuation effects and some of the symptoms for which the patient may have been prescribed the drug in the first place, so the matter is difficult to evaluate. It has been widely publicized, and legal action against the drug companies is in contemplation.

Metabolism

Fluoxetine has a very long half-life; this is a disadvantage as far as drug interactions are concerned, but means the drug could theoretically be given in one dose every few days as a 'depot antidepressant' when compliance is limited.

Safety in overdose

SSRIs are safe in overdosage. Most tricyclics, with the exception of lofepramine, are toxic, and so SSRIs are increasingly used in suicidal patients. However, although tricyclic poisoning is a contributory factor in some suicides, it has never been shown that the total death rate is greater in patients on these potentially more poisonous drugs.

Cost

SSRIs are considerably more expensive, as most are still in patent; cheap, non-brand name (generic) preparations are available for most TCAs and MAOIs.

Dosage

SSRIs have a narrower therapeutic range, and therefore the advantage of a simple standard dose regimen; this is especially useful in the elderly. However, the wide possible dose range of tricyclics can also be useful, as in permitting a very small starting dose in a patient susceptible to side-effects.

Other indications

Certain SSRIs are licensed for use in eating disorders, panic disorder, and obsessive-compulsive disorders, as well as for depressive illness. Fluoxetine has been widely used in the USA to 'enhance' mood and boost confidence in people without formal psychiatric disorder; this practice is controversial.

Antidepressants: MAOI group

MAOIs (*monoamine oxidase inhibitors*) increase brain concentrations of monoamine neurotransmitters by inhibiting the enzymes concerned in their breakdown. They are effective for depression, anxiety, and phobic states, and sometimes achieve dramatic responses in patients who have failed to respond to tricyclics.

They may have a particular place in so-called atypical depression 'with reversed biological features, e.g. increased sleep, increased appetite, mood reactivity, and rejection sensitivity' (Butler *et al.*, 2006). The *BNF* recommends that 'MAOIs should be tried in any patients who are refractory to treatment with other antidepressants as there is occasionally a dramatic response' (http://www.bnf.org/bnf/bnf/51/3341.htm?q=%22maois%22), although this advice is, sadly, seldom followed in practice.

Box 23.4 MAOI Antidepressants

Generic name	Proprietary name
Isocarboxazid	Marplan
Moclobemide	Mannerix
Phenelzine	Nardil
Tranylcypromine	Parnate

In addition to their anticholinergic side-effects (similar to those described above for the tricyclics), MAOIs may cause potentially dangerous interactions with sympathomimetic drugs (including common-cold remedies) and tyramine-containing foods (Box 23.5), which must therefore be avoided. Such interactions produce headache and palpitations; rarely, they can produce a hypertensive crisis that may lead to stroke or sudden death. In order to do so, however, the departure from the advice above must be very gross and repeated. A single indiscretion would usually not produce any adverse effect.

Patients on MAOIs should be given a card listing the items to avoid. It is probable that the risks have been overestimated, and that these effective drugs have been underused as a result. The most recently introduced MAOI, moclobemide, is less prone to cause food and drug interactions because it is selective for the MAO-A isoform, which is found in the liver as opposed to the gut. It can be used on a trial basis: patients who respond somewhat to it can then be tried on a 'proper', full-strength MAOI.

Box 23.5   Interactions with MAOI

Foods   Cheese (strong), red wine (especially Chianti), beer (strong),
            game, yeast, smoked fish, Marmite, Bovril.
Drugs   SSRIs, amphetamines, L-dopa, fenfluramine, local anaesthetics,
            ephedrine, triptans

Other antidepressant drugs

When the last edition of this book was coming out, antidepressants new to the market included *Venlafaxine* (see below) and *Nefazadone*. However, *Nefazodone* had to be withdrawn after a few years, because of liver toxicity. This should stand as a further warning, as if any were needed, against hasty prescription of new medications. (The wise psychiatrist will wait a few years while other doctors try out new drugs on their patients.) Nevertheless, the field of antidepressant prescribing seems to continue to be a 'dedicated follower of fashion'; the latest SSRI or other compound being likely to be widely adopted if it is innocuous and skillfully marketed.

Flupenthixol, which has somewhat confusingly been renamed flupentixol, is mainly used as an antipsychotic drug – most frequently as the long-acting depot injection Modecate. However, low doses (1–3 mg daily) are given by mouth as an antidepressant medication. It can be a useful adjunct when there has been a partial response to other forms of antidepressant treatment.

Tryptophan is a precursor of the amines and is thought to be low in depression. It was a popular adjuvant treatment in depression some years ago, but had to be withdrawn because of eosinophilia-myalgia syndrome. This was probably due to contamination of supplies with yeast. It is now available again; it should be initiated under specialist supervision.

Venlafaxine has been successfully marketed as 'a *serotonin noradrenaline reuptake inhibitor* or *SNRI*', although, of course, it shares this characteristic with other existing drugs. However, it has fewer sedative and antimuscarinic effects than the TCAs. The Committee on Safety of Medicine (CSM) recommends that venlafaxine be initiated and maintained by specialists only, and avoided in patients with heart disease, electrolyte imbalance, and hypertension.

Mirtazepine, a presynaptic α2-antagonist, increases brain noradrenaline and serotonin functionality. It is markedly sedative; it is useful in anxiety for that reason, but it also seems to be an effective antidepressant. Other drugs include *reboxetine* and *duloxetine*.

Benzodiazepines

Benzodiazepines were widely prescribed in the 1960s and 1970s as anxiolytics and hypnotics. For a while, they were perceived as 'wonder drugs' against neurosis, with no side-effects or addiction potential, in contrast to their predecessors, the barbiturates. In the 1980s, however, because of concern about their inappropriate use for people with social and interpersonal problems rather than true psychiatric disorder, and because of the emerging risk of dependence, prescription of benzodiazepines was discouraged, psychological techniques of anxiety management being recommended as an alternative.

Current CSM advice is that

1. Benzodiazepines are indicated for the short-term relief (2–4 weeks only) of anxiety that is severe, disabling, or subjecting the individual to unacceptable distress, occurring alone or in association with insomnia or short-term psychosomatic, organic, or psychotic illness.

2. The use of benzodiazepines to treat short-term 'mild' anxiety is inappropriate and unsuitable.

3. Benzodiazepines should be used to treat insomnia only when it is severe, disabling, or subjecting the individual to extreme distress.

Box 23.6 Benzodiazepines in Common Use

Generic name

Alprazolam
Chlordiazepoxide
Diazepam
Flurazepam
Nitrazepam
Lorazepam
Temazepam

It is important to realize that the CSM's sensible and cautious advice does not constitute a ban on benzodiazepines. The pendulum has, however, swung perhaps a little too far, and, at present, benzodiazepines as effective remedies for short-term anxiety are probably underused. Excessive prescription should certainly be avoided, but some authorities consider that these drugs remain a reasonable long-term treatment for a small minority of chronically anxious patients. Intensive effort to wean all long-term users off benzodiazepines is not automatically justified.

Further concern about benzodiazepines stems from their popularity with drug misusers. Intravenous injection of the gel from temazepam capsules became prevalent and caused gangrene of the limbs; these capsules have therefore been withdrawn.

Indications

- short-term treatment of *pathological anxiety*

- short-term treatment of *insomnia*

- *adjunctive treatment of psychosis and acute behavioural disturbance* in inpatient settings

- *alcohol withdrawal states* (e.g. DTs) and *detoxification*

- *status epilepticus*

- *muscle spasticity*
- *anaesthetic premedication*
- sedation in *terminal illness*.

Pharmacology

Benzodiazepines probably act through modification of the GABA and glycine neurotransmitter systems in the limbic system and spinal cord.

Administration

Benzodiazepines for anxiety or insomnia are most effective if taken only when required, rather than on a fixed-dose regimen, and only for a few weeks at a time. Intramuscular, intravenous, and rectal preparations are available for emergency use.

Unwanted effects

Benzodiazepines, even in overdose, are not toxic. Apart from drowsiness, they may have a few unwanted effects in the young, healthy person, but the elderly may experience marked side-effects of which the neurological and psychiatric ones are most important. These include *confusion, depression, drowsiness, amnesia, impaired psychomotor performance including an effect on driving, ataxia, dysarthria, and headache.* Some subjects experience 'paradoxical' effects of *excitement, aggression,* or *insomnia.* Benzodiazepines potentiate the effects of alcohol and other cerebral depressants.

Use in *pregnancy* should be avoided. In late pregnancy, benzodiazepines can cause the 'floppy infant syndrome' of hypotonia, respiratory embarrassment, and hypothermia, and the baby may develop withdrawal symptoms after delivery. Benzodiazepines readily enter breast milk.

Tolerance and dependence may develop with regular use. *Psychological dependence* is common. *Physical dependence* develops in around 20 per cent of those who take benzodiazepines long-term. Suddenly stopping the drugs in such patients causes a withdrawal syndrome of insomnia, tremor, fits, anorexia, vomiting, sweating, and cramps.

This syndrome, which is most often seen after the withdrawal of a short-acting drug such as *alprazolam, lorazepam,* or *temazepam,* may be mistaken for recurrence of the original anxiety for which the drug was prescribed. Withdrawal symptoms can be avoided by tapering the drug gradually, while introducing psychological anxiety management techniques. Some authorities recommend converting the benzodiazepine-dependent patient to the equivalent dose of *diazepam*, which can then be reduced by 1 mg per week over a period of 1–12 months.

Choice of drug

Many benzodiazepines are available. They vary in potency and duration of action, but many are metabolized to the same compound, *oxazepam*, and are to some extent interchangeable. The same compound can often be used in low dose to treat anxiety and in higher dose to induce sleep. Longer-acting ones can be given in a single nighttime dose to provide an immediate hypnotic effect followed by an anxiolytic effect next day. The shorter-acting ones are suitable for insomnia, which is not accompanied by daytime anxiety, or for phobic anxiety related to specific situations.

Other drugs for anxiety and insomnia

Various alternatives to the benzodiazepines are available as hypnotics and/or anxiolytics, although all have unwanted effects of their own. *Antidepressants* are often used to treat chronic anxiety or anxiety mixed with depression. *Trimipramine*, *trazadone*, and *mirtazepine* are suitable. Some immediate benefit may occur due to the sedative action, and gradual further improvement should follow over several weeks. Other options include *beta-blockers* such as *propranolol*, effective mainly for the physical symptoms of anxiety; *antipsychotics* such as *chlorpromazine* in low dose; antihistamines such as *promethazine*, and newer preparations such as *buspirone*.

For insomnia, long-established remedies include *chloral hydrate* and *promethazine*; newer drugs include *zopiclone*. Hypnotics are recommended for occasional use only; dealing with the cause of the insomnia is a better alternative to drugs. Causes include noise, discomfort, a restless partner, worry, shift work, travel, excess alcohol or caffeine intake, or unrealistic expectations about the amount of sleep required.

Barbiturates, once widely used as hypnotics and anxiolytics before benzodiazepines became available, are now obsolete as psychotropic drugs because of the high risk of dependence and high toxicity in overdose.

Mood stablizers

These drugs are used as prophylactic medication in bipolar affective disorder. That is, they are given long-term in order to reduce the frequency, duration, and severity of further episodes of affective disorder, whether manic or depressive. The drugs do have slight effectiveness in the acute episode, and are usually started during it; however, they are not strong enough to be relied on by themselves for treatment of acute episodes, needing to be supplemented by major tranquillizers and/or benzodiazepines.

The main drugs in use in the UK are lithium and certain drugs originally marketed as anticonvulsants but that have been found to have effectiveness in this area; these include sodium valproate, carbamazepine, and, to some extent, lamotrigine and other newer agents.

Lithium

Lithium is the lightest of the alkali metals. It was the first drug found to be effective as a mood stabilizer. It remains the standard treatment in the UK for probably the majority of psychiatrists. In the USA, under medico-legal pressure, it is less frequently used as a first-line treatment because of concerns about renal and other long-term effects (see below).

Indications

• *Prophylaxis of recurrent episodes of affective disorder*, when these are sufficiently frequent or disabling to justify long-term continuous drug treatment. In the past, lithium has been used mainly in bipolar disorder, being effective in reducing both frequency and severity of episodes. Lithium is now increasingly used in prophylaxis of recurrent unipolar depression also.

• *Adjunctive treatment of episodes of mania and depression.*

• *Schizo-affective disorder.*

Administration

Although any of lithium's soluble salts could potentially be used, only the carbonate (tablets) and citrate (liquid) are marketed. The most practical formulations are modified release tablets, allowing once daily dosage. Because bioavailability varies greatly between different brands, the prescriber should specify the brand.

Therapeutic effect is related to serum lithium level. The therapeutic range is 0.4–1.0 mmol/l. Levels of 0.8–1.0 mmol/l were traditionally recommended for prophylaxis, but these would now be regarded as higher than necessary for satisfactory maintenance of the majority of patients. The aim is to keep patients well on the minimum dose, which is achieved by frequent monitoring of the clinical state, and by regular blood tests.

Lithium has a narrow therapeutic margin, and there is individual variation in the dosage needed to produce a given serum level, so regular measurements are required. Blood for serum lithium should be taken 8 hours after the last dose. This usually means first thing in the morning after the regular nighttime dose. Blood tests may be weekly for, say, the first 4 weeks of therapy, and eventually patients can be maintained satisfactorily on a blood test every year. The blood test should include thyroid function tests and urea and electrolytes, to make sure that the thyroid and kidneys are not being affected.

Patients should carry a lithium card and be advised to maintain good fluid intake, without huge fluctuations in the amount of salt they consume. If they become unwell, they should seek medical advice and inform the doctor that they are taking lithium.

Extra tests should be performed in the event of a change in the preparation or in dosage, if symptoms suggesting lithium toxicity develop, if intercurrent illness develops, or at prescription of additional drugs, which may interact, especially diuretics.

If a patient has remained free of depression or mania for some years, it is reasonable to try gradual withdrawal of lithium, as the illness may have undergone natural remission.

Unwanted effects

- Relatively harmless: *nausea, mild diarrhoea, fine tremor* (which can be treated by a beta-blocker), *weight gain, oedema,* and *exacerbation of psoriasis.*

- Acute symptoms suggesting *lithium intoxication: vomiting, diarrhoea, coarse tremor, drowsiness, vertigo, dysarthria,* and *cardiac arrhythmia.* This condition is serious and, if such symptoms develop, lithium should be stopped immediately and blood taken for estimation of the serum level.

- Long-term effects of gradual onset: *hypothyroidism* (affecting 3 per cent of patients per year; it is usually reversible when the drug is stopped, and treatable with thyroxine if lithium is continued); rarely, *thyrotoxicosis*; and histological and functional changes in the *kidney*, of uncertain significance.

Case example

A postgraduate student, 23 years old, presented with an episode of psychotic depression which responded well to inpatient treatment, but he developed a manic illness some months later. He was started on lithium, but stopped taking it after a few days, complaining of tremor; he had also, through a doctor relative, found out about its unwanted effects, and felt that these had not been properly discussed with him. He declined other mood stabilizers, as he had become distrustful.

He recovered, but had a further severe manic episode 1 year later. This time, he responded only slowly to antipsychotic medication, and valproate was added with gradual success.

He then took valproate for several years; he continued to have affective episodes approximately annually, although they were less severe and could be managed without inpatient admission. He came to accept the medication as the price of his mental stability.

Lithium should be used only in low dose, and under frequent supervision, in patients with *cardiac or renal impairment, thyroid disease, diabetes insipidus, Addison's disease,* or *obesity,* or on *diuretic therapy*. Neurological impairment after combined dosage with lithium and haloperidol in high dose has been reported. Use in *early pregnancy* is teratogenic, the most common foetal malformation affecting the tricuspid valve of the heart. This and other deformities can be detected by ultrasound. After the first trimester, lithium is believed to be safe, and may need to be continued in women with severe manic-depressive illness, although the drug should be stopped for a few days at the time of delivery because of the risk of toxicity. Lithium enters breast milk.

Other mood stabilizers

Carbamazine

Carbamazine is widely used as an anticonvulsant and for other indications such as atypical facial pain. It is an alternative for prophylaxis of affective disorder, being more effective or better tolerated than lithium in some patients. As with lithium, regular measurements of serum levels are necessary to make sure they are within the therapeutic range. In resistant cases, lithium and carbamazepine can be used together. It can cause or exacerbate blood (e.g. leucopenia), liver, and skin conditions; monitoring of full blood count, liver and renal function tests, and blood level of the drug is necessary.

Valproate

Valproate is also used. This can be either the sodium salt, or semi-sodium. Again monitoring of blood levels is required.

Lithium, carbamazepine, and valproate, are all supported by evidence of effectiveness in prevention of relapse (Geddes and Briess, 2006); olanzepine has recently been licensed for this indication also.

Other drugs

Specialized drugs used, for example, in dementia and substance misuse are discussed in the chapters concerned.

References

Butler, R. et al. (2006). Depressive disorders. Clinical Evidence (15th edn), pp. 1366–1406. London: BMJ Books. http://www.clinicalevidence.com/ceweb/conditions/meh/1003/1003_14.jsp.

Geddes, J. and Briess, D. (2006). Bipolar disorder. Clinical Evidence (15th edn), pp. 1295–1314. London: BMJ Books. http://www.clinicalevidence.com/ceweb/conditions/meh/1014/1014.jsp.

National Institute for Health and Clinical Excellence (NICE). Depression in children and young people http://www.nice.org.uk/page.aspx?o=cg028niceguidelineword.

National Institute for Health and Clinical Excellence (NICE). Depression Management of depression in primary and secondary care http://www.nice.org.uk/page.aspx?o=cg023 niceguidelineword.

National Institute for Health and Clinical Excellence (NICE). Schizophrenia: Full guideline http://www.nice.org.uk/page.aspx?o=289559.

Further reading

British National Formulary. Published in frequently updated editions by British Medical Association and Royal Pharmaceutical Society of Great Britain.

Maudsley Prescribing Guidelines (2005). London: Dunitz.

24 Electroconvulsive therapy (ECT) and psychosurgery

Electroconvulsive therapy (ECT) was introduced by Cerletti in Italy in 1938. It involves production of a fit by passing an electric current through the brain. ECT today is carried out under a short general anaesthetic, and a muscle relaxant is given to reduce the intensity of the fit. Modern ECT machines deliver brief square-wave (not sine-wave) pulses of electricity and allow the 'dose' to be individually adjusted for the patient.

However, ECT has recently tended to arouse controversy. Some pressure groups have demanded a ban on its use. Most psychiatrists, however, while acknowledging and to some extent sharing these reservations, nevertheless consider it a highly effective treatment which they sometimes need to prescribe – albeit reluctantly – in certain severe mental illnesses. However, today, it seems to be needed much less frequently. I am responsible for a highly morbid and deprived catchment area, yet I have needed to prescribe it only twice in the last 3 years. Colleagues in elderly psychiatry prescribe it more frequently.

Hughes' Outline of Modern Psychiatry, Fifth Edition. David Gill.
© 2007 John Wiley & Sons, Ltd   ISBN 9780470033920

Indications

Depressive illness is the main indication. An MRC research study in 1965 showed that ECT is superior to antidepressant drugs for treating severe depression. Most depressed patients, however, are given drugs as the first-line treatment, ECT being reserved for use in the following circumstances:

* when life is threatened by *suicidality*

* when life and health are threatened by *refusal of food and drink*

* when antidepressant *drugs have failed*

* when antidepressant *drugs are contraindicated* for medical reasons, such as cardiac arrhythmia

* when unwanted effects of medication in the *elderly*, including some with cognitive impairment, may make drug treatment slower and riskier

* when a quick response is required, as in *post-natal depression.*

ECT is very occasionally used for inpatients with severe *schizophrenia*, especially *catatonic schizophrenia*, or *mania* that has not responded to intensive drug treatment. This indication is uncommon in the UK, although it remains prevalent in developing countries.

Mode of action

This is unknown, but may relate to alterations in neurotransmitter sensitivity. ECT causes many physiological changes, including slowing of the EEG, and increased secretion of sympathetic amines, prolactin, and other pituitary hormones, but none of these correlate reliably with clinical response. Some sceptics claim that ECT is effective just because it results in confusion, which makes the patient forget depressing thoughts.

Production of an adequate fit, arbitrarily defined as a generalized tonic-clonic seizure lasting at least 25 seconds, appears to be necessary for a good clinical effect. The minimum size of electrical stimulus required to cause a fit varies a great deal between patients, and is influenced by many factors including age, medication, and previous exposure to ECT. Ideally, the stimulus should be individually adjusted to be slightly above the individual's seizure threshold. If the stimulus is too low, no fit occurs; if too high, marked confusion may follow the treatment.

Medications with anticonvulsant effects, such as benzodiazepines, should be stopped before treatment.

Research studies comparing real ECT with 'pseudo-ECT', in which an anaesthetic and muscle relaxant are given but no electric shock, shows that real ECT is more effective in the treatment of depression but 'pseudo-ECT' has some clinical benefit too (Butler *et al.*, 2006). This suggests that factors such as the complexity and mystique of the treatment, the extra medical and nursing attention, and/or the anaesthetics are partly responsible for the therapeutic effect.

Efficacy and prediction of response

About 80 per cent of severe depressive episodes respond well to ECT in the short term. Features predicting a good response – which are essentially markers of a severe depressive illness in a previously healthy person – include retardation, guilt, delusions, early morning waking, symptoms worse in the mornings, short duration of illness, and stable premorbid personality.

Milder depression tends not to respond well, especially if mixed with neurotic symptoms and poorly adjusted premorbid personality, and ECT would not now be used in this situation.

About two-thirds of patients given ECT for depression will relapse within 6 months unless given maintenance treatment with an antidepressant drug or lithium.

Timing and number of treatments

ECT is usually given twice a week for depressive illness, and more frequent administration has no advantage. The number of treatments required in a course of ECT varies considerably, although typically it is 6–10. There is usually a transient improvement for a few hours after each application, which gradually becomes sustained.

Most depressive illnesses are episodes of a recurrent condition, often requiring prophylactic treatment. This is usually with medication, but there are very occasional patients whom only 'maintenance' ECT administered every few weeks can keep from relapse.

Practicalities of treatment

Treatment is best carried out in a specially equipped ECT suite within a psychiatric unit. Inpatient admission is usual for the first course, but outpatient ECT is feasible for patients in good general health, who can be trusted not to eat or drink on the morning of treatment, and not to drive or cycle home immediately afterward. The treatment is carried out by a psychiatrist, a nurse, and an anaesthetist. Physical examination must be performed before the course begins, in order to exclude the contraindications listed below.

Contraindications

- *Anaesthetic contraindications* include severe respiratory or cardiac disease.

- Another contraindication is *organic brain disease* of a kind in which increased cerebral blood flow would be dangerous, such as cerebral aneurysm, or conditions involving raised intracranial pressure. Other forms of organic brain disease, including dementia, epilepsy, and a past history of head injury, do not necessarily rule out the use of ECT, but do carry an increased risk of confusion after treatment.

These contraindications are relative, not absolute, and may need to be balanced against the risk to life posed by severe depression when deciding whether ECT is justified. Pregnancy is not a contraindication, nor is old age.

Bilateral versus unilateral ECT

The electrodes may be applied to both sides of the head (bilateral ECT), which is the standard treatment, or to the non-dominant side only (unilateral ECT). Bilateral ECT produces greater memory loss and confusion, but is more effective in that fewer treatments per course are needed for a therapeutic effect. Bilateral ECT is therefore preferred when a rapid response is required, but patients prone to marked cognitive impairment may be better treated with unilateral ECT.

Unwanted effects

- *Memory impairment*: transient memory impairment, both retrograde and anterograde, is frequent after each application, but usually settles within a few hours. ECT as used now does not seem to cause persisting memory problems. A small number of chronic ex-asylum patients may have had large numbers of treatments many years ago, and here a link to memory problems is more plausible. The whole question is of course confounded by the memory problems that accompany severe depressive illness, with or without ECT.

- *Confusion*: mild transient confusion after treatment is frequent. If a severe confusional state develops, ECT should be discontinued, and evidence for organic brain disease sought.

- *Anaesthetic complications.*

- *Fractures*: this is not a hazard if the fit is adequately modified by a muscle relaxant.

- *Mania* may be precipitated when ECT is given to patients with bipolar affective disorder in the depressed phase.

Mortality is 1 per 50 000 treatments, almost always from anaesthetic complications.

Consent for ECT

Most patients who have ECT do so voluntarily. (Indeed, the last two patients I have prescribed it for actually asked for it, after long inpatient stays without improvement.) Patients are required to sign a consent form before treatment. This should be preceded by a full explanation of the procedure, reinforced by an information leaflet.

Some patients refuse, or are unable to give, informed consent. If such patients appear to be in urgent need of ECT, they may be treated as an emergency under common law. However, it is much more usual to apply Section 3 of this act, and to seek the necessary second opinion from a doctor appointed by the Mental Health Act Commission.

Myths

Many patients are horrified when ECT is first suggested. The public perception, reinforced by certain sections of the media, is of 'unmodified' ECT as it used to be given 50 years ago without an anaesthetic. There were frequent physical complications such as broken teeth and bones, plus the dehumanizing character of the experience; for example, patients were often treated one after another in a public ward, with no privacy and no tranquillizing medication.

Modern administration of ECT is very different; patients are anaesthetized, treated, and recovered in privacy, and complications are rare. Many patients who have been successfully treated with ECT ask for further such treatment if their illness recurs. Research has shown that over half the patients who have had ECT consider it less unpleasant than going to the dentist.

NICE reviewed ECT in 2003 (NICE, 2003), and 'recommended that electro-convulsive therapy (ECT) is used only to achieve rapid and short-term improvement of severe symptoms after an adequate trial of other treatment options has proven ineffective and/or when the condition is considered to be potentially, life-threatening, in individuals with:

- severe depressive illness

- catatonia

- a prolonged or severe manic episode.'

This is uncontroversial and in line with modern practice. NICE more controversially opined that 'it is not recommended as a maintenance therapy in depressive illness'. However, maintenance ECT, other treatments having failed, seems to be the only way to keep a tiny number of patients (a handful per district) out of hospital.

The Royal College of Psychiatrists produces guidance on the commissioning and operation of a high-quality ECT service (Royal College of Psychiatrists, 2005).

For the future

Developments may include the use of gentler forms of stimulus such as transcranial magnetic stimulation (Schulze-Rauschenbach *et al.*, 2005).

Psychosurgery

Psychosurgery is brain surgery carried out to relieve a patient's suffering by changing mood or behaviour. Latest UK figures indicate that only seven operations were done for the 2-year period 2004–5 (Schulze-Rauschenbach *et al.*, 2005). It has thus become a near obsolete-treatment, probably carried out for only the most intractable cases of obsessive-compulsive disorder.

The history of psychosurgery serves to illustrate the way that the relative influences of the biological and the psychological approaches to psychiatry have varied over time. During the early decades of the twentieth century, psychological theories predominated, in particular the various schools of psychoanalysis.

However, their results in the treatment of psychiatric patients proved disappointing, particularly in relation to the rapid progress being made in other branches of medicine.

This led to a renewed search for what became known as physical treatments (including convulsive therapy, either electrically or chemically induced; psychosurgery; insulin coma; and electrosleep). Of these methods, only ECT has been shown to be effective in prospective, randomized, controlled trials, and the rest have now fallen out of use. Psychiatrists' enthusiasm for these and other unproven physical treatments, often used without informed consent, was a major reason for the emergence of the 'antipsychiatry' movement in the 1960s.

Moniz introduced psychosurgery in Portugal in 1935. During the next 20 years, many patients in mental hospitals all over the world underwent lobotomy, entailing large-scale, blind destruction of brain tissue. Some responded well, but others gained no benefit, suffered marked unwanted effects, or even died. The introduction in the 1950s of an effective antipsychotic drug (chlorpromazine) was followed by a secular decline in psychosurgery.

It is conceivable that psychosurgery may return in the future in a modified form, with the more precise use, for example, of fine electrodes precisely implanted and available for 'deep brain stimulation' (DBS).

References

Butler, R. et al. (2006). Depressive disorders. *Clinical Evidence* (15th edn), pp. 1366–1406. London: BMJ Books. http://www.clinicalevidence.com/ceweb/conditions/meh/1003/1003_19.jsp.

NICE (National Institute for Health and Clinical Excellence) (2003). Electroconvulsive therapy (ECT). http://www.nice.org.uk/page.aspx?o=TA059guidance.

Royal College of Psychiatrists (2005). *The ECT Handbook* (2nd edn). http://www.rcpsych.ac.uk/publications/collegereports/cr/cr128.aspx.

Schulze-Rauschenbach, S. C., Harms, U., Schlaepfer, T. E. et al. (2005). Distinctive neurocognitive effects of repetitive transcranial magnetic stimulation and electroconvulsive therapy in major depression. *Br J Psychiatry* **186**, 410–416.

Video

A video demonstrating the practical administration of ECT is available from the Royal College of Psychiatrists, 17 Belgrave Square, London SW1X 8PG, UK.

25 Organization of services

Introduction

Writing about UK psychiatric services is difficult – it is like trying to hit a moving target. There is constant change, and increasing differences between England, Wales, Scotland, and Northern Ireland. Recently, 'modernization' seems to have been viewed by the government as the same thing as improvement. Huge amounts of money have been wasted on extra administrators, 'management consultants', and bumbling attempts to set up a national NHS information technology network without a clear idea of what it is for. The latest 'good ideas' have been introduced into clinical practice without proper trial, and without adequate resources (i.e. '*from existing resources*').

In spite of these continuing top–down difficulties imposed on the system, psychiatry remains an enthralling specialty. Surviving in it depends on a continuing interest in patients as individuals, and also on the ability to work as part of a team – because it is through teams that psychiatry is now generally practised. These teams are largely based in the community. I will start with a description of the community mental health team, as this seems likely – at any rate, for the time being – to remain the foundation stone of psychiatric services. However, it is first necessary to say a few words about the historical background, as otherwise it is difficult to understand the pattern of existing mental health services.

Hughes' Outline of Modern Psychiatry, Fifth Edition. David Gill.
© 2007 John Wiley & Sons, Ltd   ISBN 9780470033920

Background and history

Psychiatric disorders require different systems of care from physical ones, because many psychiatric disorders are chronic, impair patients' ability to meet their own practical and social needs, and may tend to evoke rejection or ridicule from other people, rather than understanding and sympathy.

Until the 'asylum movement' of the eighteenth and nineteenth centuries, most mentally ill and mentally handicapped people were looked after by their relatives, with private nursing at home (see *Jane Eyre*, 1847), or in a private 'madhouse' for the minority who could afford it. Some were rejected by their families to become 'vagrants' and be put in the workhouse, or possibly taken in by religious or charitable institutions.

Asylums (hospitals for the mentally ill and mentally handicapped), set up with the help of charitable support amid much initial enthusiasm, were large impressive buildings usually sited in the countryside with their own gardens and farms. However, in the absence of any really effective treatments for psychiatric illness until the mid-twentieth century, their wards soon became overcrowded, and standards and morale declined. Long-stay patients, including many who would not be considered to merit even a brief psychiatric hospitalization nowadays, became apathetic and lacking in simple skills of daily living ('institutionalized'). A major stigma was attached to admission.

The gradual closure of asylum beds began in the 1950s, was accelerated in the 1960s and 1970s by several scandals and a fashionable 'anti-psychiatry' movement, and has continued to the present day under government policy of 'community care'.

In the 1970s, many modern inpatient units attached to district general hospitals (DGH units) were built to replace the old mental hospitals. DGH units offered the advantages of enabling psychiatric services to be integrated with medical and surgical ones, close to main centres of population. However, the typical DGH unit environment, with its compact unlocked wards, proved unsuitable for certain patients such as the behaviourally disturbed, and accumulation of 'new long-stay' cases soon caused blocked beds.

The more recent trend has been development of community mental health centres, plus crisis teams, and assertive outreach teams, with the aim of reducing inpatient admissions further still. In the context of managerial reorganization of the NHS as a whole, profound organizational changes to psychiatric services have been introduced. Debate continues as to which model is best, and what future policy should be.

Community care

Community care involves treating patients as far as possible in their own homes, with emphasis on a prompt, individualized, multidisciplinary response to problems. Community care is recommended on the grounds that it is as effective as hospital care, is preferred by patients and their families, minimizes the stigma of mental illness, and prevents institutionalization. These are real advantages, provided the systems are well organized, and adequately funded; good community care is not necessarily cheaper than hospital care.

Proper funding and good collaboration between the different professional groups is essential for good community mental health care. Unfortunately, staff shortages and vacancies, and morale problems are frequently reported, especially in deprived urban areas with high morbidity. Introduction of the 'care programme approach' (see below) was partly to try to make sure that the care of individual patients was properly organized so as to withstand such difficulties.

Community care for patients with long-term mental illness used to be the responsibility of local authority social services departments, but these have now, to a greater or lesser extent, been merged into community mental health teams in many areas. Each patient must have an individual needs assessment, and then appropriate services are arranged, although clients with sufficient financial means may have to contribute to the cost of these.

Social workers and community psychiatric nurses (CPNs) now work in similar ways ('generically') as care coordinators. As well as general support and advocacy, the care coordinator provide advice about the following:

- *Financial benefit entitlements.*

- *Employment:* this includes sheltered employment, or a gradual return to the work routine through activities in the voluntary sector.

- *Accommodation:* this means *residential and nursing homes* care for people with mental health problems, not only the elderly. *Supported accommodation,* including *group homes, hostels,* and other forms of accommodation, may be provided by health services, social services, or the voluntary sector, with varying degrees of resident or non-resident supervision. Such accommodation might be a group of self-contained flats, with a warden present during the day, and telephone support during the night. The *supported lodgings* scheme allows social services to pay landlords extra in exchange for some care of their tenants. *Private rented accommodation* is home to many with chronic mental illness; some of the landlords involved may be open to criticism, but their tenants might otherwise be homeless.

• *Day centres* provide a focus for regular supervision, activities, and rehabilitation.

The psychiatric multidisciplinary team

The multidisciplinary team consists of one or more members of each professional group involved in psychiatric patient care: doctors, nurses, clinical psychologists, social workers, and occupational therapists. Much good work is also done by less qualified *support workers*, who are cheaper to employ and who therefore have more time than other specialists to forge enduring relationships with individual patients.

Teams for general adult psychiatry are usually responsible for a given sector, defined geographically (for example, by postcode) or by GP. Other teams, often covering a wider area, deal with specialties such as old-age psychiatry, child psychiatry, learning disability, substance misuse, forensic psychiatry, psycho-therapy, and rehabilitation.

A *community mental health team* may be based in a hospital, a health centre, a converted house, or a purpose-built unit within the community served. Each team member is involved in assessment and management of referred patients, contributing both from their professional viewpoint and from their personal knowledge of the patient. It is usual to have a weekly team meeting, at which new referrals are discussed and progress or problems with existing patients are shared and reviewed.

Social workers in the teams used to be employed and managed by local author-ity departments of social services, leading to potential problems, as most of the rest of the team were employed by health services. Recently, there have been moves to bring all staff under the same management.

Each team may have up to 500 patients on the books at any one time; day-to-day clinical management of most of them is carried out by non-medical team members. Ultimate responsibility for patient care remains with the consultant, if the patient is seeing a psychiatrist. If the patient is seeing only a member of the team, and is not seeing a psychiatrist, responsibility lies with the team manager and/or the referring GP.

The role of the psychiatrist in the team is not only to have a caseload, but also to be a resource for the rest of the team: he must be approachable and available for advice and discussion, and able to work flexibly. Fitting in patients for consultation as soon as problems start to develop is particularly appreciated, and probably reduces everyone's workload in the long run.

In some areas, community mental 'resource centres' have been set up by social service departments with input from the voluntary sector, especially mental health charities.

Psychiatry in primary care

A quarter or more of consultations in primary care (general practice) appear to have a substantial psychological component, although the patient's presenting complaint is usually a somatic one and the underlying emotional disturbance may not be recognized by the doctor. Mixed neurotic symptoms, often accompanied by social or interpersonal problems, predominate. About 90 per cent of patients with psychiatric disorder are managed solely in primary care, and many episodes resolve quickly without specific treatment, or with brief counselling; some general practices employ their own counsellors.

Some patients require psychotropic drug therapy, and antidepressants, although often prescribed in lower doses and for shorter courses than most psychiatrists would recommend, are effective. However, in many milder cases, they are probably acting as placebos. Benzodiazepines are recommended for short periods only, but many GPs now avoid prescribing them at all.

GPs are also involved, in collaboration with psychiatric and social services, in the care of those with more severe illnesses such as schizophrenia and affective disorder, which require long-term medication and supervision. Besides being providers of primary mental health care, GPs are involved in shaping local psychiatric services.

At the time of the preparation of the previous edition of this book, 'fundholding GPs' were being introduced; the idea was that they would have a budget to purchase the services they considered necessary, including mental health services, for their patients. Political changes caused fundholding to be jettisoned, although, as is the way with the NHS, it now seems to be coming back under a different name, *practice-based commissioning*.

At the time of writing, it is difficult to predict the real impact of these changes. In principle, any move to build up primary care, which provides 90 per cent of NHS care, but gets only 10 per cent of the budget, has the potential to benefit low-tech specialties such as mental health care, and prevent further waste of money in the modern overspecialized and overtechnical general hospital. It will probably accelerate the trend to base CPNs and other mental health care staff at least partly in GP health centres.

There is a dynamic tension here between the possible benefits of such changes, and the real concern about such specialist resources being directed toward the 'worried well', and away from patients with severe chronic psychiatric illness.

One problem, which is unlikely to be solved completely by the changes proposed, is the apparently unlimited demand for 'counselling'. Some areas are trying out 'graduate mental health-care workers', that is, graduates who have received a modicum of training in CBT, as a way of trying to satisfy this demand.

Inpatient services

Despite the national reduction in psychiatric bed numbers, there is still a need for some inpatient facilities, whether in a mental hospital, a DGH unit, or a community unit. Separate wards usually exist for the following:

• *Acute admissions in general adult psychiatry* (usually patients aged 18–65). Sometimes there is a separate *intensive care unit* for severely disturbed patients.

• *Acute admissions in old-age psychiatry* (patients over 65 or 75). There may be separate wards for functional illness, and for assessment of dementia cases.

Other facilities are required, such as *residential/long-stay rehabilitation*, but these may not always be provided by the NHS 'in-house'.

Facilities vary from area to area; some rehabilitation hostels and schemes are run by local authorities or by charitable organizations. It follows in these cases that admission to them is according to their assessment, not by that of psychiatric services. This can lead to delay, if the latter have a different view. Just as the psychiatrist does not have direct authority over the non-medical members of the community mental health team, so the health service cannot direct outside agencies to accept patients, for example, for rehabilitation.

• Various types of *supported accommodation* are provided by social services and other organizations such as charities and housing associations. They allow patients to be discharged from hospital who would otherwise be unable to cope on their own.

- The NHS still seems to suffer from the fond delusion that the need for *long-stay beds* has somehow been abolished by the closure of the old psychiatric hospitals, but a small number of patients in each area still do require this. At the moment, at any rate in England, the need is met by patients generally being placed in private nursing homes or hospitals.

More specialized inpatient units exist to cover a wider population, such as a health region. These deal with, for example, *forensic cases (secure units), drug and alcohol misuse, adolescent psychiatry, mother and baby care,* and *eating disorders.*

Outpatient clinics

Psychiatric outpatient clinics, mainly conducted by the medical members of the team, exist for assessment and treatment of new referrals, and for follow-up of patients recently discharged from inpatient care. Many milder patients do not require indefinite clinic follow-up, but can be discharged to GP care with recommendations for future management. Patients who have had psychosis or bipolar affective disorder, among others, should remain in long-term follow-up.

Some clinic sessions, often supervised by specialist nurses, are dedicated to particular patient groups, such as those on long-term medication with lithium, depot antipsychotics, or clozapine. Computer registers to monitor the frequency of patient attendance, prescribing activity, and performance of relevant laboratory tests are a useful aid to managing such clinics and reviewing their performance.

Crisis and home treatment

Home treatment has been developed as an alternative to inpatient care for acute cases. This involves the '*crisis intervention*' model, in which members of the multidisciplinary team visit the patient, and the family, at frequent intervals, sometimes several times per day. The clinical experience is that such crisis teams can reduce hospital admissions and are popular with patients. However, they depend on having adequate staffing, good morale, and good relations with other parts of the service such as community mental health teams and inpatient units.

Crisis teams can screen new inpatient admissions, to see whether they can be avoided; attend Mental Health Act assessments, to see whether a potential 'section' can be handled in a different way; and attend inpatient ward rounds, to see whether patients can be given early discharge into their care. This represents another step in the general shift toward providing interventions in patients' homes, as in domiciliary assessment of new referrals and regular visits by CPNs to monitor patients who need long-term care.

Day hospitals

Many acutely ill patients can be managed in a day hospital as an alternative to admission, and day hospitals can also provide a useful period of follow-up care for those recently discharged but still needing intensive support. They offer medical and nursing care, occupational therapy, psychological treatments, and social work. The day hospital is regarded as an essential part of a fully developed mental health service, but the work it does to some extent overlaps with the currently more fashionable crisis team.

Resource centres and day centres

Mental health services have been slimmed down to the most efficient and effective service models in treatment of acute illness, but a proportion of chronically ill or recovering patients still need to have somewhere to go for social contact, meals, and other activities such as rehabilitation and education. This is often provided by resource centres, which may or may not be linked, geographically and organizationally, to mental health services.

Assertive outreach teams

Assertive outreach teams practise a type of psychiatric care for clients with multiple complex needs. It involves, for example, seeking out someone who fails to attend an appointment, and frequent visits in the long term. It is more expensive than standard care, but can serve to improve outcomes in 'revolving door' patients with poor compliance.

Recovery and rehabilitation

The modern idea of rehabilitation is helping patients in the community, with any kind of mental health problem, gradually return to normal functioning. The currently fashionable *recovery model* emphasizes positive aspects of individual patients, building strengths, so that they recover their full potential even though they need continuing support from mental health services.

This stands in complete contrast to the old idea of rehabilitation, which was restricted to severely affected psychotic patients. That old idea conjures up pictures of the long-stay 'back wards' of the old psychiatric hospitals, where deteriorated patients with schizophrenia would be rewarded with cigarettes, in return for performing simple tasks such as self-care. Such programmes of 'token economy' would, of course, now be regarded as unethical.

Rehabilitation aims to reduce disablement, or better still to prevent it, through early intervention, and to improve social functioning and quality of life. This might involve a worthwhile occupation and a stable social network, preferably involving the family, in addition to psychiatric symptom control. Individual programmes take account of each patient's impairments, positive attributes, and likely future environment. Progress toward agreed goals is often achieved gradually. Rehabilitation is part of everyday care, not something to be seen as separate.

Many patients have always done well, and there is the potential to improve outcomes and functioning for most patients through appropriate rehabilitation – in particular, *vocational rehabilitation* (http://www.vocationalrehabilitationassociation.org.uk/); that is, getting patients back to work so that they can benefit from the positive effects of having routine, social contact, and from improved self-esteem and self-confidence (and possibly improved finances, although the extremely complex benefit system may provide perverse incentives against paid work).

Old-fashioned 'sheltered employment' is now uncommon, but there are various schemes in different areas that seek to encourage people with health problems to get back to work; the Disability Employment Adviser at the job centre can help. Doing college courses or voluntary work can be very helpful first steps in rehabilitation.

In the case of patients who have an existing job, *graduated return to work programmes* can be very helpful in returning patients to work. In the case of neurotic symptoms such as anxiety and depression, we should be moving toward a presumption that they do not prevent work once the acute stage is passed. Patients do lose confidence, but prolonged absence can result in a vicious cycle and become a self-fulfilling prophecy; the well-known *therapeutic benefits of work* and the converse *risks to health of not working* are increasingly recognized.

Working patients who become unwell have legal rights that may protect their employment under the Disability Discrimination Act.

Severe, prolonged psychiatric illness, notably chronic schizophrenia, may lead to loss of daily living skills and/or socially undesirable behaviour. The result may be breakdown of family relationships, homelessness, poverty, and unemployment. However, it is clear that some patients in the past have developed these associated problems at least partly because they coincided with expectations of society and of services.

The care programme approach

The care programme approach (CPA) aims to improve delivery of services to psychiatric patients. After a formal assessment of their medical and social needs, patients and carers are invited to take part in drawing up written, individual care plans. These might include statements about the frequency of outpatient reviews, medication, home visits by the CPN, and/or social work interventions with the family. The resulting document is signed by those responsible. Regular review meetings follow. Although several members of the multidisciplinary team are likely to be involved, the plan must specify a named 'key worker' to coordinate the care and be the first point of contact in a crisis.

Two 'tiers' of the CPA exist, *enhanced* – in which the patient typically will have both a psychiatrist and a *care coordinator*, typically a social worker or CPN – and *standard*, in which the patient just sees one professional; typically, they just attend psychiatric outpatients. Enhanced cases are more complex and severe; the care coordinator may have approximately 20 at any one time. There are written risk assessments and regular CPA review meetings with care coordinator, consultant psychiatrist, patient, family, and other involved parties. Standard cases are less severe, and their care is less complex. No special paperwork is required, as the risk assessment is held to be implicit in the standard notes and letters.

Non-NHS health-care facilities

Although most psychiatric services are provided by the NHS, some care is purchased from other providers. For example, there are *private psychiatric hospitals*, including some set up for profit, and some non-profit-making institutions. The NHS often purchases services from both types in areas where it cannot itself meet demand. 'Difficult-to-manage' patients, especially the acutely psychotic and potentially violent; those suffering the chronic effects of brain injury; and special groups such as patients with eating disorders or puerperal illnesses, are among those most frequently placed in the private sector. Many private wards offer higher levels of staffing and tighter physical security than most modern NHS facilities.

Another example of purchased services comes from the *voluntary sector*: this receives public monies to provide services; thus, a charity may receive social services or health funds in order to provide 'meals on wheels' or a day centre.

Psychological treatments, such as counselling, and various forms of alternative or complementary medicine, are frequently purchased by patients directly. The practitioners consulted may or may not be properly trained and accredited, and patients may not reveal this information unless sensitively asked.

Further reading

Kent, A. and Burns, T. (2005). Assertive community treatment in UK practice. *Adv Psychiatr Treat* **11**, 388–397.

26 The Mental Health Act 1983

Introduction

The majority of patients admitted to psychiatric hospitals are voluntary or informal. The Mental Health Act 1983 (henceforth called 'the Act') is concerned with the minority who are unwilling to accept hospitalization or treatment that others consider essential. It applies to England and Wales. Scotland and Northern Ireland have separate legislation.

The government recently published a Bill that proposes, among other highly controversial measures, preventive detention of those with 'dangerous and severe personality disorder', and detention of those with substance misuse only (who are explicitly excluded from the current Act). Perhaps as an illustration of how centralized health care has become, conferences, courses, and publications on 'implementing the Bill' have been popular, even though it is self-evidently impossible to 'implement' something which, as a Bill, is just a proposal before Parliament rather than an actual law. Most mental health professionals and organizations expressed opposition to these proposals. At the time of writing, plans for an Act are on hold. Accordingly, few changes are currently necessary to the version of this chapter in the previous edition.

Hughes' Outline of Modern Psychiatry, Fifth Edition. David Gill.
© 2007 John Wiley & Sons, Ltd   ISBN 9780470033920

Background

Patients in hospital under the Act may be described as 'detained' or 'sectioned'. The general aims of the Act are as follows:

• to provide appropriate care for the mentally disordered

• to safeguard those who are not mentally disordered against wrongful detention.

Informed use of this legislation should achieve the best possible compromise between preserving freedom and human rights, on the one hand, and protecting both patients and society, on the other hand. The Act gives no authority over those who do not suffer from mental disorder. It cannot be used to enforce treatment for physical illness, unless the physical illness is believed to be causing mental disorder. In a life-threatening situation, emergency treatment may be enforced under common law without applying the Act first.

The following summary applies to the legislation for England and Wales. Other countries have separate legislation. The Act is applied in the light of an official code of practice that gives helpful practical guidance on many of the clinical dilemmas which arise.

The Act uses the following four broad diagnostic categories of mental disorder:

• *mental illness*, which it does not define

• *severe mental impairment*: a state of arrested or incomplete development of mind that includes significant impairment of intelligence and social functioning and is associated with abnormally aggressive or seriously irresponsible conduct

• *mental impairment*: as above, with the addition of the phrase, 'not amounting to severe mental impairment'

• *psychopathic disorder*: persistent disorder or disability of mind (whether or not including significant impairment of intelligence) that results in abnormally aggressive or seriously irresponsible conduct.

Antisocial or immoral conduct, sexual deviancy, and misuse of alcohol or drugs are explicitly excluded as grounds for detention (in contrast to the bad old days, when, for example, young women who had illegitimate children were sometimes detained on the spurious grounds of 'moral insanity'). However, mental disorders caused by substance misuse, such as alcoholic hallucinosis and amphetamine psychosis, are covered by the Act in the usual way.

Compulsory admission

For most 'sections', an *application* is made by either an *approved social worker* (ASW) employed by local authority social services, or by the *nearest relative*, on the basis of one or more *medical recommendations*, for the admission of the patient to an approved hospital. In order to prevent collusion within families, the code of practice recommends that an ASW, rather than a relative, be the applicant, and this is almost always the case.

Section 2: Admission for assessment

Patient: must have a *mental disorder* and detention must be necessary for his/her own health or safety or for the protection of others.
Applicant: ASW/nearest relative.
Medical recommendations: two – one must be approved under Section 12 of the Act and is usually a *psychiatrist*; the other doctor is usually the patient's *GP*.
Duration: up to *28 days*.
Right of appeal: to a Mental Health Review Tribunal within the first *14 days*; the nearest relative also has the power to discharge the patient from the Section.

Section 3: Admission for treatment

Patient: must have a *mental disorder* as for Section 2, but if the disorder is *psychopathic disorder* or *mental impairment*, there are further requirements that treatment must be considered likely to *alleviate or prevent deterioration* of the condition. This section permits *treatment*, as well as detention, against the patient's will.
Duration: up to *6 months* and then renewable; it must be reviewed before expiry.
Right of appeal: to a Mental Health Review Tribunal within the first *6 months*, and then once within each renewal period. Review by a tribunal is automatically carried out after 6 months if the patient has not already applied for a hearing. Renewal is appropriate if treatment is likely to alleviate, or prevent

deterioration in, the patient's condition, or (for mental illness or severe mental impairment) the patient, if discharged, would be unlikely to be able to care for himself or obtain the care he needs, or to guard himself against serious exploitation. The nearest relative can also apply for discharge.

Section 4: Emergency admission

Patient: as above for Section 2.
Application: nearest relative/ASW.
Recommendation: any one registered medical practitioner, who must have seen the patient within the past 24 hours.
Duration: up to 72 *hours.*
Right of appeal: none.

Section 4 is rarely used in practice; it is potentially open to abuse and the code of practice advises that it should be applied only when Section 2 would involve unreasonable delay. Section 4 can be converted into Section 2 by adding another doctor's recommendation.

Patients already in hospital

Both Sections 2 and 3 can be applied to patients already in hospital. In emergencies, it is possible to use Section 5 as follows:

Section 5(2) (application in respect of a patient already in hospital): a voluntary patient can be detained on the recommendation of one doctor, normally the responsible consultant or named deputy, for up to 72 hours.
Section 5(4) (nurses' holding power): a voluntary patient can be detained by a registered mental nurse for up to 6 hours until a doctor is found.

Section 5 may be converted into Section 2 or Section 3 by the appropriate medical and social work opinions.

Patients in the community

Section 17

Section 17 gives a detained patient leave of absence from hospital, for either a predetermined period or an open-ended trial of suitability for discharge. The responsible medical officer can impose any conditions considered necessary in the interests of the patient or for the protection of others, such as administration of depot injections by the community nurse. Patients can be recalled to hospital for health reasons, but the power of recall lapses if not used within 6 months.

Guardianship

A lesser known and possibly underused section of the Act allows a patient over 16 years old who is suffering from mental disorder to be placed under the supervision of a guardian, either a named individual or the local social services authority. Recommendation is made by two doctors, one approved, and the application is made by the nearest relative or an approved social worker. The order lasts 6 months and may be renewed for a further 6 months in the first instance and subsequently for 1 year at a time. A guardian may, for example, require the patient to reside at a specified place (not a hospital); give access, at the patient's residence, to any doctor, approved social worker, or other specified person; or attend at specified places and times for medical treatment, occupation, education, and training (but cannot compel the patient to accept the treatment offered).

Relatives

The Act defines the nearest relative from a set list, beginning with spouse, child, parent, and sibling in that order. Elder relatives take precedence in each category, as do relatives who live with or care for the patient. Cohabitees can be designated nearest relatives in some circumstances. The nearest relative has the power to discharge a patient from Section 2. Section 3 cannot be applied if the nearest relative objects, but an objection can be overruled by a county court if considered unreasonable. A relative is not legally permitted to consent to treatment on behalf of an adult patient, so consent from the nearest relative does not remove the necessity to apply the Act.

Approved social workers (ASWs)

ASWs have been approved, after specific training, as competent to deal with mental disorder. Only ASWs (not other social workers) can make application under the Act, and local authorities have a statutory obligation to provide an ASW service. ASWs have a responsibility to ensure that hospital admission is the most appropriate way of dealing with the case. When the nearest relative rather than an ASW makes the application for admission, the hospital managers must request a social work report as soon as possible.

Police powers

Section 136 allows a police constable who finds a person apparently suffering from mental disorder in a place to which the public has access to remove him/ her to a place of safety for assessment by an ASW, who would usually request medical examination by a police surgeon and a psychiatrist. The person must appear in immediate need of care and control, and detention must appear necessary in the person's own interests or for the protection of others. Although Section 136 lasts up to 72 hours, good practice requires it to be cancelled after the professional assessment and, if necessary, replaced by Section 2 or 3.

Section 135 allows a constable, on a magistrate's warrant, to enter premises to remove a patient to a place of safety for up to 72 hours, if there is reasonable cause to suspect that a person suffering from mental disorder is being ill-treated or neglected, is not under proper control, or is unable to care for himself/herself and is living alone. It is used infrequently, as the constable in such a situation traditionally 'smells gas' and effects an entry under common law.

Mentally abnormal offenders

Several sections of the Act deal with mentally disordered offenders. These sections are mainly applied after consultation with colleagues such as a forensic psychiatrist or a probation officer. Compulsory psychiatric treatment under the Act cannot be given in the prison setting, but only after transfer to a psychiatric hospital.

Accused persons

Section 35 remands an accused person awaiting trial or sentence to a specified hospital for *observation*, on evidence from one doctor of reason to suspect mental disorder; in practice, it is mainly used for the preparation of psychiatric reports. *Section 36* remands a person accused of an imprisonable offence to hospital for *treatment*, on the evidence of two doctors, one of whom will be in charge of treatment. The patient must have a mental illness or severe mental impairment.

Both Sections 35 and 36 last *28 days*, renewable at 28-day intervals up to *12 weeks*.

Sentenced persons

Section 37 permits a court to order hospital admission (or, occasionally, guardianship) for a patient who has committed an imprisonable offence, and who is suffering from mental disorder of a nature or degree that makes this course appropriate. It is imposed as a 'disposal', that is, instead of, for example, a prison sentence. Two doctors, one approved, must give evidence. It lasts up to 6 months, and may be renewed, appeal to a Mental Health Review Tribunal being allowed in the second 6 months.

Section 38 (interim hospital order) allows a trial of psychiatric treatment for *3 months* when a full Section 37 may be inappropriate.

A *restriction order (Section 41)* can be applied, in addition to Section 37, for serious cases in which the patient may not be given leave, transferred, or discharged without permission from the Home Secretary (in practice, a particular branch of the Home Office) in order to protect the public. The Home Secretary may sometimes come under pressure from MPs or members of the public in relation to individual patients on restriction orders.

Section 47 (transfer of a sentenced prisoner) and *Section 48 (transfer of other prisoners, including those remanded)* to hospital are by order of the Home Secretary, on two medical recommendations. A restriction on discharge may be added (*Section 49*) and applies until the end of the sentence with remission. The patient may appeal to a tribunal in the first 6 months.

Consent to treatment

Somewhat paradoxically, many detained patients consent to have treatment once they are 'sectioned', but others do not. *Section 58 (treatment requiring consent or a second opinion)* covers the use of ECT in detained patients, and administration of drugs when a particular medication is being continued longer than 3 months. Administration of such treatment requires that *either* the patient consented and this has been certified as 'informed' by the responsible medical officer or an independent doctor; *or* an independent doctor has certified that the patient has not given consent or is not capable of understanding the nature, purpose, and likely effects of the treatment, but that, having regard to the likelihood of its alleviating or preventing deterioration of his/her condition, the treatment should be given. The independent doctor must consult two other staff members, one a nurse and the other neither a doctor nor a nurse.

Section 57 (treatment requiring consent and *a second opinion)* covers the special conditions regulating two treatments that have often given rise to ethical concern: *psychosurgery* and *surgical implantation of hormones to reduce male sexual drive.* Here, the patient's informed consent is not sufficient on its own (whether the patient is detained or voluntary). It must be supported by an independent doctor appointed by the Mental Health Act Commission, and two other non-medical appointed persons who have certified in writing that the patient is capable of understanding the nature, purpose, and likely effects of the proposed treatment and has consented to it. This occasionally gives rise to situations where a patient consents to, or even requests, a particular treatment (for example, hormone treatment of a sex offender), but the commission refuses.

Section 62 (urgent treatment), a treatment normally restricted under Sections 57 or 58, may be given to a detained patient without obtaining formal consent or a second opinion in an emergency, such as ECT to save the life of a seriously dehydrated depressed patient. In practice, such treatment would often be given under common law.

Information for detained patients

Section 132 specifies the duties of hospital managers to inform detained patients as soon as possible, both orally and in writing, about their legal position and their rights of appeal.

Detained patients' rights of appeal

There is an initial right of appeal to the *hospital managers*: unless there has been procedural irregularity, it is unusual for managers to overrule clinicians.

Subsequent appeal is to a *Mental Health Review Tribunal* of three members: a lawyer (the chairperson), a doctor, and a layperson. Tribunals may discharge detained patients if they consider them no longer dangerous or no longer suffering from mental disorder. They may also recommend leave of absence or transfer to another hospital. Under certain sections, patients have the right of application to a tribunal. Review by a tribunal is mandatory at specified intervals for some of the longer treatment sections, such as Section 3, and must be requested by the hospital managers if the patient has not already exercised the right to a tribunal hearing.

Patients may be eligible for legal aid to assist them in preparing a case and obtaining an independent medical opinion, and to cover the cost of legal representation.

Mental Health Act Commission

This is a special multidisciplinary body, its members including doctors, nurses, social workers, lawyers, and laypersons. Its function is to see that detained patients are being cared for appropriately and that the Mental Health Act is being properly applied. Members visit every psychiatric unit in the country once or twice a year, and every Special Hospital at least once a month, to see detained patients, ensure the staff are adhering to the principles of the Act, and consider any complaints that have arisen. Appointed members provide independent second opinions.

Further reading

Bluglass, R. (1983). *A Guide to the Mental Health Act*. Edinburgh: Churchill Livingstone.

Department of Health and Welsh Office (1999). *Code of Practice: Section 118 of the Mental Health Act 1983*. http://www.dh.gov.uk/assetRoot/04/07/49/61/04074961.pdf.

Jones, R. (Ed.) (1999). *Mental Health Act Manual* (6th edn). London: Sweet & Maxwell.

Glossary

I give below a brief list of some of the more commonly used terms in clinical psychiatry. The interested reader is referred to larger works for a fuller word list.

Long words in Greek, Latin, German, etc., are not necessarily included if they are not in common clinical use. Plain English has advantages; if someone is colour blind, it is probably better to say so, rather than that he is 'suffering from achromatopsia'.

Words are included for the various catatonic phenomena, even though these are now rarely seen in UK clinical practice, since they are of historical importance.

Certain aspects such as named syndromes (Capgras) and psychodynamic terms are also included, not because of their practical usefulness, if any, but because they are part of the language and culture of psychiatry – and because they have not yet completely disappeared from the memory banks of examination setters.

abreaction	A technique, now little used, in which the patient is administered a sedative such as a barbiturate and then interviewed, usually about difficult matters.
acculturation	The process of adapting to a different culture or environment; difficulties here need to be distinguished from mental disorder.

Hughes' Outline of Modern Psychiatry, Fifth Edition. David Gill.
© 2007 John Wiley & Sons, Ltd   ISBN 9780470033920

acetylcholine   A neurotransmitter in the brain, lack of which may contribute to memory problems.

achromatopsia   Colour blindness, innate and acquired.

acting out   A description of disturbed behaviour that is presumed to express underlying emotional conflicts. It implies that the user of the term does not think the patient should be blamed for his actions.

addiction   Psychological or physical dependence on a substance; there may be tolerance and withdrawal.

adjustment disorder   A temporary psychological reaction to external events. It goes beyond a normal reaction, and usually lasts less than 6 months.

affect   Current emotional state, at a given point, as distinct from mood, which is predominant over time. Sometimes the term is used to refer only to the outward expression of an underlying mood state, but this use is less frequent.

affect illusion   Illusions associated with changes in affect, so that, if a person is frightened, he may see a shadow as an assailant.

affective disorders   Disorders of mood.

age-associated memory impairment   The mild (normal) difficulties in memory with age; synonyms are 'benign senescent forgetfulness' and 'a senior moment'.

agitation   Excessive physical activity in association with anxiety, such as fidgeting, hand wringing, or restlessness.

agnosia   Inability to recognize objects or parts of the body, even though sensory function, such as sight and hearing, is normal; seen in dementia and stroke, among other conditions.

agoraphobia   Literally, fear of the marketplace; that is, fear of public places, or of being in circumstances from which escape might be difficult or embarrassing. It is seen in anxiety and depressive disorders, and commonly panic attacks also occur.

akathisia
Excessive motor activity due to restlessness, typically causing pacing or fidgeting. There is a psychological component of agitation also; it is usually due to psychotropic drugs, especially antipsychotics.

akinesia
Markedly reduced voluntary movement.

akinetic mutism
The patient appear to be conscious, but does not move or speak.

alexithymia
Difficulty in verbal expression of emotion.

alogia
Reduced thinking, often inferred from poverty of speech, as seen in chronic schizophrenia.

ambivalence
Contradictory feelings or thoughts about a particular issue or person; this is not in itself pathological.

amentia
Synonym for 'severe learning difficulty'.

amines
Compounds containing an amino group: some, such as adrenaline and noradrenaline, are important as neurotransmitters.

amnesia
Loss of memory, whether partial or complete, anterograde amnesia is loss of memory of things happening after the head injury or other event; retrograde amnesia is loss of memory for things that happened before.

amok
Culture-specific syndrome from Malaysia, involving an acute confusional state with violence toward others and/or suicide.

amygdala
Brain structure; part of the limbic system.

amyloid
Proteins deposited in cells in Alzheimer's disease and other diseases.

anal stage
Freud's theory of psychosexual development suggests that a child of 1–3 years is focused on defecation; however, the theory is unproven and of little clinical relevance.

anankastic personality	Synonym for 'obsessive-compulsive personality'.
anhedonia	The patient is unable to take pleasure in things he normally enjoys; it is seen in depressive states.
anima	Jung's term for someone's inner self, as distinct from the persona presented to the outside world.
anomie	Alienation from family and society, suggested by Durkheim as a factor in suicide.
anorexia nervosa	An eating disorder with morbid fear of fatness, leading to excessive dieting, exercising, self-induced vomiting, laxative misuse, etc. Patients have body image disturbance, believing they are obese when most are underweight.
anosognosia	Condition in which a stroke patient seems unaware of his disability.
anxiety	Apprehensive anticipation of danger or misfortune accompanied by a feeling of dysphoria and/or bodily symptoms such as palpitations, dizziness, hyperventilation, and faintness. Unlike fear, which can be seen as an appropriate response to a real threat, the symptoms in anxiety are out of proportion to any actual threat, if any, that is present.
apathy	Lack of feeling or initiative.
aphasia	Impaired language ability in understanding or expression.
apraxia	Impaired ability to do skilled motor activities despite intact understanding and motor function.
astasia-abasia	A form of hysterical disorder of gait.
asthenia	A general weakness or debility, without physical cause: neurasthenia denotes an illness characterized by tiredness, emotional symptoms, and reduced function, similar to 'chronic fatigue syndrome'.

asyndesis	Type of disorder of the form of thought, with loosening of association between topics – the subject jumps from one subject to another with little connection between them.
ataxia	Loss of coordination of voluntary muscular movement.
attention	The capacity to concentrate on an activity: reduced attention can be seen in easy distractibility or difficulty in completing things.
auditory hallucination	The person hears a sound that is real to him, and comes from outside the head, but there is no sensory stimulus, no real sound which others could hear.
aura	A premonitory sensation or thought that warns of an attack of migraine or epilepsy.
autochthonous delusion	A delusion that comes on suddenly, without apparent cause.
automatic obedience	Excessive compliance with an examiner's instructions; it is associated with catatonia, and is therefore now rare.
automatism	Behaviours, such as sleepwalking and epileptic movement, that appear to happen without conscious control, and are usually not recalled afterward.
avolition	Lack of drive and initiative to carry out normal activities; this is seen most commonly as a 'negative symptom' of schizophrenia.
basal ganglia	Clusters of neurons deep in the brain, involved in control of movement.
belle indifférence ('la belle indifférence')	Lack of concern about a hysterical disability.
bestiality	Sexual relations between a person and an animal, or the desire for them; it is a type of paraphilia.
beta-blocker	Drug that blocks the actions of adrenaline and the related noradrenaline, and is used in high blood

pressure and heart disease; it is also used to treat physical manifestations of anxiety, such as palpitations.

bizarre delusion Content of delusion obviously implausible in view of patient's background and culture.

blunted affect Reduction in range and intensity of emotional expression.

body image Sense of the self and body.

bouffée délirante French term for brief psychotic disorders.

bradykinesia Neurological term for generalized motor slowness.

bruxism Unconscious grinding of the teeth while awake or asleep; associated with mental disorder.

bulimia nervosa Eating disorder characterized by abnormal eating patterns, especially bingeing.

Capgras syndrome (illusion des sosies) Delusion that family member has been replaced by a double, usually secondary to schizophrenia or organic brain disease.

catalepsy Catatonic maintenance of abnormal body positions over an extended period of time.

cataplexy Sudden attack of muscular flaccidity, leading to collapse in association with strong emotion.

catatonic behaviour Severe, 'classical' form of schizophrenia, now rare, with motor immobility (i.e. catalepsy or stupor), negativism, mutism, posturing or stereotyped movements, and echolalia or echopraxia.

catharsis Positive resolution of emotional crisis, often by talking through the problem with the therapist.

causalgia Semi-obsolete synonym for severe pain, especially pain that cannot be explained by physical disease.

cerea flexibilitas ('waxy flexibility') This is seen in catatonic schizophrenia, and is therefore now rare; the patient's limbs can be placed in awkward positions that he will maintain as if he were made from plasticene.

chorea	Abnormal involuntary writhing movements.
circumstantiality	Speech is indirect, with irrelevant material, but the patient does get to the point in the end.
clang association	Disorder of the form of thought in which words seem to follow each other on the basis of sound or rhyme rather than meaning.
climacteric	Menopause.
clouding of consciousness	An organic mental state characterized by drowsiness and generalized impairments in cognitive functioning. It usually suggests an acute confusional state or delirium.
cognitive	To do with thought or thinking.
comorbidity	Simultaneous existence of two or more disorders, such as mental illness and substance misuse.
compensation	Either an unconscious, psychoanalytic 'defence mechanism' or a consciously desired outcome of litigation.
compulsion	Ritualistic behaviour, such as repeated cleaning, to prevent some dreaded consequence, even though the patient knows it is irrational.
concrete thinking	Focus on immediate practical matters and inability to deal with abstractions. It may be secondary to organic brain disease or schizophrenia.
confabulation	Fluctuating false memory made up by the patient to cover organic amnesia.
constricted affect	Mildly reduced range and intensity of emotional expression.
conversion	The hysterical production of neurological symptoms such as weakness or blindness.
coprolalia	Involuntary use of socially inappropriate words.
coprophagia	Eating of faeces.
Cotard's syndrome	Type of nihilistic delusion: the patient believes that he does not exist.

counter-transference	The therapist's unconscious emotional reactions to the patient, deriving from the therapist's own issues.
cretinism	Severe mental retardation due to untreated congenital thyroid deficiency.
cri du chat	Type of mental retardation, with characteristic cat-like cry; it is caused by partial deletion of chromosome 5.
culture-specific syndromes	Forms of disturbed behaviour in certain societies that are difficult to fit into psychiatric classification systems; they include amok, koro, latah, etc.
cyclothymia	Type of personality with pronounced variability of mood through depression and elation that is not severe enough to count as bipolar affective disorder.
decompensation	Loose shorthand for deterioration of symptoms and/or behaviour under stress.
defence mechanisms	In psychoanalytic theory, unconscious psychological processes that serve to protect the individual from awareness of internal or external stressors or dangers.
déjà pensé	A new thought feels familiar – feeling that one has thought the same thing before.
déjà vu	The sensation of undue familiarity with an event or a person – feeling that the same thing has happened before, etc.
delirium	Synonymous with 'acute organic brain syndrome' and 'confusional state': due to physical causes, consciousness is reduced, with disorientation, illusions, visual hallucinations, persecutory ideation, and consequent disturbed behaviour.
delirium tremens	Confusional state following sudden stoppage of drinking in a dependent subject.
delusion	A (usually) false belief that is inappropriate to the patient's religion and culture, and impervious to argument or evidence.
delusion of reference	Condition in which events or other circumstances have a particular meaning for the patient; for example, 'The

car flashed its headlights which confirms that the secret services are after me.'

delusional jealousy Delusion that one's partner is unfaithful.

delusional mood Also known as wahnstimmung, the conviction that something of special importance to the patient is about to happen.

delusional perception Normal perception that has become incorporated into a delusional system.

dementia Chronic organic mental illness, such as Alzheimer's disease, with progressive global deterioration in intellectual function.

dementia praecox Kräpelin crucially distinguished this psychotic illness ('premature dementia') from manic depressive illness (now termed 'bipolar affective disorder'). His patients had what we would now diagnose as severe schizophrenia with negative symptoms. The term dementia praecox is not now used clinically, however, as the patients do not demonstrate the modern concept of dementia.

dementia pugilistica ('punch-drunk') Parkinsonism with intellectual impairment in professional boxers and others with a history of repeated head trauma.

denial Postulated psychoanalytic defence mechanism in which certain information is repressed from consciousness.

depersonalization Sensation that one has become unreal or detached from reality, or is in a dream; can be normal (as in exhaustion or strong emotion) or associated with anxiety, hysteria, and neurological disorders.

depression Affective disorder, currently overdiagnosed, with profound, persistent sadness, unresponsive to circumstances.

derailment (loosening of associations) A disorder of the form of thought in which the patient, while speaking, keeps changing topics without obvious links, but still makes grammatical sense.

derealization	Sensation that the world has become unreal, as in depersonalization.
detachment	Personality characterized by general aloofness in personal relations.
dhat	Culture-bound syndrome (Indian males) involving complaint of losing semen in the urine.
disinhibition	Loss of normal social inhibitions as seen in intoxication, psychosis, mania, and organic disorders such as dementia and occasionally tumour.
disorientation	Loss of correct knowledge of the day, date, season, or location, due to loss of short-term memory in organic mental states. Long-term memory, as of who one is, is relatively preserved.
displacement	Postulated psychoanalytic defence mechanism in which emotions are unconsciously transferred from their original focus to some more acceptable one.
dissociation or dissociative state	State of hysteria (or conversion and dissociative disorders, to use the current term), in which the patient loses psychological function, as in *hysterical amnesia* or *psychogenic fugue*.
distractibility	Inability to attend.
doppelgänger	Phenomenon in which the patient feels that his 'double' accompanies him.
double bind	Bateson suggested that schizophrenia might be contributed to by the patient's having to respond to inconsistent communications in the family.
drive	Motivation.
dyad	Two-person relationship.
dysarthria	Speech affected by disorder of its physical organs, as in hoarseness due to laryngitis.
dyskinesia	Technically, any disorder of movement, but, in practice, used to mean involuntary muscular activity, such as the grimacing of tardive dyskinesia.

dyslexia	Reading difficulty, as in word blindness.
dysphoria	Any unpleasant mood state, such as sadness, anxiety, or irritability.
dyspraxia	Difficulty in carrying out skilled movement, suggestive of stroke or other cerebral pathology.
dystonia	Disorder of muscle tone.
écho de la pensée	See *gedankenlautwerden*.
echolalia	Automatic repetition of the last words the patient has heard.
echopraxia	Automatic mirroring of another's doings.
ego	The psychoanalytic model of the mind suggests that there are three major components: ego, id, and super-ego. The ego can be thought of as the conscious mind, the id as primitive instinct, and the superego as conscience.
ego-dystonic	Those aspects of a person he experiences as inconsistent with his personality as a whole.
elaboration	Postulated unconscious psychoanalytic process whereby details about, say, a dream are embellished.
elevated mood erotomania (de Clérambault's syndrome)	Mood is high, euphoric, or elated. Patient's delusion, usually part of schizophrenia, that another person is in love with (usually) her.
euthymic	Normal mood state.
extinction	In behaviour therapy, a reinforced operant response will gradually become extinguished if reward (reinforcement) ceases, so that Pavlov's dogs would gradually stop salivating at the sound of the bell if the bell were no longer accompanied by food.
extracampine	Hallucinations outside the possible range of sensation, such as seeing oneself from behind.

extroversion	A personality type in which energy and attention are largely directed toward the outside world.
fatuous affect	Mood state is silly and childlike; seen in schizophrenia.
first-rank symptoms	Schneider's list of the most characteristic symptoms of schizophrenia, although we now know that all of them occur to some extent in other disorders.
flashback	Recurrence of a memory, feeling, or perceptual experience from the past.
flat affect	Reduced range of emotional fluctuation.
flight of ideas	In elevated mood states, thoughts are speeded up and jump from topic to topic with no sense, perhaps linked only by a similar word sound.
flooding	Technique of behaviour therapy in which, for example, a fear of water would be treated by jumping into a swimming pool.
folie à deux	Delusions held by a strong-willed person, such as a father, can come to be held by a weaker person living with him, typically a child; so-called induced psychosis.
formal thought disorder	Shorthand for disorder of the form of thought, including *derailment* or *loosening of associations*, *Knight's move thinking*, and *word salad*.
formication	Tactile hallucination that ants are crawling on one; seen most characteristically in *delirium tremens*.
free association	Psychoanalytic technique in which the patient says whatever comes to mind.
Fregoli syndrome	Delusion secondary to schizophrenia or organic brain disease that someone threatening is somehow present in a familiar person; cf. *Capgras syndrome*.
frontal lobe syndrome	Pathology here can impair judgement, change personality, and cause disinhibition, among other features.
frotteurism	Sexual deviation involving desire to touch a non-consenting person, as on a crowded train.

gedankenlautwerden	Audible thoughts: the patient hears his thoughts spoken aloud, a Schneiderian first-rank symptom.
gegenhalten	In catatonia, the patient opposes all passive movements.
gender dysphoria	Aversion to one's biological sex, possibly with conviction that one 'should have' been born into the other biological sex.
gender identity	One's self-view as male or female.
globus hystericus	Sensation of a 'lump in the throat': seen in anxiety.
grandiosity	Idea or delusion that one has superior powers, strength, wealth, beauty, etc., as seen in mania and psychosis.
gustatory hallucination	Involves the sense of taste.
hallucination	A sensory perception that seems real to the person but that arises without external stimulus. It may occur in any sensory modality. Visual ones suggest organic states; auditory ones, mental illness, especially schizophrenia. False perceptions can occur while falling asleep (hypnagogic), dreaming, or awakening (hypnopompic), but these would not usually be termed hallucinations.
heautoscopy	The hallucination of 'seeing one's own body at a distance'.
hippocampus	Part of the limbic system that is involved in memory and emotion.
hyperacusis	Oversensitivity to noise; seen in anxiety.
hypersomnia	Excessive sleepiness.
hypnagogic hallucinations	See *hallucinations*.
hypnopompic	Referring to the state immediately preceding awakening; may include hallucinations that are of no pathological significance.
hypnopompic hallucinations	See *hallucinations*.

hypomania　Affective disorder characterized by elation, overactivity, and insomnia; insight is partially preserved; may progress to *mania*.

hysterical amnesia　Sudden loss of memory without organic cause, usually in context of psychosocial stress.

id　In Freudian theory, primitive part of the mind, source of instinct and drive.

ideas of reference　Feeling that things and events have direct reference to oneself. May reach sufficient intensity to constitute delusion.

idée fixe　See *overvalued idea*.

identification　In psychoanalysis, defence mechanism of unconsciously modelling oneself on some other person. Said to be important in personality development, especially of the *superego* (cf. conscience).

idiot savant　Person with learning difficulty who can nevertheless do elaborate arithmetic or memory tasks.

illusion　Misinterpretation of a real sensory stimulus, often coloured by emotion; for example, fear making a person see a shadow as an assailant.

imprinting　In animal behaviour, rapid learning or behavioural patterning at critical points in development. Relevance in man is unclear.

inappropriate affect　Mood incongruous to situation/thought content.

incoherence　See *word salad*.

individuation　The process by which the unique individual personality is formed.

indoleamine　Amines (e.g. serotonin) with an indole ring in their chemical structure.

initial insomnia　Difficulty in falling asleep.

insight　The patient's understanding of whether he is ill, his need for treatment, etc.

insomnia	Complaint of difficulty in falling or staying asleep or poor sleep quality.
instinct	Inborn drive.
intellectualization	Excessive abstract thinking to avoid difficult issues.
introspection	Examination of one's own feelings and thoughts.
introversion	Preoccupation with self rather than others and the world.
jamais vu	Abnormal feeling that something familiar has never happened before (see *déjà vu*).
Klinefelter's syndrome	Males with extra X chromosome; may include feminization, sterility, and low intelligence.
Klüver Bucy syndrome	Placidity, hyperphagia, and other features; caused by limbic system damage.
Knight's move thinking	A disorder of the form of thought with unusual though fathomable associations between ideas; cf. *derailment of thought* or *loosening of associations*.
koro	Culture-bound syndrome (China): panic from fear that penis has retracted into abdomen, and that this will be fatal.
Korsakoff's syndrome	Amnesia (especially short-term memory) and confabulation in chronic alcoholism. Personality and long-term memory are relatively preserved.
kuru	In New Guinea, a prion disease, spongiform encephalopathy transmitted (formerly) by cannibalism.
la belle indifférence	See *belle indifférence*.
labile affect	Abnormally unstable, sudden, rapid shifts in affect.
latah	Culture-bound syndrome (Malaysia) said to involve automatic obedience, echolalia, and echopraxia.
latent content	In psychoanalysis, unconscious meaning, especially relating to dreams.
learned helplessness	Proposed animal model of depression (Seligman); subjects repeatedly exposed to adverse treatment adopt

withdrawn and apparently helpless presentation; relevance to human condition uncertain.

learning disability   Below-average IQ (<70 or below), together with impaired social functioning.

libido   Sex drive.

Lilliputian hallucinations   Objects seem reduced in size, but otherwise normal; said to be characteristic of **delirium tremens**.

logorrhoea   Somewhat pretentious synonym for 'volubility' or 'loquacity'.

long-term memory   Includes both autobiographical (from childhood onward) and more recent memory, as for events in current affairs.

loosening of associations   See **derailment**.

magical thinking   A term that expresses well some aspects of childhood thinking, but which seems imprecise as a component of the US diagnosis of 'schizotypal disorder', a condition, much less well recognized internationally.

mania   Affective disorder with elevated mood, overactivity, and loss of insight.

mania a potu   A disputed entity, suggested as 'pathological intoxication' with alcohol, small amounts producing marked disinhibition and violence.

manifest content   In psychoanalysis, the parts of a dream one remembers, as distinct from the 'latent content' said to be revealed in analysis.

masochism   Sexual variation consisting of pleasure derived from receiving pain.

mental retardation   See **learning disability**.

middle insomnia   Waking in the night and then going back to sleep, but with difficulty.

mitgehen	Extreme form of ***mitmachen***.
mitmachen	A phenomenon of catatonia in which the patient's body can be put by the examiner into any position in spite of the instruction that the patient resist.
mood	The predominant, sustained emotional state of the subject: it is the emotional 'climate', as against the *affect*, which by extension is the emotional 'weather'.
mood-congruent	All features of an illness in line with and apparently produced by the mood; for example, a person with severe psychotic depression may have the delusion that he is an evil murderer and does not deserve to live, but when his mood has improved, the delusion gradually disappears.
negative symptoms	Characteristics of some patients with schizophrenia, including lack of initiative; reduced self care; poverty of speech, emotion, and action; lack of interest in relationships; etc.
neologism	A nonsense word made up by a patient with severe psychosis, usually part of the disorder of the form of thought.
neuroleptic malignant syndrome	Hyperpyrexia, autonomic instability, and muscular rigidity, related to the use of neuroleptic (antipsychotic) medication.
neurosis	Umbrella term for the common mental disorders such as anxiety, depression, etc.; it is distinct from psychotic disorder, as reality testing is intact.
night terrors	See ***sleep terror disorder***.
nihilistic delusion	Belief that oneself or the world does not exist; seen in severe depression.
nystagmus	Involuntary repeated movements of the eyes.
object relations	In psychoanalysis, focus on the ability to have relationships.
obsession	Repetitive unpleasant thought known to be nonsensical by patients, but that they recognize as their own thought.

Effort to stop the thoughts is accompanied by an increase in anxiety. May be accompanied by *compulsions*.

Oedipal stage In psychoanalysis, postulated stage of development between the ages of approximately 4 and 6 years when the personality develops and the relationship with the parents matures.

olfactory hallucination Involves a false taste perception; for example, patients with psychotic depression may smell their own flesh rotting.

oneiroid state Dreamlike state: the term is usually used in connection with epilepsy.

operant conditioning (instrumental conditioning) In behaviour theory, the results of the behaviour influence whether it will be repeated, reward promoting repetition, and lack of reward or punishment discouraging it.

oral stage In psychoanalysis, the postulated early stage of infant development, from birth to about 1 year when the baby is fixated on suckling.

orientation See *disorientation*.

overvalued idea A belief, usually false, that is inappropriate in view of the person's culture and background, and that is partially maintained in the face of contrary evidence and arguments, but the intensity of the holding of the belief is less than that of a delusion.

panic attacks Sudden severe attacks of anxiety that may be unexpected or produced by a known trigger, such as having to speak in public.

paranoid ideation Ideas of persecution, etc., of less than delusional intensity.

parasomnia Unusual behaviour during sleep, such as sleepwalking.

pareidolia An inconsequential stimulus mistakenly seen as real (e.g. a face in the clouds); it is not necessarily abnormal, but is seen in a variety of mental disorders.

passivity phenomena	Psychotic phenomena in which the patient believes his actions or mind is controlled by others, as in ***thought insertion*** and ***thought withdrawal***.
persecutory delusion	Patients feel they are being conspired against, etc.
perseveration	Inappropriate repetition of some behaviour, thought, or speech, even though the provoking stimulus, such as a question, has ceased. It is seen in organic disorders and schizophrenia.
personality disorder	Permanent maladaptive patterns of thinking and behaviour, present by adolescence or early adulthood, and continuing in spite of adverse experience.
phobia	Anxiety provoked by a specific object or situation, such as dogs. It may lead to avoidance of the provoking stimulus.
pressure of speech	Usually a feature of mania; the speech is loud, speeded up, and hard to interrupt.
prodrome	Premonitory sign or symptom of a developing disorder.
projection	In psychoanalysis, unconscious defence mechanism in which the difficulties in the self are projected onto others.
pseudocyesis	Phantom pregnancy.
pseudodementia	A severe mental illness, most often severe depression in the elderly, that mimics the features of dementia.
pseudologia fantastica	Exaggeration or fabrication of symptoms as in malingering and factitious disorder.
psychogenic fugue	Patient arrives in place distant from home, claiming not to know who he is, how he got there, etc. Dissociative amnesia following psychosocial stress is usual.
psychological pillow	Catatonic feature in which the patient holds his head a few inches above the bed.
psychomotor retardation	General slowing of movement and speech, typically in severe depression.

psychosis	Severe mental disorder, with *delusions* and *hallucinations*, so that the patient has lost touch with reality.
psychotic	Relating to **psychosis**.
psychotropic medication	Drugs affecting the mental state; in effect, drugs used in the treatment of mental disorder.
reaction formation	In psychoanalysis, unconscious defence mechanism in which a person behaves in a way that is the opposite of his inner self.
regression	Return to immature patterns of behaviour under stress.
reinforcement	Refers to the central principle of behaviour theory, which is that a behaviour is reinforced if it is rewarded.
residual phase	For example, a psychotic episode can respond to treatment and symptoms such as delusions and hallucinations disappear, but the patient may still be left with chronic schizophrenia with negative symptoms.
seasonal affective disorder	Depressive illness mainly during winter; responds to standard treatment for depression.
secondary gain	External gain from any illness, such as attention, benefits, and release from unpleasant responsibilities.
sensitiver Beziehungswahn	See **ideas of reference**.
shaping	Type of behaviour therapy in which behaviours are rewarded according to how similar they are to that desired; used in learning disability.
sick role	Identity adopted by an individual as a 'patient', displaying expected dependent behaviours (mechanical).
sleep terror disorder	Otherwise known as **night terrors**: seen in children, it is like waking from a nightmare, except that no dream can be recalled.

somatic delusion	Delusion about the body; for example, the bowels have turned to stone.
splitting	Mental mechanism in which the self or others are viewed as either good or bad; it is seen, for example, in patients with personality disorder, who skilfully divide staff teams and set them against each other in an effort to avoid dealing with their own issues.
stereotyped movements	Repetitive and unrewarding behaviours such as rocking, tapping, etc.
Stockholm syndrome	Condition in which a hostage or other vulnerable person seems, paradoxically, to display loyalty toward the hostage taker.
structural theory	Freud's model of the mental apparatus composed of *id*, *ego*, and *superego*.
stupor	A state of unresponsiveness with immobility and mutism.
suggestibility	Uncritical compliance or acceptance of a proposition.
superego	In psychoanalysis, part of the mental make-up, similar to conscience, and formed by identification with parents and others in early life.
systematic desensitization	Behaviour therapy for anxiety, especially phobias, by making a hierarchy of anxiety-provoking stimuli; the patient then encounters them progressively, starting with the easiest, until they no longer produce anxiety.
tactile hallucination	False perception of being touched, as in *formication* (see *delirium tremens*).
tangentiality	Oblique or irrelevant replies, which may not answer the question properly. Cf. *circumstantiality*.
tardive dyskinesia	Involuntary movement disorder, with mouth and facial movements, truncal movements, or athetoid limb movements.

termination	The process of ending in psychotherapy.
therapeutic community	Residential group therapy in which patients encourage each other to function within norms and deal with issues.
thought blocking	Delusion that the patient's thoughts are stopped, apparently by an outside agency; in schizophrenia, a Schneiderian first-rank symptom.
thought broadcasting	The delusion that the patient's thoughts are being broadcast; in schizophrenia, a Schneiderian first-rank symptom.
thought disorder	Disorder of the form of thought in which connections between thoughts are disrupted.
thought insertion	Delusion that thoughts, not one's own, are being inserted into one's mind; in schizophrenia, a Schneiderian first-rank symptom.
thought withdrawal	Delusion that thoughts are being removed from one's mind; in schizophrenia, a Schneiderian first-rank symptom.
tic	Involuntary, quick, stereotyped movement or vocalization.
token economy	Application of operant conditioning to the management of, say, a rehabilitation unit, with tokens (for tangible rewards) given for task performance; there are obvious ethical problems here, and the method is now less used.
tolerance	In substance misuse, as the effect of the given dose of a substance gets less, the patient tends to increase the dose.
transvestism	Sexual pleasure from dressing and/or appearing as a member of the opposite sex.
trichotillomania	Habit of pulling out one's hair.
visual hallucination	Hallucination involving sight; it may consist of formed images, such as of people, or of unformed images, such

as flashes of light. Visual hallucinations should be distinguished from illusions, which are misperceptions of real external stimuli.

word salad Severe disorder of the form of thought, in which speech consists of an unintelligible mixture of words, syllables, or even sounds.

zoophilia Sexual interest in or activity with animals.

Index

Hughes' Outline of Modern Psychiatry, Fifth Edition. David Gill.
© 2007 John Wiley & Sons, Ltd   ISBN 9780470033920